Anatomic ACL Reconstruction

Editors

FREDDIE H. FU
VOLKER MUSAHL

CLINICS IN SPORTS MEDICINE

www.sportsmed.theclinics.com

Consulting Editor
MARK D. MILLER

January 2013 • Volume 32 • Number 1

ELSEVIER

1600 John F. Kennedy Blvd. ● Suite 1800 ● Philadelphia, Pennsylvania 19103

http://www.theclinics.com

CLINICS IN SPORTS MEDICINE Volume 32, Number 1
January 2013 ISSN 0278-5919, ISBN-13: 978-1-4557-7331-2

Editor: David Parsons

Clinics in Sports Medicine (ISSN 0278-5919) is published quarterly by Elsevier Inc., 360 Park Avenue South, New York, NY 10010-1710. Months of issue are January, April, July, and October. Business and Editorial Offices: 1600 John F. Kennedy Blvd., Ste. 1800, Philadelphia, PA 19103-2899. Customer Service Office: 3251 Riverport Lane, Maryland Heights, MO 63043. Periodicals postage paid at New York, NY and additional mailing offices. Subscription prices are $324.00 per year (US individuals), $503.00 per year (US institutions), $160.00 per year (US students), $367.00 per year (Canadian individuals), $608.00 per year (Canadian institutions), $223.00 (Canadian students), $446.00 per year (foreign individuals), $608.00 per year (foreign institutions), and $223.00 per year (foreign students). Foreign air speed delivery is included in all *Clinics* subscription prices. All prices are subject to change without notice. **POSTMASTER:** Send address changes to *Clinics in Sports Medicine*, Elsevier Health Sciences Division, Subscription Customer Service, 3251 Riverport Lane, Maryland Heights, MO 63043. Customer Service (orders, claims, online, change of address): Elsevier Health Sciences Division, Subscription Customer Service, 3251 Riverport Lane, Maryland Heights, MO 63043. Tel: 1-800-654-2452 (U.S. and Canada); 314-447-8871 (outside U.S. and Canada). Fax: 314-447-8029. E-mail: journals customerservice-usa@elsevier.com (for print support); journalsonlinesupport-usa@elsevier.com (for online support).

Reprints. For copies of 100 or more of articles in this publication, please contact the Commercial Reprints Department, Elsevier Inc., 360 Park Avenue South, New York, NY 10010-1710. Tel.: 212-633-3812; Fax: 212-462-1935; E-mail: reprints@elsevier.com.

Clinics in Sports Medicine is covered in *MEDLINE/PubMed (Index Medicus) Current Contents/Clinical Medicine, Excerpta Medica,* and *ISI/Biomed.*

Printed and bound by CPI Group (UK) Ltd, Croydon, CR0 4YY

Transferred to digital print 2012

Contributors

CONSULTING EDITOR

MARK D. MILLER, MD
S. Ward Casscells Professor of Orthopaedic Surgery, University of Virginia; Team Physician, James Madison University, Harrisonburg, Charlottesville, Virginia

GUEST EDITORS

FREDDIE H. FU, MD, DSc(Hon)
David Silver Professor and Chairman, Department of Orthopaedic Surgery, Center for Sports Medicine, School of Medicine, University of Pittsburgh, Pittsburgh, Pennsylvania

VOLKER MUSAHL, MD
Assistant Professor, Department of Orthopaedic Surgery, Center for Sports Medicine, School of Medicine, University of Pittsburgh, Pittsburgh, Pennsylvania

AUTHORS

MATTIAS AHLDÉN, MD
Department of Orthopaedics, Sahlgrenska University Hospital/Mölndal, Sahlgrenska Academy, University of Gothenburg, Mölndal, Sweden

DANIEL ANDERSSON, MD
Department of Orthopaedics, Sahlgrenska University Hospital, Mölndal, Sweden

DAISUKE ARAKI, MD, PhD
International Research Associate, Department of Orthopaedic Surgery, School of Medicine, University of Pittsburgh, Pittsburgh, Pennsylvania; Clinical Fellow, Department of Orthopaedic Surgery, Graduate School of Medicine, Kobe University, Kobe, Japan

O.R. AYENI, MD, MSc, FRCSC
Assistant Professor, Division of Orthopaedic Surgery, McMaster University Medical Center, McMaster University, Hamilton, Ontario, Canada

MICHAEL G. BARAGA, MD
Assistant Professor, Department of Orthopaedic Surgery, Miller School of Medicine, University of Miami, Miami, Florida

ASHEESH BEDI, MD
Assistant Professor, MedSport, Department of Orthopaedic Surgery, University of Michigan, Ann Arbor, Michigan

M. BHANDARI, MD, PhD, FRCSC
Professor, Division of Orthopaedic Surgery, McMaster University, Hamilton, Ontario, Canada

TOMMASO BONANZINGA, MD
Laboratorio di Biomeccanica e Innovazione Tecnologica, Istituto Ortopedico Rizzoli, Bologna, Italy

KARL F. BOWMAN Jr, MD
Sports Medicine Fellow, Department of Orthopaedic Surgery, UPMC Center for Sports Medicine, Pittsburgh, Pennsylvania

CONSTANCE R. CHU, MD
Albert Ferguson Endowed Chair, Professor of Orthopaedic Surgery and Bioengineering, Director, Cartilage Restoration Center, Vice Chair, Translational Research, University of Pittsburgh Medical Center, Pittsburgh, Pennsylvania

M.R. DENKERS, MD, FRCSC
Assistant Professor, Division of Orthopaedic Surgery, Hamilton General Hospital, McMaster University, Hamilton, Ontario, Canada

VICTORIA B. DUTHON, MD
Senior Resident, Department of Orthopaedic Surgery, Orthopaedic Surgery and Traumatology, University Hospital of Geneva, Genève, Switzerland

N. EVANIEW, MD
Resident, Division of Orthopaedic Surgery, McMaster University Medical Center, McMaster University, Hamilton, Ontario, Canada

NICOLE A. FRIEL, MD
Resident, Department of Orthopaedic Surgery, University of Pittsburgh Medical Center, University of Pittsburgh, Pittsburgh, Pennsylvania

FREDDIE H. FU, MD, DSc(Hon)
David Silver Professor and Chairman, Department of Orthopaedic Surgery, Center for Sports Medicine, School of Medicine, University of Pittsburgh, Pittsburgh, Pennsylvania

ALBERTO GRASSI, MD
Laboratorio di Biomeccanica e Innovazione Tecnologica, Istituto Ortopedico Rizzoli, Bologna, Italy

JAMES J. IRRGANG, PhD, PT, ATC, FAPTA
Associate Professor, School of Health and Rehabilitation Sciences; Associate Professor and Director of Clinical Research, Department of Orthopaedic Surgery, School of Medicine, University of Pittsburgh, Pittsburgh, Pennsylvania

SALLY JÄRVELÄ, MD, PhD
Department of Orthopaedics and Traumatology, Tampere University Hospital, Tampere, Finland; Ylojarvi, Finland

TIMO JÄRVELÄ, MD, PhD
Sports Clinic, Hospital Mehiläinen; Medical Faculty, Tampere University, Tampere, Finland

JÓN KARLSSON, MD, PhD
Department of Orthopaedics, Sahlgrenska University Hospital/Mölndal, Sahlgrenska Academy, University of Gothenburg, Mölndal, Sweden

HIROMI KAZUSA, MD
Graduate Student, Department of Orthopaedic Surgery, Integrated Health Sciences, Institute of Biomedical & Health Sciences, Hiroshima University, Minami-ku, Hiroshima, Japan

JONG-MIN KIM, MD
Department of Orthopedic Surgery, Asan Medical Center, University of Ulsan College of Medicine, Seoul, Korea

NICOLA LOPOMO, PhD
Laboratorio di Biomeccanica e Innovazione Tecnologica, Istituto Ortopedico Rizzoli; Laboratorio di NanoBiotecnologie-NaBi, Istituto Ortopedico Rizzoli, Bologna, Italy

C. BENJAMIN MA, MD
Department of Orthopaedic Surgery, Orthopaedic Institute, University of California San Francisco, San Francisco, California

ROBERT A. MAGNUSSEN, MD
Assistant Professor, Department of Orthopaedic Surgery, The Ohio State University College of Medicine, Columbus, Ohio

MAURILIO MARCACCI, MD
Professor, Laboratorio di Biomeccanica e Innovazione Tecnologica, Istituto Ortopedico Rizzoli, Bologna, Italy

GIULIO MARIA MARCHEGGIANI MUCCIOLI, MD
Laboratorio di Biomeccanica e Innovazione Tecnologica, Istituto Ortopedico Rizzoli, Bologna, Italy

BART MULLER, MD
Research Fellow, Department of Orthopaedic Surgery, UPMC Center for Sports Medicine, University of Pittsburgh, Pittsburgh, Pennsylvania; PhD Candidate, Department of Orthopaedic Surgery, Orthopaedic Research Center Amsterdam, Amsterdam, The Netherlands

VOLKER MUSAHL, MD
Assistant Professor, Department of Orthopaedic Surgery, Center for Sports Medicine, School of Medicine, University of Pittsburgh, Pittsburgh, Pennsylvania

ATSUO NAKAMAE, MD, PhD
Assistant Professor, Department of Orthopaedic Surgery, Integrated Health Sciences, Institute of Biomedical & Health Sciences, Hiroshima University, Minami-ku, Hiroshima, Japan

PHILIPPE NEYRET, MD
Professor and Chief, Department of Orthopaedic Surgery, Hôpital de la Croix-Rousse, Lyon, France

MITSUO OCHI, MD, PhD
Professor and Chairman, Department of Orthopaedic Surgery, Integrated Health Sciences, Institute of Biomedical & Health Sciences, Hiroshima University, Minami-ku, Hiroshima, Japan

R. OGILVIE, MD, FRCSC
Associate Clinical Professor, Division of Orthopaedic Surgery, McMaster University, Ancaster, Ontario, Canada

D.C. PETERSON, MD, FRCSC
Associate Professor, Division of Orthopaedic Surgery, Department of Surgery, McMaster University Medical Center, McMaster University, Hamilton, Ontario, Canada

STEPHEN J. RABUCK, MD
Assistant Professor, Department of Orthopaedic Surgery, Center for Sports Medicine, School of Medicine, University of Pittsburgh, Pittsburgh, Pennsylvania

KRISTIAN SAMUELSSON, MD, PhD
Department of Orthopaedics, Sahlgrenska University Hospital/Mölndal, Sahlgrenska Academy, University of Gothenburg, Mölndal, Sweden

ELVIRE SERVIEN, MD, PhD
Professor, Department of Orthopaedic Surgery, Hôpital de la Croix-Rousse, Lyon, France

CECILIA SIGNORELLI
Laboratorio di Biomeccanica e Innovazione Tecnologica, Istituto Ortopedico Rizzoli, Bologna, Italy; Dipartimento di Bioingegneria, Politecnico di Milano, Milano, Italy

SCOTT TASHMAN, PhD
Associate Professor, Director, Orthopaedic Biodynamics Laboratory, Department of Orthopaedic Surgery, School of Medicine; Associate Professor, Department of Bioengineering, School of Engineering, University of Pittsburgh, Pittsburgh, Pennsylvania

ANDREA VISANI, MD
Laboratorio di Biomeccanica e Innovazione Tecnologica, Istituto Ortopedico Rizzoli, Bologna, Italy

ROBIN V. WEST, MD
Associate Professor, Department of Orthopaedic Surgery, Center for Sports Medicine, School of Medicine, University of Pittsburgh, Pittsburgh, Pennsylvania

TIMOTHY S. WHITEHEAD, FRACS
Orthopaedic surgeon, OrthoSport Victoria, Richmond, Australia; Musculoskeletal Research Centre, Faculty of Health Sciences, LaTrobe University, Bundoora, Australia; Orthopaedic Department, Austin Health, Heidelberg, Australia

MOHAMMAD A. YABROUDI, MS, PT
Doctoral Student, School of Health and Rehabilitation Sciences; Department of Orthopaedic Surgery, School of Medicine, University of Pittsburgh, Pittsburgh, Pennsylvania

STEFANO ZAFFAGNINI, MD
Laboratorio di Biomeccanica e Innovazione Tecnologica, Istituto Ortopedico Rizzoli, Bologna, Italy

Contents

Acute anterior cruciate ligament (ACL) tears are most frequently sustained by young, physically active individuals. ACL injuries are seen at high incidence in adolescents and young adults performing sports and occupational activities that involve pivoting. Young women participating in pivoting sports have a 3 to 5 times higher risk of ACL injury than men. Studies show that ACL injury increases osteoarthritis (OA) risk with symptomatic OA appearing in roughly half of individuals 10–15 years later. Because the majority of patients sustaining acute ACL tears are younger than 30, this leads to early onset OA with associated pain and disability during premium work and life growth years between ages 30 and 50. Effective strategies to prevent ACL injury and to reduce subsequent OA risk in those sustaining acute ACL tears are needed.

Graft healing and maturation are important considerations during the rehabilitation process. Histologic studies have identified the stages of graft healing following anterior cruciate ligament (ACL) reconstruction. Correlations between histology and radiographic findings have allowed for the development of noninvasive methods to assess graft maturity. Important information regarding graft vascularity and incorporation of the graft to host bone can be obtained from imaging modalities. The role of noninvasive means in the evaluation of patients following ACL reconstruction continues to develop as these powerful tools evolve.

MRI has led to significant advancement in diagnosis of soft tissue injuries. Previous technology has been limited to morphologic diagnosis and static images. Recent advances allow high-resolution images with shorter acquisition time and compositional analysis of tissues. Static, unloaded, and morphologic examination became dynamic, loaded, and biochemical analyses. This article focuses on the use of advanced MRI techniques in the evaluation of anterior cruciate ligament (ACL) injury and its surgical outcome. Up-to-date applications of quantitative MRI and kinematic analysis of ACL injuries and reconstructed knees are reviewed.

the development of symptomatic ACL-deficient degenerative arthrosis. Validated and reproducible examination maneuvers are necessary for accurate diagnosis and appraisal of surgical interventions. Appropriately powered expertise-based trials should be emphasized to minimize bias, enhance validity, and reduce crossover. Best practice rehabilitation protocols can guide postoperative care while minimizing heterogeneity within studies. Functional outcome scores should be sensitive, responsive, and able to reliably detect small changes.

According to the 20 prospective, randomized studies found from the English literature and included into this review, 6 studies (30%) did not find any significant differences in the clinical results between double-bundle and single-bundle anterior cruciate ligament reconstructions. However, 14 studies (70%) reported significantly better results with the double-bundle technique than with the single-bundle technique. In addition, none of the studies found that the single-bundle technique had better results in any of these evaluations than the double-bundle technique.

Operative reconstruction of a torn anterior cruciate ligament (ACL) has become the most broadly accepted treatment. An important, but underreported, outcome of ACL reconstruction is graft failure, which poses a challenge for the orthopedic surgeon. An understanding of the tendon-bone healing and the intra-articular ligamentization process is crucial for orthopedic surgeons to make appropriate graft choices and to be able to initiate optimal rehabilitation protocols after surgical ACL reconstruction. This article focuses on the current understanding of the tendon-to-bone healing process for both autografts and allografts and discusses strategies to biologically augment healing.

Many surgeons intend to replicate the native anterior cruciate ligament (ACL) as much as possible, aiming at anatomic ACL reconstruction. An outline of new surgical preferences is starting to form; orthopedic surgeons have shifted their preferences in arthroscopic technique, graft type, and fixation during the past decade. The days of simple silk suturing of the native ACL stump to the femoral periosteum are over. Today, knee surgeons performing ACL reconstruction have a wide array of technical considerations, graft choices, and fixation techniques at hand that enable them to specifically tailor each reconstruction to each patient's anatomy and specific needs.

causes of failure, including graft failure, loss of motion, extensor mechanism dysfunction, osteoarthritis, and infection. The etiology of graft failure is discussed in detail with a particular emphasis on failure after anatomic anterior cruciate ligament reconstruction.

CLINICS IN SPORTS MEDICINE

FORTHCOMING ISSUES

April 2013
Blunt Trauma Injuries in the Athlete
Thomas M. DeBerardino, MD,
Guest Editor

July 2013
MRI in Sports Medicine
Timothy G. Sanders, MD, *Guest Editor*

October 2013
Unicompartmental Knee Arthroplasty
Kevin Plancher, MD, and
Albert Dunn, DO, *Guest Editors*

RECENT ISSUES

October 2012
Rotator Cuff Surgery
Stephen F. Brockmeier, MD, *Guest Editor*

July 2012
Spinal Injuries in the Athlete
Pierre A. d'Hemecourt, MD, and
Lyle J. Micheli, MD, *Guest Editors*

April 2012
Leg Pain in the Running Athlete
Alexander K. Meininger, MD, *Guest Editor*

January 2012
Sports-Related Injuries of the Meniscus
Peter R. Kurzweil, MD, *Guest Editor*

Foreword

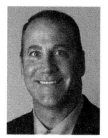

Mark D. Miller, MD
Consulting Editor

Dr Freddie Fu, who has taught us all the concept of "Anatomic" ACL reconstruction, recently hosted a worldwide symposium on this topic. In true Dr Fu fashion, he spared no expense and invited a veritable Who's Who of experts from around the globe to discuss this topic. The conference was well attended, but I think this is such an important topic that I wanted to help share this information with other sports medicine providers. Dr Fu teamed up with Dr Volker Musahl, also at the University of Pittsburgh, to put together this treatise. All aspects of ACL anatomy, biomechanics, examination, imaging, reconstruction, biology, and rehabilitation are included. It is interesting that we thought that we had "solved" the ACL problem less than a decade ago and now we have all been humbled as we tumbled back down the learning curve. But, as Dr Fu has once again confirmed—restoring normal anatomy usually results in the best results in orthopedic surgery. Congratulations to Drs Fu and Musahl—now let's start climbing back up that curve!

Mark D. Miller, MD
S. Ward Casscells Professor of Orthopaedic Surgery
University of Virginia
James Madison University
400 Ray C. Hunt Drive, Suite 330
Charlottesville, VA 22908-0159, USA

E-mail address:
MDM3P@hscmail.mcc.virginia.edu

Clin Sports Med 32 (2013) xiii
http://dx.doi.org/10.1016/j.csm.2012.10.002
0278-5919/13/$ – see front matter © 2013 Published by Elsevier Inc.

sportsmed.theclinics.com

Preface

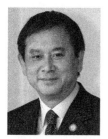 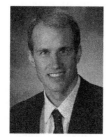

Freddie H. Fu, MD, DSc   Volker Musahl, MD
Guest Editors

Anatomic ACL reconstruction has long been a topic of interest but even more so over the past 10 years. Several recent editorials have been devoted to the increasing number of research articles published on this topic. Although research articles sometimes reveal conflicting results, it has been established that ACL reconstruction should be anatomic (ie, reproduce native insertion site anatomy and tension pattern, and individualized surgery).

At the recent Panther Global Summit (Pittsburgh, PA, USA, August 25-27, 2011), 24 of 28 (85%) experts utilize anatomic techniques for ACL reconstruction. This is in contrast to 10 years ago when the predominant technique utilized was the transtibial technique. Anatomic ACL reconstruction includes the study, preservation, and reconstruction of ACL footprint anatomy. The ultimate goal of ACL reconstruction surgery is to prevent the development of osteoarthritis. This may involve measures such as anatomic surgery, disease-modifying treatments, and longer time to return to play following ACL reconstruction surgery to allow for adequate healing of the reconstructed ACL.

This issue of *Clinics in Sports Medicine* is dedicated to anatomic ACL reconstruction. We are delighted to have such a diverse group of authors who each have a unique perspective on the field. Fifteen topics that we believe are essential for understanding the concept of anatomic ACL reconstruction are discussed. The focus of this issue is on practical guides and surgical techniques, instructing how to make a difference in anatomic ACL reconstruction.

In the first section of this issue of *Clinics in Sports Medicine*, the development of knee osteoarthritis following ACL injury is discussed by Constance Chu. Stephen Rabuck discusses ACL healing and advances in imaging that may ultimately lead to better understanding of the safe return to full activity criteria. Benjamin Ma discusses different methods of quantitative MRI and its role in assessing osteoarthritis. Asheesh Bedi discusses current concepts on ACL graft healing and biologics.

The next section focuses on biomechanics, knee kinematics, and the pivot shift. Mattias Ahlden discusses rotatory knee laxity following ACL reconstruction. Scott Tashman reviews the role of functional, dynamic stereo radiography in assessing kinematics of the ACL reconstructed knee. There are several new developments in

Clin Sports Med 32 (2013) xv–xvi
http://dx.doi.org/10.1016/j.csm.2012.10.001
0278-5919/13/$ – see front matter © 2013 Elsevier Inc. All rights reserved.

the field of quantitative assessment of the pivot shift. Stefano Zaffagnini discusses inertial sensors for noninvasive quantification of the pivot shift.

The practice of evidence-based medicine to improve outcome for patients following ACL reconstruction is described by Olufemi Ayeni. Timo Jarvela discusses outcomes of studies with level I evidence to compare single-bundle versus double-bundle ACL reconstruction. Krisitan Samuelsson provides a global perspective on surgeons' preferences on ACL reconstruction technique.

The final section of this issue of *Clinics in Sports Medicine* focuses on surgical techniques. Mitsuo Ochi discusses developing and refining techniques for ACL augmentation. Philippe Neyret provides history and current concepts of extra-articular surgery for the restoration of knee laxity. Robin West discusses anatomic ACL reconstruction utilizing the quadriceps tendon. James Irrgang reviews principles in rehabilitation after ACL reconstruction. Timothy Whitehead illustrates the reasons for failure of anatomic ACL reconstruction.

We would like to sincerely thank all the authors for their excellent contribution to this issue of *Clinics in Sports Medicine*. This issue presents current knowledge in biology of healing and development of osteoarthritis, biomechanics and quantitative laxity assessment, imaging, and evidence-based medicine. Global trends are illustrated, and the section on surgical techniques provides the reader with a practical guide for anatomic ACL reconstruction. The goal of anatomic ACL reconstruction is to ultimately improve patient outcome.

Freddie H. Fu, MD, DSc
Volker Musahl, MD
Department of Orthopaedic Surgery
University of Pittsburgh
3471 Fifth Avenue, Suite 1011
Pittsburgh, PA 15213, USA

E-mail address:
ffu@upmc.edu (F.H. Fu)

The Role of ACL Injury in the Development of Posttraumatic Knee Osteoarthritis

Nicole A. Friel, MD, Constance R. Chu, MD*

KEYWORDS

- ACL • ACL reconstruction • Cartilage • Posttraumatic osteoarthritis

KEY POINTS

- Acute ACL tears commonly occur in young, physically active individuals under age 30.
- ACL injury increases osteoarthritis risk resulting in early onset OA during prime work and life years between ages 30 and 50.
- Effective strategies to prevent ACL injury and to reduce OA risk after ACL tear are needed.

The anterior cruciate ligament (ACL) a relatively common injury in young, physically active individuals. ACL injuries are seen at high incidence in adolescents playing sports that involve pivoting, such as football, soccer, basketball, and team handball. Young women have a 35 times higher risk of ACL injury than do men when participating in these sports.[1–3] Most patients with acute ACL tears are younger than 30 at the time of their injury. As such, ACL injuries result in early onset osteoarthritis (OA) were associated with pain, functional limitations, and decreased quality of life.[4] The reported incidence of posttraumatic osteoarthritis (PTOA) following ACL injury as high as 87%.[5,6] By comparison, the prevalence of OA in all adults older than 45 years of age was 19.2%, as reported by the Framingham Osteoarthritis Study, and 27.8%, as reported by the Johnston County Osteoarthritis Project.[7] It has also been estimated that an ACL rupture ages the knee by 30 years.[1] Variations in the incidence of PTOA may be due to different methods used to evaluate patients, various surgical techniques, the time interval between surgery and reconstruction, and the duration of follow-up after ACL injury. In addition, clinical symptoms do not always correlate with imaging or physical assessments, resulting in many areas of ongoing debate in the management of ACL injuries. Management

Department of Orthopaedic Surgery, University of Pittsburgh Medical Center, University of Pittsburgh, 200 Lothrop Street, Pittsburgh, PA 15213, USA
* Corresponding author.
E-mail address: chucr@upmc.edu

Clin Sports Med 32 (2013) 1–12
http://dx.doi.org/10.1016/j.csm.2012.08.017
0278-5919/13/$ – see front matter © 2013 Elsevier Inc. All rights reserved.

of a torn ACL ranges from nonoperative treatment to reconstructive surgery. The primary goals of ACL reconstruction are to restore knee stability, allowing the patient to resume his or her preinjury activities. ACL reconstruction has not been shown to delay later development of PTOA. Study results vary, with reports showing decreased, equal, or even increased levels of PTOA in patients who have had ACL reconstruction. As such, there is high need for improved understanding of OA development after ACL injury to inform development of strategies to reduce OA risk in this population.

BIOMECHANICS AND BASIC SCIENCE OF PTOA

The mechanism responsible for cartilage breakdown and progression to OA following ACL injury is multifactorial and not completely understood. The development of OA after ACL injury may be the result of the initial injury to the subchondral bone and hyaline cartilage. At the time of injury, the high force of the trauma disrupts the intra-articular structures.[8] Occult osteochondral lesions, or bone bruises, as measured on magnetic resonance imaging (MRI), occur in 80%–90%[9] of patients with an acute ACL injury, most commonly on the posterolateral tibial plateau and the anterolateral femoral condyle. These lesions suggest that articular cartilage sustains a considerable mechanical impact at the time of injury.[10]

In addition to initial trauma, the lack of a functionally normal ACL leads to chronic changes in the static and dynamic loading of the knee and increased forces on the cartilage and other joint structures.[11] Therefore, subsequent intra-articular injuries occur over time, especially to the cartilage and the meniscus. These lesions play a role in the development of OA, as seen in many studies that show higher rates of OA in patients with concomitant intra-articular injuries.

ACL reconstruction, or even the historically performed ACL repair, has been postulated to prevent OA by restoring the biomechanical stability of the knee joint. Although ACL reconstruction does improve knee stability in ACL deficient knees, it does not restore *normal* knee kinematics.[12] While ACL reconstruction has not been shown to prevent PTOA, there is substantial interest in whether more anatomical reconstruction techniques will restore knee kinematics and reduce OA risk.

Despite the ability of ACL reconstruction to reduce knee instability, the incidence of posttraumatic OA remains high. ACL disruption initiates a cascade of pathogenic processes. Lohmander and colleagues[13] have shown repeatedly an increased turnover of the cartilage proteoglycan aggrecan and type II collagen within days and weeks following joint injuries. In a histologic study of cartilage biopsies at the time of ACL reconstruction, there is histologic evidence of degeneration and a persistent increase in collagenase cleavage and denaturation of type II collagen, occur within a year of ACL injury that is associated with an early transient increase in the total content of proteoglycan, similar to that seen in idiopathic OA.[14]

Any injury to the knee joint, including ACL rupture, alters in levels of synovial fluid of compounds that may contribute to joint degeneration. Multiple inflammatory cytokines, or biomarkers, such as tumor necrosis factor-alpha, interleukin-1 (IL-1β), and IL-6, are upregulated after joint injury.[15–20] Although these studies show a wide variation in the time periods in which these inflammatory cytokines remain elevated, it is consistent that cytokines are elevated immediately following injury and likely persist for a prolonged period of time. Furthermore, if ACL surgery is pursued, the joint is again traumatized, resulting in prolonged joint inflammation with a postoperative hemarthrosis. The cytokines involved in this inflammation have been associated with cartilage destruction and have been identified as inhibitors to chondrogenesis.

RISK FACTORS FOR PTOA

In an effort to reduce the incidence or progression of PTOA, the identification of risk factors associated with the development of this disabling process would be beneficial. Candidate risk factors for PTOA include the following:

- Neuromuscular factors
- Meniscus status
- Body mass index (BMI)
- Chondral damage
- Age
- Graft choice
- Time interval between injury and surgical intervention.

Nonsurgical Versus Surgical Management

ACL injury dramatically increases OA risk, the surgical objectives of ACL reconstruction are to reestablish function and to prevent instability that can result in added repetitive damage to the articular cartilage and other soft tissues.[21,22] However, no studies show that ACL reconstruction can prevent PTOA.

Before the advent of ACL reconstruction, when ACL injuries were more often treated nonoperatively, 1 study[23] showed that at 14 years after injury, one-third of ACL ruptures treated without repair or reconstruction demonstrated joint space narrowing or unequivocal OA. In this study, 86% of these patients had removal of 1 or both menisci at the time of surgery, and 75% of patients returned to the previous sport. In a retrospective cohort clinical study with longer follow-up, Nebelung and Wuschech[24] evaluated 19 Olympic athletes who sustained an ACL injury and were treated without reconstruction. All athletes returned to high-level activity, but at the 20-year follow-up, 95% of the knees showed severe symptoms of OA and instability, and more than 50% had undergone total joint replacement after 35 years.

Van der Hart and colleagues[25] concluded that bone-patellar tendon-bone ACL reconstruction does not prevent the occurrence of radiological OA after 10 years, as 45% of patients had radiographic OA per the Kellgren-Lawrence grading scale versus 3% on the contralateral knee. In a study of radiological outcome of patients who had undergone ACL reconstruction in comparison to a group of nonoperatively treated patients, at 17 to 20 years after injury, both groups showed degenerative changes on radiographs.[26] Half of the patients treated with ACL reconstruction had mild degenerative changes and 16.5% had severe OA. However, in nonoperatively treated patients there were no normal knees and 56% of the patients had severe OA. The authors concluded that reconstruction of ACL cannot prevent OA but may lead to a lower prevalence of its onset. Potter and colleagues,[10] following both nonoperative and reconstructive treatments by MRI, found an increased risk of cartilage degeneration of the medial tibial plateau and patella in nonsurgical patients compared to the surgically treated patients. Kessler and colleagues[27] also compared nonoperative versus reconstructive treatment of arthroscopically confirmed ACL ruptures, observing that ACL reconstructed patients had significantly better knee stability but more OA. However, the authors excluded 2 important groups of patients: patients with concomitant injuries (to the meniscus, cartilage, or other ligaments) and patients who required revision operation within the study period. Nonoperative management of ACL injury results in a significantly higher rate of meniscal lesions requiring later surgery than surgically treated ACL injury. However, this study did not incorporate the degree of OA in the knees with secondary meniscal tears, which may have changed their conclusions regarding the rate of OA.

This highlights the heterogeneity of people, treatments and assessments in ACL injury. It is possible that some patients with characteristic injury patterns are better candidates for surgery than others. For example, it is unclear what secondary damage occurs when ACL injuries are treated nonoperatively. Removing the variable of meniscal injury provides a more homogeneous population of patients with isolated ACL injuries. Hoffelner and colleagues[28] found that athletes with an isolated ACL rupture had no increased risk for the development of PTOA after ACL reconstruction in the long term when compared to the uninjured contralateral knee. This offers several interpretations. It lends support to ACL reconstruction in this population, because surgery may prevent secondary meniscal and chondral injuries that advance OA. Further, there is an increased rate of reconstruction after a period of nonoperative treatment, which may be considered an argument in favor of primary ACL reconstruction. Conversely, if a patient is willing to modify activities to avoid instability primary nonoperative treatment, may be preferable. Neuman and colleagues[29] reported low rates of OA after ACL injured patients who agree to moderate their level of activity to avoid reinjury.

Daniel and colleagues[30] concluded that patients who had undergone reconstruction had a higher level of arthrosis by radiograph and bone scan evaluation. Although this study does show significant results, it is not without limitations, because the more severely injured knees (ie, concomitant injuries) were more often reconstructed. The authors state that an increased incidence of degenerative joint disease in patients with reconstructed knees can in part be explained by a higher incidence of meniscal surgery in the patients who have undergone knee reconstruction. However, a comparison of bone scan scores for patients who did not have meniscal surgery revealed a greater incidence of arthrosis in patients who had reconstructed knees.

Meniscus Status

The status of the meniscus is a critically important factor in the development of OA after injury to the ACL. Multiple studies have reported that meniscal injury, meniscus surgery, or meniscectomy at the time of ACL repair or reconstruction increases OA risk.[1,6,21,23–25,29–46]

A recent systematic review,[47] including 31 different studies, reported meniscal injury and meniscectomy as the most frequently reported risk factors. The status of the meniscus has been identified as the most important factor for developing posttraumatic OA after an ACL injury regardless of whether the patient undergoes ACL surgery or nonoperative treatment.[21] Wu and colleagues[45] compared radiographic findings of patients at 10 years postoperatively, dividing the patients into 2 different groups: those with an intact meniscus at the time of ACL reconstruction and those who underwent concomitant meniscectomy at the time of ACL reconstruction. Two of 25 patients with intact menisci had radiographic OA, whereas 9 of 9 patients undergoing meniscectomy had radiographic OA. Thus, the authors noted that the meniscus should be repaired, not removed, whenever possible. Lohmander and colleagues[1] found a very high prevalence of radiographic knee OA, pain, and functional limitations in young women who sustained an ACL tear during soccer play 12 years earlier. The authors note that ACL-injured players who also underwent meniscus surgery had a higher prevalence (69%) of radiographic knee OA than those without such surgery (39%). Similarly, von Porat and colleagues[44] evaluated male soccer players, with a higher percentage (59%) of radiographic OA in patients who had meniscal injury compared to those with an isolated ACL injury (31%). Li and colleagues[48] found that 24 of 37 (65%) patients who underwent concurrent meniscectomy developed radiographic OA, differing from the 72 of 212 (34%) patients who did not undergo concurrent meniscectomy but developed radiographic OA. The authors further evaluated patients who had undergone prior meniscectomy, noting that 16 of 19 (84%) patients who had undergone prior meniscectomy developed evidence of radiographic OA. In perhaps the most striking example, Nakata and colleagues[6] found that degenerative joint disease changes were present in 13 of 15 (87%) meniscectomized knees, whereas those changes were seen in only 12 of 46 knees (26%) with intact or repaired meniscus.

In an interesting study,[49] a population of men and women with OA underwent MRI, in which 49 of the 265 participants were found to have loss of ACL integrity. Remarkably, ACL deficiency increased the risk for cartilage loss of the medial tibiofemoral compartment; however, following adjustment for the presence of medial meniscal tears, there was no increased risk for cartilage loss. Based on this study, it seems that increased risk for cartilage loss is mediated by concomitant meniscus pathology in those with OA.

Findings of increased OA associated with meniscus injury may be explained by decreased stability and altered contact mechanics of the knee after partial or total meniscectomy.[48] Further, it is possible that the decreased tibiofemoral joint space associated with a meniscectomy can change the relationship of the patellar to the femoral trochlea, causing patellofemoral cartilage degeneration.[38]

The injured meniscus is addressed with meniscal repair or partial meniscectomy rather than complete meniscectomy. In recent years, even though partial rather than total meniscectomies have been performed, the incidence of OA associated with ACL surgery remains high, especially in comparison to ACL surgery with no meniscal damage. Meniscus repair in the presence of ACL injury is also common, as results have shown a lower incidence of OA in ACL-reconstructed patients with repaired menisci compared to those with partial meniscectomies.[50]

Body Mass Index

BMI is well known to be associated with onset and progression of knee OA in patients without ACL rupture.[51] Not surprisingly, multiple studies have found that patient BMI is correlated with joint space narrowing or OA following injury to the ACL.[22,23,27,48]

Bowers and colleagues[52] aimed to identify demographic and anthropometric risk factors for intra-articular injuries observed during ACL reconstruction and found that height, weight, and BMI are significant risk factors for injuries to articular surfaces and menisci as observed during ACL reconstruction. Although the authors did not correlate any of their findings to the development of OA, other studies have supported that intra-articular injuries (ie, meniscus and cartilage) are risk factors for the development of OA. The authors, therefore, hypothesize that athletes could possibly reduce risk of certain intra-articular pathologies with maintenance of lower body weight and BMI and thus potentially improve long-term functional outcomes after ACL reconstruction.

Chondral Damage

Damage to the cartilage at the time of injury has been suggested as another risk factor for PTOA. Through evaluation of the articular cartilage during arthroscopy, Ichiba and Kishimoto[36] found that the "cartilage-damaged" group had an increase in OA scores compared to the "no cartilage-damage" group. In another study, when the tibiofemoral and patellofemoral joints are analyzed separately, chondral lesions were shown as risk factors for the development of OA in both joint compartments.[38] Conversely, Li and colleagues[48] found that chondrosis in the lateral compartment was not significantly associated with knee OA, whereas patellofemoral chondrosis was significantly associated with knee OA.

Multiple different theories exist regarding the relationship between chondral damage and OA. Damage to the articular cartilage at the time of trauma may lead directly to OA. Similarly, instability after ACL injury with recurrent episodes of pivot shifting may increase cartilage damage and result in the development of OA.[53] Chondral injuries also produce a biochemical cascade, with increased concentrations of chondrodestructive cytokines and decreased concentration of chondroprotective cytokines compared to the contralateral knee.[54]

The relationship between occult osteochondral lesions, or bone bruises, and articular cartilage damage is unclear. Bone bruises occur in 80%–90%[9] of patients with an acute ACL injury, most commonly on the posterolateral tibial plateau and the anterolateral femoral condyle. Potter and colleagues[10] showed that the size of the bone marrow edema pattern was associated with cartilage degeneration from baseline through the third year. However, other studies show no correlation between bone bruise and cartilage degeneration or OA. Hanypsiak and colleagues[33] concluded that the presence of a bone bruise at the time of initial injury did not significantly alter the patient-oriented outcome or predict OA.

Age

Not surprisingly, age has been identified as a risk factor for the development of PTOA.[22,27,43,55–57] In 1 study,[38] age at the time of surgery proved to be a predictor for patellofemoral OA, but not for tibiofemoral OA.

Factors including chondrocyte senescence and preexisting joint degeneration increase the possibility of developing OA. In other words, because OA is a process not only of degeneration but also of mechanical wear and remodeling, the balance between anabolic and catabolic processes decrease with age. Age is often overlooked in ACL studies, however, because most patients who undergo ACL reconstruction are young.

Graft Choice

With improvements in surgical technique, there have been several graft choices, from allograft to autograft, and from bone-patellar tendon-bone to hamstring. Differences in opinion regarding graft choice indicate the lack of research identifying the optimal graft choice. Although most studies report outcomes of ACL reconstruction based on their preferential graft choice, a few studies have identified a superior graft choice for the prevention of PTOA.

Pinczewski and colleagues[58] found a trend toward increasing osteoarthritic changes in both the bone-patellar tendon-bone and the hamstring tendon graft cohorts between 2 and 10 years. However, the percentage of patients with normal (**International Knee Documentation Committee** grade A) radiographs decreased by 19% in the hamstring tendon group and 34% in the bone-patellar tendon-bone group. Three other studies also reported similar results,[38,48,59] in which the use of a bone-patellar tendon-bone graft was associated with an increased prevalence of OA compared to a hamstring tendon graft.

Time Interval between Injury and Surgical Intervention

Controversy exists regarding the timing of ACL reconstruction in patients who have chosen operative intervention. Because one of the goals of ACL reconstruction is to prevent secondary meniscal or chondral injuries, many argue that ACL surgery should not be delayed unnecessarily. Studies have shown that early reconstruction of the ACL reduces the development of OA when compared with late reconstruction.[37,38,43,60]

Keays and colleagues[38] concluded that a time delay between injury and surgery may be a predictor for tibiofemoral OA. Seon and colleagues[43] established that OA developed in 52% of those who underwent reconstruction more than 6 months after the initial injury. Additionally, 4 of 5 cases of advanced degenerative OA had developed in patients who had their reconstruction more than 2 years after the initial injury, suggesting that not only does a longer interval between injury and surgery increase the risk of OA but it also increases its severity. Especially in individuals intent on continuing activities that involve sidestepping or pivoting, early ACL reconstruction is advocated before episodes of giving way occur.[37] In a review of knee radiographs of 77 patients, Kullmer and colleagues[60] found that patients with acute ACL tears had a lower degree of OA on the day of surgery compared to the patients with chronic insufficiency, but the postoperative increase was identical in both groups.

WHERE DO WE GO FROM HERE?

Surgical techniques have improved, including the advent of arthroscopic surgery and the abandonment of repair for the improved reconstructive procedures. Preservation of meniscal tissues is of the utmost importance, in which total meniscectomies are nearly nonexistent, and partial meniscectomies or meniscal repair have been the treatment of choice for concomitant meniscal injury. Early rehabilitation, both preoperatively and postoperatively, has improved outcomes. Despite these changes in operative management, PTOA continues to be present after ACL and other joint injuries. New strategies are needed to delay or prevent the onset (of premature osteoarthritis) after ACL injury.

ADDRESSING THE BIOCHEMISTRY

From a biochemical standpoint, the ultimate method of preventing PTOA after ACL injury may be prevention of the inflammation that occurs acutely after injury. The majority of research in disease-modifying OA drugs focuses on the later stages of joint degeneration. However, in the case of PTOA, in which there is a clear precipitating event, a unique opportunity arises to intervene early in the acute posttraumatic period.[61] Prevention of the cascade of destructive processes within the joint may one day play a greater role. The use of antagonists to inflammatory cytokines such as tumor necrosis factor-alpha and IL-1 may be able to promote cartilage repair and/or restore joint homeostasis in the acute injury phase.

REHABILITATION

Whether a patient is treated nonoperatively or with ACL reconstruction, rehabilitation is an integral part of the treatment program. Rehabilitation techniques have evolved substantially over the past several decades, and the use of rehabilitation programs has become widely accepted. The goals of both nonoperative and postoperative rehabilitation include return of neuromuscular control, strength, power, and lower extremity functional symmetry.[62] Depending on the patient (high-level athlete vs a more sedentary individual), the rehabilitation protocol can be modified based on the individual patient's goals, resources, and response to treatment.

PREVENTION

Prevention of ACL injury is the number 1 approach to prevent PTOA. To reduce the risk of this injury, a large number of research studies are currently being conducted to identify ways to reduce the rate of ACL injuries and to improve rehabilitation after the injury.[63] Currently, neuromuscular training is the most effective tool to reduce the incidence of ACL injuries.[64] In a nonrandomized prospective study, female athletes enrolled in a neuromuscular and proprioceptive performance program saw in subsequent years, an 88% and 75% decrease, respectively, in ACL injury compared to the age-matched and skill-matched controls. A systemic review of the effectiveness of all ACL injury prevention training programs[65] found that a significant reduction in the risk of ACL rupture in the prevention group, with the number needed to treat as low as 5 in 1 study.

SUMMARY

Anterior cruciate ligament tear accelerates joint degeneration and leads to osteoarthritis in a high proportion of patients. While successful in stabilizing ACL deficient knees, ACL reconstruction has not been shown to conclusively reduce OA risk. Altered biomechanics, age, meniscal status, cartilage and other joint tissue injury, as well as patient factors contribute to accelerated development of OA after ACL injury. The injury typically occurs in teenagers and young adults resulting in early onset disability. Post-traumatic OA after ACL injury illustrates the concept that modifiable extrinsic factors play a substantial role in OA development.[61] As such, improved understanding of the factors leading to early onset OA after ACL injury will be important to development of new disease modifying strategies to delay or prevent development of not just PTOA but potentially also other forms of OA.

REFERENCES

1. Lohmander LS, Ostenberg A, Englund M, et al. High prevalence of knee osteoarthritis, pain, and functional limitations in female soccer players twelve years after anterior cruciate ligament injury. Arthritis Rheum 2004;50:3145–52.
2. Griffin LY, Albohm MJ, Arendt EA, et al. Understanding and preventing noncontact anterior cruciate ligament injuries: a review of the Hunt Valley II meeting, January 2005. Am J Sports Med 2006;34:1512–32.
3. Piasecki DP, Spindler KP, Warren TA, et al. Intraarticular injuries associated with anterior cruciate ligament tear: findings at ligament reconstruction in high school and recreational athletes. An analysis of sex-based differences. Am J Sports Med 2003;31:601–5.
4. Lohmander LS, Englund PM, Dahl LL, et al. The long-term consequence of anterior cruciate ligament and meniscus injuries: osteoarthritis. Am J Sports Med 2007;35:1756–69.
5. Shelbourne KD, Stube KC. Anterior cruciate ligament (ACL)-deficient knee with degenerative arthrosis: treatment with an isolated autogenous patellar tendon ACL reconstruction. Knee Surg Sports Traumatol Arthrosc 1997;5:150–6.
6. Nakata K, Shino K, Horibe S, et al. Arthroscopic anterior cruciate ligament reconstruction using fresh-frozen bone plug-free allogeneic tendons: 10-year follow-up. Arthroscopy 2008;24:285–91.
7. Lawrence RC, Felson DT, Helmick CG, et al. Estimates of the prevalence of arthritis and other rheumatic conditions in the United States. Part II. Arthritis Rheum 2008;58:26–35.

8. Roos H, Lindberg H, Gardsell P, et al. The prevalence of gonarthrosis and its relation to meniscectomy in former soccer players. Am J Sports Med 1994;22: 219–22.

9. Nishimori M, Deie M, Adachi N, et al. Articular cartilage injury of the posterior lateral tibial plateau associated with acute anterior cruciate ligament injury. Knee Surg Sports Traumatol Arthrosc 2008;16:270–4.

10. Potter HG, Jain SK, Ma Y, et al. Cartilage injury after acute, isolated anterior cruciate ligament tear: immediate and longitudinal effect with clinical/MRI follow-up. Am J Sports Med 2012;40:276–85.

11. Andriacchi TP, Mundermann A, Smith RL, et al. A framework for the in vivo pathomechanics of osteoarthritis at the knee. Ann Biomed Eng 2004;32: 447–57.

12. Papannagari R, Gill TJ, Defrate LE, et al. In vivo kinematics of the knee after anterior cruciate ligament reconstruction: a clinical and functional evaluation. Am J Sports Med 2006;34:2006–12.

13. Lohmander LS, Ionescu M, Jugessur H, et al. Changes in joint cartilage aggrecan after knee injury and in osteoarthritis. Arthritis Rheum 1999;42:534–44.

14. Nelson F, Billinghurst RC, Pidoux I, et al. Early post-traumatic osteoarthritis-like changes in human articular cartilage following rupture of the anterior cruciate ligament. Osteoarthritis Cartilage 2006;14:114–9.

15. Cuellar VG, Cuellar JM, Golish SR, et al. Cytokine profiling in acute anterior cruciate ligament injury. Arthroscopy 2010;26:1296–301.

16. Cuellar JM, Scuderi GJ, Cuellar VG, et al. Diagnostic utility of cytokine biomarkers in the evaluation of acute knee pain. J Bone Joint Surg Am 2009;91: 2313–20.

17. Cameron ML, Fu FH, Paessler HH, et al. Synovial fluid cytokine concentrations as possible prognostic indicators in the ACL-deficient knee. Knee Surg Sports Traumatol Arthrosc 1994;2:38–44.

18. Elsaid KA, Fleming BC, Oksendahl HL, et al. Decreased lubricin concentrations and markers of joint inflammation in the synovial fluid of patients with anterior cruciate ligament injury. Arthritis Rheum 2008;58:1707–15.

19. Irie K, Uchiyama E, Iwaso H. Intraarticular inflammatory cytokines in acute anterior cruciate ligament injured knee. Knee 2003;10:93–6.

20. Higuchi H, Shirakura K, Kimura M, et al. Changes in biochemical parameters after anterior cruciate ligament injury. Int Orthop 2006;30:43–7.

21. Meunier A, Odensten M, Good L. Long-term results after primary repair or non-surgical treatment of anterior cruciate ligament rupture: a randomized study with a 15-year follow-up. Scand J Med Sci Sports 2007;17:230–7.

22. Lebel B, Hulet C, Galaud B, et al. Arthroscopic reconstruction of the anterior cruciate ligament using bone-patellar tendon-bone autograft: a minimum 10-year follow-up. Am J Sports Med 2008;36:1275–82.

23. McDaniel WJ Jr, Dameron TB Jr. The untreated anterior cruciate ligament rupture. Clin Orthop Relat Res 1983;(172):158–63.

24. Nebelung W, Wuschech H. Thirty-five years of follow-up of anterior cruciate ligament-deficient knees in high-level athletes. Arthroscopy 2005;21:696–702.

25. van der Hart CP, van den Bekerom MP, Patt TW. The occurrence of osteoarthritis at a minimum of ten years after reconstruction of the anterior cruciate ligament. J Orthop Surg Res 2008;3:24.

26. Mihelic R, Jurdana H, Jotanovic Z, et al. Long-term results of anterior cruciate ligament reconstruction: a comparison with non-operative treatment with a follow-up of 17-20 years. Int Orthop 2011;35:1093–7.

27. Kessler MA, Behrend H, Henz S, et al. Function, osteoarthritis and activity after ACL-rupture: 11 years follow-up results of conservative versus reconstructive treatment. Knee Surg Sports Traumatol Arthrosc 2008;16:442–8.

28. Hoffelner T, Resch H, Moroder P, et al. No increased occurrence of osteoarthritis after anterior cruciate ligament reconstruction after isolated anterior cruciate ligament injury in athletes. Arthroscopy 2012;28:517–25.

29. Neuman P, Englund M, Kostogiannis I, et al. Prevalence of tibiofemoral osteoarthritis 15 years after nonoperative treatment of anterior cruciate ligament injury: a prospective cohort study. Am J Sports Med 2008;36:1717–25.

30. Daniel DM, Stone ML, Dobson BE, et al. Fate of the ACL-injured patient. A prospective outcome study. Am J Sports Med 1994;22:632–44.

31. Cohen M, Amaro JT, Ejnisman B, et al. Anterior cruciate ligament reconstruction after 10 to 15 years: association between meniscectomy and osteoarthrosis. Arthroscopy 2007;23:629–34.

32. Fink C, Hoser C, Hackl W, et al. Long-term outcome of operative or nonoperative treatment of anterior cruciate ligament rupture–is sports activity a determining variable? Int J Sports Med 2001;22:304–9.

33. Hanypsiak BT, Spindler KP, Rothrock CR, et al. Twelve-year follow-up on anterior cruciate ligament reconstruction: long-term outcomes of prospectively studied osseous and articular injuries. Am J Sports Med 2008;36:671–7.

34. Hart AJ, Buscombe J, Malone A, et al. Assessment of osteoarthritis after reconstruction of the anterior cruciate ligament: a study using single-photon emission computed tomography at ten years. J Bone Joint Surg Br 2005;87:1483–7.

35. Hertel P, Behrend H, Cierpinski T, et al. ACL reconstruction using bone-patellar tendon-bone press-fit fixation: 10-year clinical results. Knee Surg Sports Traumatol Arthrosc 2005;13:248–55.

36. Ichiba A, Kishimoto I. Effects of articular cartilage and meniscus injuries at the time of surgery on osteoarthritic changes after anterior cruciate ligament reconstruction in patients under 40 years old. Arch Orthop Trauma Surg 2009;129:409–15.

37. Jomha NM, Borton DC, Clingeleffer AJ, et al. Long-term osteoarthritic changes in anterior cruciate ligament reconstructed knees. Clin Orthop Relat Res 1999;358: 188–93.

38. Keays SL, Newcombe PA, Bullock-Saxton JE, et al. Factors involved in the development of osteoarthritis after anterior cruciate ligament surgery. Am J Sports Med 2010;38:455–63.

39. Maletius W, Messner K. Eighteen- to twenty-four-year follow-up after complete rupture of the anterior cruciate ligament. Am J Sports Med 1999;27:711–7.

40. Pritchard JC, Drez D Jr, Moss M, et al. Long-term followup of anterior cruciate ligament reconstruction using freeze-dried fascia lata allografts. Am J Sports Med 1995;23:593–6.

41. Reid JS, Hanks GA, Kalenak A, et al. The Ellison iliotibial-band transfer for a torn anterior cruciate ligament of the knee. Long-term follow-up. J Bone Joint Surg Am 1992;74:1392–402.

42. Salmon LJ, Russell VJ, Refshauge K, et al. Long-term outcome of endoscopic anterior cruciate ligament reconstruction with patellar tendon autograft: minimum 13-year review. Am J Sports Med 2006;34:721–32.

43. Seon JK, Song EK, Park SJ. Osteoarthritis after anterior cruciate ligament reconstruction using a patellar tendon autograft. Int Orthop 2006;30:94–8.

44. von Porat A, Roos EM, Roos H. High prevalence of osteoarthritis 14 years after an anterior cruciate ligament tear in male soccer players: a study of radiographic and patient relevant outcomes. Ann Rheum Dis 2004;63:269–73.

45. Wu WH, Hackett T, Richmond JC. Effects of meniscal and articular surface status on knee stability, function, and symptoms after anterior cruciate ligament reconstruction: a long-term prospective study. Am J Sports Med 2002; 30:845–50.
46. Yamaguchi S, Sasho T, Tsuchiya A, et al. Long term results of anterior cruciate ligament reconstruction with iliotibial tract: 6-, 13-, and 24-year longitudinal follow-up. Knee Surg Sports Traumatol Arthrosc 2006;14:1094–100.
47. Oiestad BE, Engebretsen L, Storheim K, et al. Knee osteoarthritis after anterior cruciate ligament injury: a systematic review. Am J Sports Med 2009;37:1434–43.
48. Li RT, Lorenz S, Xu Y, et al. Predictors of radiographic knee osteoarthritis after anterior cruciate ligament reconstruction. Am J Sports Med 2011;39: 2595–603.
49. Amin S, Guermazi A, Lavalley MP, et al. Complete anterior cruciate ligament tear and the risk for cartilage loss and progression of symptoms in men and women with knee osteoarthritis. Osteoarthritis Cartilage 2008;16:897–902.
50. Aglietti P, Zaccherotti G, De Biase P, et al. A comparison between medial meniscus repair, partial meniscectomy, and normal meniscus in anterior cruciate ligament reconstructed knees. Clin Orthop Relat Res 1994;307:165–73.
51. Englund M, Lohmander LS. Risk factors for symptomatic knee osteoarthritis fifteen to twenty-two years after meniscectomy. Arthritis Rheum 2004;50:2811–9.
52. Bowers AL, Spindler KP, McCarty EC, et al. Height, weight, and BMI predict intra-articular injuries observed during ACL reconstruction: evaluation of 456 cases from a prospective ACL database. Clin J Sport Med 2005;15:9–13.
53. Droll KP, Marks P. Risk factors in developing osteoarthritis in the anterior cruciate deficient knee. Univ Toronto Med J 1999;76:70–9.
54. Marks PH, Donaldson ML. Inflammatory cytokine profiles associated with chondral damage in the anterior cruciate ligament-deficient knee. Arthroscopy 2005; 21:1342–7.
55. Asano H, Muneta T, Ikeda H, et al. Arthroscopic evaluation of the articular cartilage after anterior cruciate ligament reconstruction: a short-term prospective study of 105 patients. Arthroscopy 2004;20:474–81.
56. Strand T, Molster A, Hordvik M, et al. Long-term follow-up after primary repair of the anterior cruciate ligament: clinical and radiological evaluation 15-23 years postoperatively. Arch Orthop Trauma Surg 2005;125:217–21.
57. Segawa H, Omori G, Koga Y. Long-term results of non-operative treatment of anterior cruciate ligament injury. Knee 2001;8:5–11.
58. Pinczewski LA, Lyman J, Salmon LJ, et al. 10-year comparison of anterior cruciate ligament reconstructions with hamstring tendon and patellar tendon autograft: a controlled, prospective trial. Am J Sports Med 2007;35:564–74.
59. Jarvela T, Paakkala T, Kannus P, et al. The incidence of patellofemoral osteoarthritis and associated findings 7 years after anterior cruciate ligament reconstruction with a bone-patellar tendon-bone autograft. Am J Sports Med 2001; 29:18–24.
60. Kullmer K, Letsch R, Turowski B. Which factors influence the progression of degenerative osteoarthritis after ACL surgery? Knee Surg Sports Traumatol Arthrosc 1994;2:80–4.
61. Chu CR, Williams AA, Coyle CH, et al. Early diagnosis to enable early treatment of pre-osteoarthritis. Arthritis Res Ther 2012;41:212–22.
62. Myer GD, Paterno MV, Ford KR, et al. Neuromuscular training techniques to target deficits before return to sport after anterior cruciate ligament reconstruction. J Strength Cond Res 2008;22:987–1014.

63. Butler RJ, Minick KI, Ferber R, et al. Gait mechanics after ACL reconstruction: implications for the early onset of knee osteoarthritis. Br J Sports Med 2009;43: 366–70.
64. Hurd WJ, Chmielewski TL, Snyder-Mackler L. Perturbation-enhanced neuromuscular training alters muscle activity in female athletes. Knee Surg Sports Traumatol Arthrosc 2006;14:60–9.
65. Sadoghi P, von Keudell A, Vavken P. Effectiveness of anterior cruciate ligament injury prevention training programs. J Bone Joint Surg Am 2012;94:769–76.

Anterior Cruciate Ligament Healing and Advances in Imaging

Stephen J. Rabuck, MD[a],*, Michael G. Baraga, MD[b],
Freddie H. Fu, MD[a]

KEYWORDS

- Anterior cruciate ligament • Healing • Imaging • Magnetic resonance imaging
- Plain radiography • Computed tomography • Vascularization • Maturation

KEY POINTS

- Graft maturity undergoes a process of "ligamentization," which can be correlated with magnetic resonance imaging findings.
- The process of graft maturation includes early, remodeling, and maturation phases.
- Cross-sectional imaging provides the most complete assessment of graft healing within tunnels.
- Tunnel healing appears to lag behind graft maturation.

INTRODUCTION

Advances in imaging have provided clinicians with powerful, noninvasive methods to assess the progress of a patient in the healing process. Magnetic resonance imaging (MRI) has been used to assess the healing process of articular cartilage, menisci, and ligamentous structures.[1–3] The utility of these tools in anterior cruciate ligament (ACL) reconstruction continues to evolve as clinicians attempt to understand the impact of graft healing on patient outcomes. Perhaps most importantly in ACL reconstruction is the ability for a graft to tolerate the required forces for a patient to return to sport. There is tremendous variability in the literature regarding return to sport following ACL reconstruction, with reports ranging from 33% to 92%.[4,5] This variability suggests patients may be returning to sport before the reconstructed ACL is able to tolerate the forces necessary to do so. Ideally a patient would return to sport once the reconstructed ACL had matured. As a result, methods to assess graft maturity and healing

Funding sources: There were no funding sources for this study.
Conflict of interest: The authors report no conflict of interest.
[a] Department of Orthopaedic Surgery, University of Pittsburgh Medical Center, Pittsburgh, PA, USA; [b] UHealth Sports Medicine, Department of Orthopaedic Surgery, University of Miami Miller School of Medicine, Miami, Florida, USA
* Corresponding author. Department of Orthopaedic Surgery, University of Pittsburgh Medical Center, Center for Sports Medicine, 3200 South Water Street, Pittsburgh, PA 15203.
E-mail address: rabucksj@upmc.edu

Clin Sports Med 32 (2013) 13–20
http://dx.doi.org/10.1016/j.csm.2012.08.003
0278-5919/13/$ – see front matter © 2013 Elsevier Inc. All rights reserved.

are important clinical tools in assessing which stage each individual has reached in the progression of graft healing and maturation. These tools may also be helpful in developing physical therapy protocols and deciding when an athlete is allowed to return to sport.

GRAFT MATURATION

The "ligamentization" process, by which an ACL graft undergoes healing and remodeling, has been studied histologically in animal models and, to a lesser degree, in humans. Numerous animal studies have shown a process involving revascularization, cell repopulation, and metaplasia of the tendon tissue to a ligamentous appearance.[6,7] Although the ligamentization process in animals has correlated well with human studies, the time frame in which this process occurs has been shown to take longer in humans.

The stages of graft healing and maturation have been divided into early, remodeling, and maturation, although there does not seem to be a consensus on the timing of these stages.[8–12] Studies have shown increasing vascularity in the early phase, establishing the groundwork for graft remodeling and healing. This increase in vascularity will slowly decrease as remodeling progresses toward a tissue that histologically resembles the native ACL. Although visualization under light microscopy provides direct information regarding revascularization, studies on ACL graft healing in humans are difficult to perform, given their invasive nature and the need to remove tissue from the reconstructed ACL. MRI provides a noninvasive means to evaluate revascularization, as represented by an increased signal intensity of the graft and periligamentous tissue.

Studies have shown that MRI may be used to determine graft vascularity by correlating to signal intensity. Several studies have described methods to assess graft vascularity using MRI. On proton density (PD)-weighted sequences, an increase in signal appears to correlate with increased vascularity (**Fig. 1**). Graft signal will then

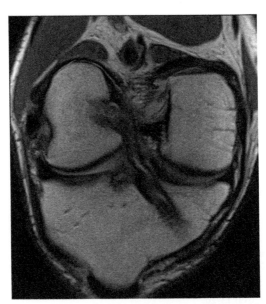

Fig. 1. Magnetic resonance image of immature ACL reconstruction 6 months postoperatively, with high signal consistent with vascularization of the ACL graft.

decrease as the graft matures (**Fig. 2**). Ntoulia and colleagues[13] studied this finding in human subjects undergoing autograft bone-patellar tendon-bone ACL reconstruction. Contrast-enhanced MRI was used to evaluate graft vascularity by calculating the Enhancement Index (ratio between the signal-to-noise quotient [SNQ] after contrast and before contrast). Thirty-two male patients were evaluated at postoperative day 3, as well as 6 and 12 months after surgery. No increase in graft signal intensity was seen 3 days after surgery. The intra-articular graft site showed significant enhancement at 6 months, with no significant increase at 12 months.

Gohil and colleagues[14] used MRI to evaluate the effects a remnant-sparing minimal debridement technique may have on revascularization in subjects undergoing autologous hamstring ACL reconstruction. The investigators reported earlier revascularization in the minimal debridement group at 2 months in comparison with standard reconstruction techniques. Although histologic studies have confirmed the presence of a vascularized graft as early as 3 weeks, the findings of these studies correlate with the increase in vascularity described in histologic studies.[11]

MRI has also been useful in comparing healing between autograft and allograft tissue. Marumatsu and colleagues[15] compared remodeling between autogeneic and allogeneic bone-patellar tendon-bone grafts in patients undergoing ACL reconstruction. Contrast-enhanced MRI was performed at 1, 4, 6, and 12 months after surgery, with occasional MRIs obtained up to 72 months after. An SNQ was calculated as described by Weiler and colleagues.[16] Autografts were shown to have increased signal intensity as early as 1 month after surgery, whereas no change was seen in the allograft group at the same time point. Autografts were also shown to reach peak revascularization early at 4 to 6 months after surgery. Allografts on the other hand showed increasing SNQ values 12 to 24 months after surgery, indicating a slower onset and rate of vascularization.

Weiler and colleagues[16] were able to correlate an increase in vascularity with decreased mechanical properties in a sheep model of ACL reconstruction. The investigators studied sheep undergoing autogenous Achilles tendon ACL reconstruction at

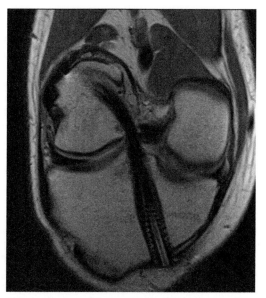

Fig. 2. Magnetic resonance image of ACL reconstruction 10 months postoperatively, with low signal consistent with maturation of the ACL graft.

time intervals of 6, 12, 24, 52, and 104 weeks postreconstruction. Both contrast and noncontrast enhanced MRI, as well as histologic evaluation, were used to study graft vascularity, which correlated with higher signal intensity. The specimens were also tested for biomechanical properties at the time of sacrifice. The investigators were able to identify an inverse relationship between the signal intensity of the graft and its biomechanical properties, noting that grafts tested during the early remodeling with high vascularity were significantly weaker than grafts implanted at time zero. This finding may help explain why allografts exhibit a higher retear rate than autografts, given their delayed revascularization.

Although evaluation using an SNQ from contrast-enhanced MRI seems promising, the signal intensity can be affected by unrelated factors such as scanner characteristics and image-acquisition techniques. Graft impingement has also been described as a possible cause of increased graft signal intensity. Fleming and colleagues[17] evaluated the use of alternative parameters, independent of acquisition characteristics. These investigators hypothesized that graft volume would reflect the structural properties, and T2 mapping would also provide information as it relates to collagen and water content. A significant correlation was shown between graft volume and load to failure. Normalizing for T2 relaxation time made this correlation stronger.

TUNNEL HEALING

The process of graft maturation and healing requires incorporation of the newly reconstructed ACL graft into the host bone. The time required for this process to take place can vary depending on the graft used as well as host factors. Noninvasive means to assess the progress of graft healing may play an important role in individualizing rehabilitation and return to sport. The noninvasive modalities most commonly used include plain radiographs, computed tomography (CT), and MRI.

Plain Radiographs

Routine follow-up after ACL reconstruction often includes radiographic evaluation. Anteroposterior and lateral radiographs can be used to not only assess tunnel position, integrity, and position of fixation devices but also as an evaluation for signs of graft incorporation within tunnels.[18–20]

Tunnel widening is one of the most commonly encountered parameters used to evaluate graft incorporation (**Fig. 3**). Correlations have been drawn between the documented delay in graft incorporation on histologic examination and an increased incidence of tunnel widening in allograft ACL reconstructions.[21] Tunnel widening has been implicated in delayed incorporation, maturation, and graft laxity.[18,22–24] However, the clinical significance of tunnel widening has come into question as small studies have shown no difference in outcomes for those cases with tunnel widening.[25,26]

Another radiographic parameter used to assess graft incorporation and tunnel healing is the development of a cortical rim. Histologic examination has demonstrated a thickened cortical rim in specimens with graft incorporation.[22] Radiographic evaluation has shown a correlation between the histologic findings of graft incorporation and development of a cortical rim on imaging.[23,24] In addition, clinical studies at 5-year follow-up have shown radiographic findings to correlate with good outcomes.[20]

Plain radiographs are commonly obtained in follow-up, and pose minimal risk to patients because they require limited radiation exposure and are relatively inexpensive. However, plain radiography is limited in its ability to assess tunnel healing, and in cases

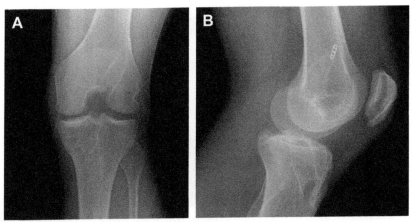

Fig. 3. Anteroposterior (*A*) and lateral (*B*) radiographs of a patient following failure of primary ACL reconstruction, with evidence of tunnel widening.

where further detail is necessary, especially when examining the femoral tunnel, advanced imaging such as CT and MRI more reliably assess graft incorporation.[20]

Computed Tomography

Assessment of ACL graft with CT scanning has taken on an important role in anatomic reconstruction of the ACL. This modality allows for assessment of anatomic placement of the ACL graft, as bony landmarks that identify the native anatomy have recently been recognized. On the medial wall of the lateral femoral condyle, the lateral intercondylar ridge identifies the anterior border of the anatomic position of the ACL (**Fig. 4**) and can be assessed for tunnel position in anatomic ACL reconstruction.[27]

When assessing graft incorporation on a CT scan, cross-sectional area and the development of a cortical rim have become recognized measures of graft incorporation for both soft-tissue and osseous grafts in animal models.[22,28] Cross-sectional imaging has demonstrated decreases in cross-sectional area to correlate well with histologic examination showing osteointegration of the graft within the tunnel.[22,23] In addition, graft bone plug incorporation and bridging trabeculae or the development of a cortical rim for soft-tissue grafts can be assessed with cross-sectional imaging.[28]

Magnetic Resonance Imaging

MRI is a powerful tool that not only provides information regarding osseous morphology and development but also changes in vascular supply. As discussed previously, the ACL graft undergoes a predictable sequence of graft maturation, which can be followed using MRI.[3] The changes in graft structure are not limited to the intra-articular portion of the graft, but perhaps more importantly can be followed for the portions of the graft within the femoral and tibial tunnels.

Maturation of the graft within the tunnel appears to lag behind the intra-articular graft. In a study of 32 patients undergoing ACL reconstruction evaluated up to 12 months postoperatively by Ntoulia and colleagues,[13] graft maturation appeared to occur most rapidly for the intra-articular portion, and be delayed for the graft adjacent to fixation devices located within the tunnel.

An important benefit of MRI in the evaluation of tunnel healing is that information on graft vascularity can be obtained while evaluating cross-sectional imaging of tunnel

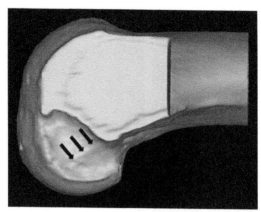

Fig. 4. Computed tomography scan of the medial wall of the lateral femoral condyle, identifying anatomic landmarks for ACL reconstruction including the lateral intercondylar ridge (arrows).

diameter and osteointegration. Cross-sectional imaging provides more reliable information of tunnel diameter, and MRI is superior to plain radiographs for the assessment of tunnel diameter.[20] Decreases in tunnel diameter on MRI have been correlated with increased osteointegration and vascularity.[20]

The additional information obtained with MRI can also assess the influence of graft-fixation devices on healing within the tunnel. Although this information can be used to guide rehabilitation and clinical decision making, further outcomes studies are necessary to assess the role of advanced imaging in patient care.

SUMMARY

Recent literature has shown noninvasive methods used to assess graft maturity to correlate with histologic findings. The importance of allowing adequate graft healing must be considered as the current understanding of anatomic ACL reconstruction continues to evolve. Graft forces across an anatomically positioned ACL reconstruction may exceed those of a maturing graft. The literature has shown a predictable sequence of graft maturation through early, remodeling, and mature phases. This graft maturation appears to precede tunnel incorporation and maturation on MRI; however, further studies are necessary to better assess tunnel incorporation. Additional information can be obtained from plain radiographs and CT, with improved assessment of trabeculae and bony incorporation. As the use of imaging expands, the role for these tools in assessing patients' progress through rehabilitation and timing their return to sport may also expand. With this information, clinicians may use these tools to minimize the risk of graft failure on return to sport and improve patients' outcomes following ACL reconstruction.

REFERENCES

1. Choi JY, Ha JK, Kim YW, et al. Relationships among tendon regeneration on MRI, flexor strength, and functional performance after anterior cruciate ligament reconstruction with hamstring autograft. Am J Sports Med 2012;40(1): 152–62.

2. Frobell RB, Le Graverand MP, Buck R, et al. The acutely ACL injured knee assessed by MRI: changes in joint fluid, bone marrow lesions, and cartilage during the first year. Osteoarthritis Cartilage 2009;17(2):161–7.
3. White LM, Kramer J, Recht MP. MR imaging evaluation of the postoperative knee: ligaments, menisci, and articular cartilage. Skeletal Radiol 2005;34(8): 431–52.
4. Langford JL, Webster KE, Feller JA. A prospective longitudinal study to assess psychological changes following anterior cruciate ligament reconstruction surgery. Br J Sports Med 2009;43(5):377–8.
5. Nakayama Y, Shirai Y, Narita T, et al. Knee functions and a return to sports activity in competitive athletes following anterior cruciate ligament reconstruction. J Nihon Med Sch 2000;67(3):172–6.
6. Amiel D, Kleiner JB, Roux RD, et al. The phenomenon of "ligamentization": anterior cruciate ligament reconstruction with autogenous patellar tendon. J Orthop Res 1986;4(2):162–72.
7. Arnoczky SP, Tarvin GB, Marshall JL. Anterior cruciate ligament replacement using patellar tendon. An evaluation of graft revascularization in the dog. J Bone Joint Surg Am 1982;64(2):217–24.
8. Abe S, Kurosaka M, Iguchi T, et al. Light and electron microscopic study of remodeling and maturation process in autogenous graft for anterior cruciate ligament reconstruction. Arthroscopy 1993;9(4):394–405.
9. Claes S, Verdonk P, Forsyth R, et al. The "ligamentization" process in anterior cruciate ligament reconstruction: what happens to the human graft? A systematic review of the literature. Am J Sports Med 2011;39(11):2476–83.
10. Falconiero RP, DiStefano VJ, Cook TM. Revascularization and ligamentization of autogenous anterior cruciate ligament grafts in humans. Arthroscopy 1998; 14(2):197–205.
11. Rougraff BT, Shelbourne KD. Early histologic appearance of human patellar tendon autografts used for anterior cruciate ligament reconstruction. Knee Surg Sports Traumatol Arthrosc 1999;7(1):9–14.
12. Sanchez M, Anitua E, Azofra J, et al. Ligamentization of tendon grafts treated with an endogenous preparation rich in growth factors: gross morphology and histology. Arthroscopy 2010;26(4):470–80.
13. Ntoulia A, Papadopoulou F, Ristanis S, et al. Revascularization process of the bone-patellar tendon-bone autograft evaluated by contrast-enhanced magnetic resonance imaging 6 and 12 months after anterior cruciate ligament reconstruction. Am J Sports Med 2011;39(7):1478–86.
14. Gohil S, Annear PO, Breidahl W. Anterior cruciate ligament reconstruction using autologous double hamstrings: a comparison of standard versus minimal debridement techniques using MRI to assess revascularisation. A randomised prospective study with a one-year follow-up. J Bone Joint Surg Br 2007;89(9):1165–71.
15. Muramatsu K, Hachiya Y, Izawa H. Serial evaluation of human anterior cruciate ligament grafts by contrast-enhanced magnetic resonance imaging: comparison of allografts and autografts. Arthroscopy 2008;24(9):1038–44.
16. Weiler A, Peters G, Maurer J, et al. Biomechanical properties and vascularity of an anterior cruciate ligament graft can be predicted by contrast-enhanced magnetic resonance imaging. A two-year study in sheep. Am J Sports Med 2001;29(6):751–61.
17. Fleming BC, Vajapeyam S, Connolly SA, et al. The use of magnetic resonance imaging to predict ACL graft structural properties. J Biomech 2011;44(16): 2843–6.

18. Hoher J, Moller HD, Fu FH. Bone tunnel enlargement after anterior cruciate ligament reconstruction: fact or fiction? Knee Surg Sports Traumatol Arthrosc 1998; 6(4):231–40.
19. L'Insalata JC, Klatt B, Fu FH, et al. Tunnel expansion following anterior cruciate ligament reconstruction: a comparison of hamstring and patellar tendon autografts. Knee Surg Sports Traumatol Arthrosc 1997;5(4):234–8.
20. Lajtai G, Schmiedhuber G, Unger F, et al. Bone tunnel remodeling at the site of biodegradable interference screws used for anterior cruciate ligament reconstruction: 5-year follow-up. Arthroscopy 2001;17(6):597–602.
21. Fahey M, Indelicato PA. Bone tunnel enlargement after anterior cruciate ligament replacement. Am J Sports Med 1994;22(3):410–4.
22. Matsumoto T, Kubo S, Sasaki K, et al. Acceleration of tendon-bone healing of anterior cruciate ligament graft using autologous ruptured tissue. Am J Sports Med 2012;40(6):1296–302.
23. Sasaki K, Kuroda R, Ishida K, et al. Enhancement of tendon-bone osteointegration of anterior cruciate ligament graft using granulocyte colony-stimulating factor. Am J Sports Med 2008;36(8):1519–27.
24. Webster KE, Chiu JJ, Feller JA. Impact of measurement error in the analysis of bone tunnel enlargement after anterior cruciate ligament reconstruction. Am J Sports Med 2005;33(11):1680–7.
25. Clatworthy MG, Annear P, Bulow JU, et al. Tunnel widening in anterior cruciate ligament reconstruction: a prospective evaluation of hamstring and patella tendon grafts. Knee Surg Sports Traumatol Arthrosc 1999;7(3):138–45.
26. Ma CB, Kawamura S, Deng XH, et al. Bone morphogenetic proteins-signaling plays a role in tendon-to-bone healing: a study of rhBMP-2 and noggin. Am J Sports Med 2007;35(4):597–604.
27. Ferretti M, Ekdahl M, Shen W, et al. Osseous landmarks of the femoral attachment of the anterior cruciate ligament: an anatomic study. Arthroscopy 2007;23(11): 1218–25.
28. Gulotta LV, Kovacevic D, Ying L, et al. Augmentation of tendon-to-bone healing with a magnesium-based bone adhesive. Am J Sports Med 2008;36(7):1290–7.

Quantitative MRI of the ACL-Injured and Reconstructed Knee

Jong-Min Kim, MD[a], C. Benjamin Ma, MD[b],*

KEYWORDS

- Knee reconstruction • MRI • ACL injury • Knee

KEY POINTS

- MRI has led to significant advancement in diagnosis of soft tissue injuries.
- Recent advances in MRI allow high-resolution images with shorter acquisition time and compositional analysis of tissues. Static, unloaded, and morphologic examination became dynamic, loaded, and biochemical analyses.
- Up-to-date applications of quantitative and kinematic analysis of ACL-injured and reconstructed knees are reviewed.

INTRODUCTION

Evaluations of anterior cruciate ligament (ACL)-injured and reconstructed knees have focused mainly on radiographic evaluations, subjective and objective scoring systems, and stability assessed with instruments such as KT-1000 (MEDmetric, San Diego, CA). These modalities are helpful in evaluating the current status and clinical function of each patient. However, they do not provide information on early or subtle changes in adjacent articular cartilage and knee kinematics that may influence treatment plan and long-term prognosis following ligament injuries.

Late complications of ACL injury, such as cartilage degeneration, were considered to be a consequence of long-standing functional deficit of the ACL itself. Contrary to this expectation, several studies reported that several cases resulted in degenerative arthritis, even after ACL-reconstruction surgery.[1–4] These results indicate that initial injury to cartilage and underlying bony architecture may contribute substantially to the long-term outcomes following ACL injuries. Moreover, there needs to be better evaluation of surgical success because knee kinematics or cartilage health may not be restored despite surgical reconstructions. It is important to detect the extent of injury to tissues other than ACL as early as possible to properly guide the patients

[a] Department of Orthopedic Surgery, Asan Medical Center, University of Ulsan College of Medicine, Seoul, Korea; [b] Department of Orthopaedic Surgery, University of California San Francisco, Orthopaedic Institute, 1500 Owens street, San Francisco, CA 94158, USA
* Corresponding author.
E-mail address: maben@orthosurg.ucsf.edu

Clin Sports Med 32 (2013) 21–36
http://dx.doi.org/10.1016/j.csm.2012.08.004
0278-5919/13/$ – see front matter © 2013 Elsevier Inc. All rights reserved.

and obtain satisfactory outcomes. Recent advances in MRI enable physicians to make accurate morphologic assessment on injured structures and to precisely quantify changes in biochemical composition of cartilage and knee kinematics.

QUANTITATIVE MRI

MRI techniques have evolved over the past 2 to 3 decades to improve detection of minor changes in morphology of soft tissues as well as bony structures of knee joint. Various sequences, such as fat-suppression techniques, two-dimensional (2D) and three-dimensional (3D) fast spin echo, spoiled gradient-echo, driven equilibrium Fourier transform, dual echo steady state, and balanced steady-state free precession imaging have been used to delineate articular cartilage of knee joint.[5] Scoring systems were also devised to accommodate these changes in semiquantitative fashion, including whole-organ MRI score (WORMS),[6] the Boston-Leeds osteoarthritis knee score (BLOKS),[7] and the knee osteoarthritis scoring system (KOSS).[8] High sensitivity and specificity have been reported with these techniques.[9]

However, early phenomenon of cartilage breakdown does not always manifest as morphologic change. Earlier events of cartilage degeneration that precede morphologic change are known to be changes in its biochemical composition.[10] Detection of early biochemical changes in cartilage is amenable with the recent development in MRI techniques. This article addresses some of the new advancements in quantitative MRI of articular cartilage and bone injuries. Recent literature and research in delayed gadolinium-enhanced MRI of cartilage (dGEMRIC), T2 mapping, T1ρ mapping, and magnetic resonance spectroscopy imaging (MRSI) on bone marrow edema-like lesions (BMEL) is discussed.

dGEMRIC

Articular cartilage consists of water, chondrocytes, and extracellular matrix composed of collagen fibrils and proteoglycan, which contains negatively charged glycosaminoglycan (GAG) molecules. Decrease in GAG content is known to be an early event of cartilage breakdown.[10] When anions such as gadolinium diethylenetriaminepentaacetic acid (Gd-DTPA)$^{2-}$ enter a joint, they distribute in cartilage inversely to the amount of GAG (**Fig. 1**). In other words, the more damaged the articular cartilage is, the higher is the concentration of Gd-DTPA^{2-} in the area. The gadolinium-enhanced

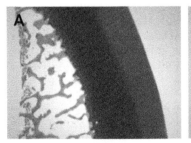 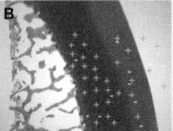

Fig. 1. (A) Toluidine blue, a cationic dye used to visualize GAG, shows two distinct regions in histologic section: one staining light purple, indicating low GAG, and the other staining dark purple, indicating high GAG concentration. (B) The relative distribution of mobile ions. Due to the GAG's negative charge, cations are more concentrated in cartilage than in the surrounding synovial fluid and are more concentrated in the high GAG than in the low GAG region. Conversely, the higher GAG, the less concentrated the anions.

measurement of tissue T1 values (T1Gd or dGEMRIC index) represents the amount of GAG in cartilage. Low T1Gd index is commonly observed in the area of cartilage degeneration.

Application in ACL Injuries

In an observational longitudinal study, cartilage GAG content after ACL injury was evaluated using dGEMRIC.[11] The ACL-injured group (29 subjects) was examined by dGEMRIC at 3 weeks and 2.3 years after injury and compared with a reference cohort (24 normal subjects). T1Gd index was measured at the central weight-bearing portion of lateral and medial femoral cartilage. The healthy reference group showed higher T1Gd value than the ACL-injured group did in both medial and lateral compartments. In the ACL-injured group, the T1Gd index was lower in subjects with concomitant meniscectomy than in subjects without meniscectomy in both medial and lateral compartments. Follow-up dGEMRIC examination in the ACL-injured group showed similar T1Gd values in the medial compartment and minor but significant increase in the lateral compartment. GAG content was lower in the ACL-injured group and more pronounced with associated meniscectomy. T1Gd index was considered to be a useful early biomarker for early posttraumatic osteoarthritis (OA).

In another study, 15 subjects with unilateral ACL injury were examined using dGEM-RIC with the contralateral knee used as control.[12] The median time from injury to MRI was 82 days and the median slice of medial compartment was selected for comparison. Index comparisons were made of knee status (ACL-injured vs control group), scan order (ACL-injured first vs control first), and cartilage location (femur vs tibia). There was a significant difference in the mean dGEMRIC indices between injured and uninjured knees (**Fig. 2**). No significant effects were identified owing to test order or cartilage location.

Review

Advantages of dGEMRIC
- It is an effective demonstration of GAG changes in cartilage
- It is a well-validated method of measuring GAG level.

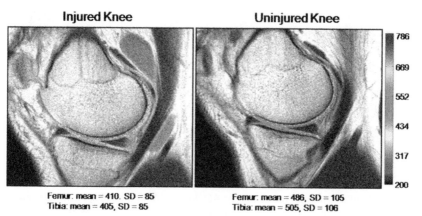

Fig. 2. T1 maps of the medial compartment of the femur and the tibia with the mean dGEMRIC indices calculated. The blue and red regions denote high and low GAG concentrations, respectively. SD, standard deviation.

Disadvantages of dGEMRIC

- It is time consuming and requires an intravenous injection of gadolinium followed by light exercise for even diffusion of contrast throughout the joint. Although there is no unanimous agreement on the time interval, about 50 to 90 minutes are needed from injection to imaging. Several hours are required to undergo the whole process, which comprises injection, joint exercise, diffusion, and image acquisition.
- It requires a two to three times higher dose of intravenous gadolinium than usual. Intravenous use of gadolinium has been implicated in the rare but fatal condition of nephrogenic systemic fibrosis for patients with renal insufficiency.

T2 MAPPING

T2 mapping measures interactions between a water molecule and surrounding macro-molecules and reflects the collagen component in the cartilage extracellular matrix. Increased interaction between water and collagen decreases T2 values. Therefore, T2 mapping is very sensitive to water and collagen changes in cartilage, which subsequently makes it suitable for early detection of degeneration. It is also sensitive to the orientation of collagen fibrils. Taking zonal variations of collagen orientation in cartilage into account, T2 mapping enables analysis of cartilage in layers. T2 values are barely influenced by GAG content in cartilage.

Application in ACL Injuries

T2 mapping has not been popularized in evaluation of ACL-injured patients. One recent longitudinal study used this technique in part to assess cartilage status of ACL-injured subjects at follow-up.[13] Forty-two knees with acute, isolated ACL injury underwent MRI at the time of injury and at yearly follow-up with a maximum of 11 years (**Figs. 3** and **4**). All subjects showed chondral damage at the time of injury. By follow-up years 7 to 11, the risk of cartilage loss for lateral femoral condyle was 50 times baseline, 30 times for patella, and 19 times for medial femoral condyle.

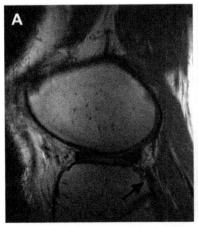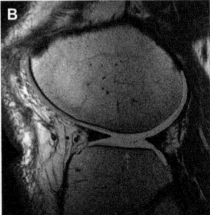

Fig. 3. A patient's MRI at 22 months after ACL injury. (*A*) The cartilage-sensitive sequence shows depression of the far posterolateral tibial plateau with cartilage loss. Focal bone formation is seen over the site of impact (*arrow*). (*B*) T2 mapping shows prolongation of T2 relaxation times over the far posterolateral tibial plateau (*solid arrow*) as well as over the central lateral tibial plateau (*dashed arrow*), an area that was not involved by the initial bone bruise.

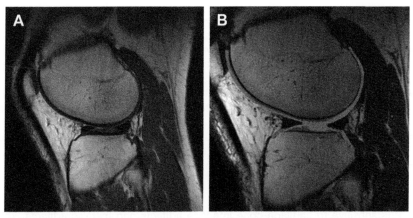

Fig. 4. The patient from Fig. 3, 4 years after injury. (*A*) Morphologic image shows depression of the far posterolateral tibial plateau. (*B*) T2 mapping shows progressive prolongation of T2 relaxation times over the central tibial plateau (*arrow*) compared with the study in **Fig. 3**.

To acquire very short T2 signal from type-I collagen of tendons, ligaments, or menisci, a specific sequence is needed. Ultrashort echo time-enhanced T2* (UTE-T2*) was used in an effort to detect early degeneration of meniscal tissue before surface breakdown.[14] The investigators compared UTE-T2* with histologic findings in 16 cadaveric menisci. UTE-T2* values tended to be lower in histologically normal menisci and higher in torn or degenerated tissues. UTE-T2* values of 10 asymptomatic subjects were compared with ACL-injured subjects with or without meniscal tear. Posteromedial meniscus UTE-T2* values in ACL-injured subjects with medial meniscus tear were 87% higher than in asymptomatic control subjects ($P<.001$). Posteromedial meniscus UTE-T2* values in ACL-injured subjects without medial meniscus tear were 33% higher than control ($P = .001$) (**Fig. 5**). The investigators stated that UTE-T2* mapping is sensitive to subclinical degeneration of meniscal tissue.

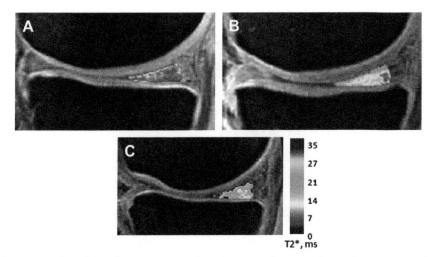

Fig. 5. UTE-T2* values of an asymptomatic patient were lower and more homogeneous (*A*) than observed in a patient without (*B*) or in a patient with tear in the medial meniscus (*C*). ms, millisecond.

Advantages of T2 mapping
- It is highly sensitive to changes in water content and orientations of collagen fibers. It has been reported to be effective in recognizing early degeneration in cartilage.[15]
- Zonal differences in density and orientation of collagen fibers in normal cartilage are readily detected. It can be advantageous in longitudinal monitoring of cartilage repair procedure.[16–19]
- It requires no additional hardware and can be easily conducted in usual, routine MRI, which makes it feasible in most current MRI machines.
- There is a relatively short scanning time.

Disadvantages of T2 mapping
- It is sensitive to cartilage-bone interface artifacts and metallic artifacts. Thus, cautious segmentation of cartilage is needed for accurate analysis.
- T2 values are not as sensitive to the degree of cartilage degeneration.[20]

T1ρ MAPPING

T1ρ mapping can measure the low-frequency interactions between spinning hydrogen proton and local macromolecular environment. Therefore, changes in local macromolecular environment, such as proteoglycan depletion, will result in changes in T1ρ values.[21] Changes in collagen content may also influence T1ρ values. Eventually, degenerated cartilage will show higher T1ρ values than normal (**Fig. 6**).

Application in ACL Injuries

Li and colleagues[22] used T1ρ and T2 mapping in an acutely ACL-injured group at the time of injury and 1 year after ACL reconstruction. They also used a control group for comparison. At baseline, posterior lateral tibial cartilage, where the bone bruises were

A healthy volunteer

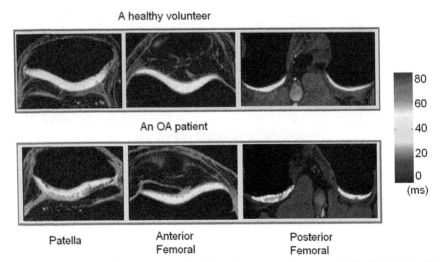

An OA patient

| Patella | Anterior Femoral | Posterior Femoral |

Fig. 6. T1ρ mapping of cartilage in a healthy volunteer and a patient with OA. Higher T1ρ values are noted in the patient with OA. ms, millisecond.

located, demonstrated elevated T1ρ value in the ACL-injured group compared with the control group. A year after ACL reconstruction, this elevation decreased but did not recover. The investigators stated that overlying cartilage (OC) may not be fully recovered in spite of resolution of the BMEL beneath it. T1ρ values in the weight-bearing portion of medial femorotibial cartilage of ACL-injured group were elevated significantly compared with normal control group at 1-year follow-up. T2 values showed no significant difference between the ACL-injured and the control group at all times. Data indicated that T1ρ may be more sensitive than T2 in detection of early cartilage degeneration with ACL injury. Subjects with medial meniscus posterior horn lesions demonstrated significantly higher T1ρ and T2 values in adjacent cartilage at both baseline and 1-year follow-up compared with subjects without medial meniscus lesions.

In another study, evaluation of BMEL and OC in nine ACL-injured and subsequently reconstructed knees were done using T1ρ mapping.[23] MRI scans were obtained at initial injury and at 0.5, 6, and 12 months after ACL reconstruction. BMELs were more frequently found in the lateral than in the medial compartment; the most common site was the lateral tibial plateau (LTP). Half of BMELs resolved in 1 year. T1ρ values in OC in the LTP were significantly higher than those in surrounding cartilage at all times (**Fig. 7**). The percent increase in T1ρ values in OC in LTP was correlated with volume of BMEL ($r = 0.74$, $P<.05$). The T1ρ values in OC remained elevated in spite of resolution of BMELs. This preliminary study led us better understanding of the extent of injury to particular tissue types and can help physicians develop long-term prognoses to these injuries.

Review

Advantages of T1ρ mapping
- T1ρ mapping is known to have higher sensitivity in detecting early events of carti-lage degeneration[24,25] and higher specificity in detecting changes in proteo-glycan content than T2-weighted imaging.[26]
- It allows measurement of proteoglycan concentration without intravenous contrast injection.

Disadvantages T1ρ mapping
- T1ρ mapping requires a special sequence with additional radiofrequency pulse that is not available for all machines.
- It takes extra time to acquire and interpret the data.
- It needs calibration between different machines to allow comparison.

BONE MARROW IMAGING

Bone bruises in acute injury show increased signal intensity in T2-weighted, fat-sup-pressed MRIs or short inversion time inversion recovery (STIR) images. This increased signal intensity is believed to represent abnormal trabeculae, bone marrow edema and necrosis, swelling of fat cells, and marrow bleeding. Bone bruises have been reported in about 48% to 85% of ACL injuries.[27–29] Although some investigators reported fairly benign end results of bone bruise with spontaneous resolution within 6 to 12 weeks,[29,30] others reported worse outcome with severe type being persistent for years and recommended stratified treatment of this common injury.[31–33] Some investigators used biopsy to determine the histopathology of bone bruise and revealed cancellous bone edema, bleeding, osteocyte necrosis, loss of proteoglycan in OC, and

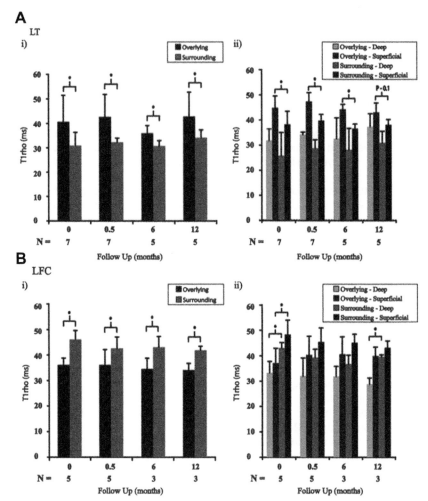

Fig. 7. Full-thickness and zonal analysis of T1ρ values for overlying and surrounding cartilage in (A) lateral tibia (LT) and (B) lateral femoral condyle (LFC). The OC in the lateral tibia shows significantly higher full-thickness T1ρ values than those of the surrounding cartilage at all time points. The deep and superficial layers of the OC are elevated T1ρ values compared with their respective layers of the surrounding cartilage at all time points. Dots denote significance at P<.05.

chondrocyte degeneration or necrosis.[34,35] Therefore, accurate quantification of bone bruise in early phase of treatment seems helpful to improve the outcome of this injury (**Fig. 8**).

Application in ACL Injuries

Proton MRSI provides a noninvasive method for quantifying metabolic changes in tissues. MRI has been used mainly in cerebral tissues and other organs, such as prostate, breast, and muscle. In bone marrow, MRSI may help quantify water and lipids in a region of interest. One study adopted MRSI to quantitatively assess BMEL and OC in OA and ACL-injured subjects.[36] Eighty healthy controls and 30 subjects (13 knee OA,

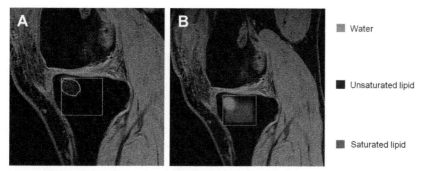

Fig. 8. (A) Bone bruise over anterior tibia. (B) Water and lipids for each voxel are estimated using a nonlinear fitting algorithm. Spectra are reconstructed and a color map is overlaid over the region of interest. There is high water content in the center of the bone bruise with unsaturated lipids over the transition area and saturated lipids over normal bone marrow.

15 ACL injury, 1 osteochondritis dissecans, 1 posterior cruciate ligament injury) with BMEL underwent 3T MRI and 3D MRSI. Significant elevation in water and unsaturated lipid and decrease in saturated lipid were observed in BMEL. The volume of elevated water significantly correlated with the volume of BMEL. The unsaturation index outside BMEL was significantly higher in ACL-injured subjects than in those with OA. MRSI seems to offer a promising tool that allows quantitative evaluation of BMEL. The investigators stated that MRSI may allow quantitative, longitudinal evaluation of traumatic and degenerative lesions of the knee. MRSI is considered to be another effective measurement of bone marrow lesion to identify recovery or deterioration.

KINEMATIC MRI

The most important aim of treatment of ACL injuries is the restoration of anteroposterior and rotatory laxity, thereby reestablishing normal knee kinematics. The determination of stability has traditionally relied on physical examination by skilled orthopedic surgeons, stress plain radiographs, laxity examination devices such as KT-1000, and sometimes gait analysis to recognize dynamic instability.[37] MRI has not been an eligible device for evluation of knee stability. However, the methods mentioned above evaluate the motion of tibia with relation to femur and do not take soft tissue mechanics (eg, menisci) into account. The current techniques also lack the precision needed for complex 3D knee motion. Most tests, such as the Lachman test, anterior drawer, or KT-1000 measurement have focused on anteroposterior laxity but not rotational laxity. Recently, the presence of associated meniscal injury is thought to influence the long-term consequence more significantly than does the ACL injury itself. The advancement of MR instruments and techniques allowed dynamic and/or quantitative analysis of knee kinematics in vivo, as well as more accurate morphologic diagnosis.

Application in ACL Injuries

Analyses of ACL-deficient knees

Several studies used MRI to quantitatively delineate knee kinematics with ACL injury. Scarvell and colleagues[38] measured the tibiofemoral (TF) contact area and flexion facet center (FFC) of 20 subjects with unilateral ACL injury under an axial load of 150 N through the knee motion arc from 0° to 90° using a closed MR scanner.

Uninjured contralateral knees served as controls. With TF contact method in healthy controls, femoral roll-back motion was identified from 0° to 30° flexion. In other words, the TF contact point moved posteriorly in both the medial and lateral tibial plateau with flexion. With further flexion to 90°, glide motion, instead of roll-back motion, occurred. This phenomenon was more pronounced in the medial compartment. ACL-injured knees showed similar roll or glide characteristics but had significantly more posterior TF contact points than normal controls. With the FFC method in healthy controls, medial FFC remained centrally located while the lateral FFC moved posteriorly at a steady rate. ACL-injured knees demonstrated a similar pattern with FFC method. The investigators were able to quantitatively describe axial rotation of the ACL-injured and healthy knees around the medially located longitudinal axis using MRI. The investigators also reported updated results.[39] Logan and colleagues[40] used 0.5 T open MRI to identify the tibiofemoral translation of medial and lateral compartments in 10 unilateral ACL-injured subjects. Image acquisition was done at 0°, 20°, 45°, and 90° of knee flexion during standing; the uninjured contralateral side served as control (**Fig. 9**). ACL-deficient knees demonstrated persistent anterior subluxation of LTP throughout the arc of motion compared with controls, whereas no significant difference was found in medial compartment between the two groups.

Some investigators reported slightly different results from the above mentioned studies. Von Eisenhart-Rothe and colleagues[41] used 0.2 T open MRI and 3D postimage processing to evaluate meniscotibial and tibiofemoral translation patterns with motion in 10 subjects with unilateral ACL injury. Contralateral healthy knees were scanned as controls. External load producing a torque of 10 N-m was applied to make isometric contraction of knee extensor and flexor, respectively. Posterior translation of femur and menisci occurred with flexion in all knees. In ACL-injured knees,

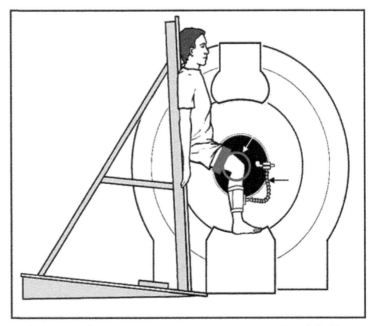

Fig. 9. Weight-bearing dynamic MRI using an open scanner. MR coil (*white arrow*). MR tracker (*black arrow*).

posterior translation of medial femoral condyle was significantly greater than that of normal knees, whereas posterior translation of medial menisci demonstrated no difference in both groups. The investigators stated that increased posterior translation with flexion in ACL-injured knees may cause greater shear force to medial meniscus and may account for the high rates of secondary medial meniscus tears in ACL-injured knees.

Shefelbine and colleagues[42] used a closed-bore MRI to investigate knee kinematics in 10 healthy volunteers and eight ACL-injured subjects. Knees were scanned at full extension and 45° flexion under a compressive load of 125 N. At extension, the position of the femur in relation to the tibia was 2.6 mm posterior in ACL-injured knees compared with contralateral normal knees. During flexion to 45°, the femur in ACL-injured knees showed anterior translation of 4.3 mm, whereas no significant anterior translation was observed in normal knees. This result seemed to illustrate pivot-shift phenomenon quantitatively. Meniscal translation, however, demonstrated no significant difference between two groups. The investigators suggested that significantly changed bone kinematics in the setting of constant meniscus kinematics might help explain increased risk of meniscal tears and subsequent cartilage injuries in chronic ACL-deficient knees.

Some investigators even used cine-phase contrast dynamic MRI to observe real-time knee kinematics.[43] They investigated anteroposterior translation and axial rotation of tibia during active quadriceps knee extension exercise in terminal 30° of motion. Significant increase in anterior translation (3.4 ± 2.8 mm) of the tibia in ACL-injured knees was found, whereas no significant difference was found in tibial rotation associated with ACL injury. The same investigators further investigated the differences between copers and noncopers.[44] Tibial positioning was not different between copers and noncopers and no changes in tibial axial rotation patterns associated with ACL injury were identified in this study.

Analyses of ACL-reconstructed knees
There are several studies that adopted MRI to evaluate knee kinematics after ACL reconstruction. Carpenter and colleagues[45] studied nine ACL-reconstructed knees and their contralateral healthy knees for control using 3.0 T closed MR scanner at full extension and 40° flexion. At full extension, ACL-reconstructed knees exhibited $3.6° \pm 4.2°$ external rotation of tibia compared with contralateral knees. The external rotation was due to anterior subluxation of medial tibial plateau. At 40° flexion, both ACL-reconstructed and contralateral knees showed 5.3° internal rotation. This study proved that ACL reconstruction restored normal kinematics in the lateral compartment but not in the medial.

Logan and colleagues[46] used 0.5 T open scanner to analyze the tibiofemoral kinematics of ACL-reconstructed knees with favorable clinical outcome. Image acquisition was done at 0°, 20°, 45°, and 90° of knee flexion during standing; the uninjured contralateral side served as control. Additional images were obtained with Lachman and reverse-Lachman stress applied manually at 20° knee flexion. With both Lachman and reverse-Lachman stress, ACL-reconstructed knees demonstrated no significant difference in tibial translation of both compartments compared with controls. During weight-bearing motion, the amount of excursion in tibiofemoral joint was similar between the two groups. However, LTP demonstrated persistent anterior subluxation throughout the arc of motion in ACL-reconstructed knees compared with controls. The investigators concluded that ACL reconstruction reduced anteroposterior instability to within normal limits but did not restore normal knee kinematics even in subjects with successful clinical outcome.

Another study compared knee kinematics after ACL reconstruction performed with anteromedial (AM) and transtibial (TT) femoral tunnel reaming using 3T MRI scanning at full extension and 30° to 40° flexion.[47] All kinematic measures measured in the AM group were similar to contralateral healthy knees. The TT group demonstrated a significantly increased amount of total tibial rotation during motion, whereas AM group did not. At full extension, the tibia was more externally rotated in the TT group than in the control group. During motion, the TT group showed greater medial tibial translation than the control group. ACL reconstruction with the AM technique was proved to better restore knee kinematics in terms of stability than the TT technique.

Kothari and colleagues[48] performed a study of the rotational kinematics of ACL-reconstructed knees with the AM technique. Six subjects with unilateral ACL injury were scanned with 3T MRI before and 8 months after surgery; contralateral healthy knees were used as controls. During MRI examinations, the knees were placed in 15° flexion and an internal-external rotation torque (3.35 Nm) was applied to the foot. In the ACL-deficient state, the differences of tibial rotation between ACL-deficient and control knees was 5.9° ± 4.1°, which decreased to −0.2° ± 6.1° after ACL reconstruction. This study demonstrated restoration of rotational stability with ACL reconstruction using AM technique. Another study recently investigated rotational kinematic using MRI of ACL-injured knees starting with the hypotheses that there is greater tibial rotation in women than in men and in ACL-deficient knees than in healthy knees.[49] Each subject underwent MRI examination with 15° knee flexion with a rotational torque applied in internal-external rotation. Healthy women had greater tibial rotation than did men. ACL-deficient male and female knees demonstrated greater tibial rotation compared with contralateral healthy knees. Kinematic MRI proved to be a reproducible method to quantify total knee rotation.

Types of MR Scanners for Kinematic MRI Analysis

Closed MRI

Advantages
- There is a long history and various sequences are available.
- It allows high-resolution and 3D analyses.
- With shorter acquisition time, it even allows a certain amount of loading, which mimics the weight-bearing condition (**Fig. 10**).

Disadvantages
- The degree of knee flexion in examination is restricted due to the size of the coil. Most examinations are limited to low flexion angles up to 45°.
- The loading conditions re nonphysiologic.

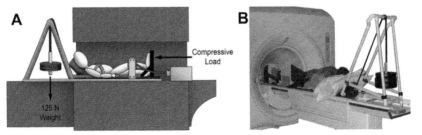

Fig. 10. (*A*) Device used to load a knee joint in a closed MR scanner. (*B*) Its application with a real patient.

Open MRI

Advantages
- It allows almost full range of motion.
- It allows standing position and physiologic loading.

Disadvantages
- It has low resolution with low magnet strength.
- Most technology is limited to a single-plane analysis and would not provide 3D data or rotational measurements.

Cine MRI

Advantages
- It offers real-time information.
- It provides dynamic analysis with a cine image of knee motion.

Disadvantages
- It is limited to single-plane analysis.
- The motion studied has to be very simple and reproducible, such as knee flexion and extension only. Complex knee motion or loading conditions are not feasible.

Review

It is evident that kinematic analysis using MRI offers noninvasive, accurate in vivo quantification of stability of knee joint. Each MRI type has its own advantages and disadvantages that physicians should be aware to properly apply this method. Kinematics MRI is an exciting field that can allow quantitative measurements of knee mechanics under load. This can allow us to better stratify the severity of knee injuries as well as outcomes following surgical treatments of ligament injuries.

SUMMARY

MRI has evolved from morphologic to a semiquantitative evaluation tool and now there is further advancement to quantitative methods. dGEMRIC is a useful, validated method for probing GAG change in cartilage but requires injection of high dose of Gd DTPA^{2-} and long image-acquisition time. T2 mapping is a relatively convenient method for detecting collagen and water changes and is particularly useful in longitudinal analysis because it allows zonal evaluation of cartilage. T1ρ mapping is a highly sensitive technique to detect early changes in GAG content, as well as collagen. Quantitative MRI will become more available and a requirement to assess cartilage health.

MRI has also been used as a dynamic, quantitative evaluation tool for knee kinematics in ACL-injured knees. It can provide precise 2D and 3D knee kinematics under load. Furthermore, the images can allow determination of soft tissue mechanics such as meniscus position and contact areas. MRI is a promising method for ACL kinematics because it provides noninvasive in vivo analysis.

REFERENCES

1. Daniel DM, Stone ML, Dobson BE, et al. Fate of the ACL-injured patient. A prospective outcome study. Am J Sports Med 1994;22(5):632–44.

2. Fithian DC, Paxton EW, Stone ML, et al. Prospective trial of a treatment algorithm for the management of the anterior cruciate ligament-injured knee. Am J Sports Med 2005;33(3):335–46.

3. Myklebust G, Holm I, Maehlum S, et al. Clinical, functional, and radiologic outcome in team handball players 6 to 11 years after anterior cruciate ligament injury: a follow-up study. Am J Sports Med 2003;31(6):981–9.

4. Myklebust G, Bahr R. Return to play guidelines after anterior cruciate ligament surgery. Br J Sports Med 2005;39(3):127–31.

5. Crema MD, Roemer FW, Marra MD, et al. Articular cartilage in the knee: current MR imaging techniques and applications in clinical practice and research. Radiographics 2011;31(1):37–61.

6. Peterfy CG, Guermazi A, Zaim S, et al. Whole-Organ Magnetic Resonance Imaging Score (WORMS) of the knee in osteoarthritis. Osteoarthritis Cartilage 2004;12(3):177–90.

7. Hunter DJ, Lo GH, Gale D, et al. The reliability of a new scoring system for knee osteoarthritis MRI and the validity of bone marrow lesion assessment: BLOKS (Boston Leeds Osteoarthritis Knee Score). Ann Rheum Dis 2008;67(2): 206–11.

8. Kornaat PR, Ceulemans RY, Kroon HM, et al. MRI assessment of knee osteoarthritis: Knee Osteoarthritis Scoring System (KOSS)—inter-observer and intra-observer reproducibility of a compartment-based scoring system. Skeletal Radiol 2005;34(2):95–102.

9. Potter HG, Linklater JM, Allen AA, et al. Magnetic resonance imaging of articular cartilage in the knee. An evaluation with use of fast-spin-echo imaging. J Bone Joint Surg Am 1998;80(9):1276–84.

10. Venn M, Maroudas A. Chemical composition and swelling of normal and osteoarthrotic femoral head cartilage. I. Chemical composition. Ann Rheum Dis 1977; 36(2):121–9.

11. Neuman P, Tjornstrand J, Svensson J, et al. Longitudinal assessment of femoral knee cartilage quality using contrast enhanced MRI (dGEMRIC) in patients with anterior cruciate ligament injury—comparison with asymptomatic volunteers. Osteoarthritis Cartilage 2011;19(8):977–83.

12. Fleming BC, Oksendahl HL, Mehan WA, et al. Delayed Gadolinium-Enhanced MR Imaging of Cartilage (dGEMRIC) following ACL injury. Osteoarthritis Cartilage 2010;18(5):662–7.

13. Potter HG, Jain SK, Ma Y, et al. Cartilage injury after acute, isolated anterior cruciate ligament tear: immediate and longitudinal effect with clinical/MRI follow-up. Am J Sports Med 2012;40(2):276–85.

14. Williams A, Qian Y, Golla S, et al. UTE-T2* mapping detects sub-clinical meniscus injury after anterior cruciate ligament tear. Osteoarthritis Cartilage 2012;20(6): 486–94.

15. Dunn TC, Lu Y, Jin H, et al. T2 relaxation time of cartilage at MR imaging: comparison with severity of knee osteoarthritis. Radiology 2004; 232(2):592–8.

16. White LM, Sussman MS, Hurtig M, et al. Cartilage T2 assessment: differentiation of normal hyaline cartilage and reparative tissue after arthroscopic cartilage repair in equine subjects. Radiology 2006;241(2):407–14.

17. Welsch GH, Mamisch TC, Domayer SE, et al. Cartilage T2 assessment at 3-T MR imaging: in vivo differentiation of normal hyaline cartilage from reparative tissue after two cartilage repair procedures—initial experience. Radiology 2008; 247(1):154–61.

18. Gobbi A, Nunag P, Malinowski K. Treatment of full thickness chondral lesions of the knee with microfracture in a group of athletes. Knee Surg Sports Traumatol Arthrosc 2005;13(3):213–21.

19. Domayer SE, Welsch GH, Nehrer S, et al. T2 mapping and dGEMRIC after autologous chondrocyte implantation with a fibrin-based scaffold in the knee: preliminary results. Eur J Radiol 2010;73(3):636–42.

20. Koff MF, Amrami KK, Kaufman KR. Clinical evaluation of T2 values of patellar cartilage in patients with osteoarthritis. Osteoarthritis Cartilage 2007;15(2): 198–204.

21. Duvvuri U, Charagundla SR, Kudchodkar SB, et al. Human knee: in vivo T1(rho)-weighted MR imaging at 1.5 T—preliminary experience. Radiology 2001;220(3): 822–6.

22. Li X, Kuo D, Theologis A, et al. Cartilage in anterior cruciate ligament-reconstructed knees: MR imaging T1{rho} and T2–initial experience with 1-year follow-up. Radiology 2011;258(2):505–14.

23. Theologis AA, Kuo D, Cheng J, et al. Evaluation of bone bruises and associated cartilage in anterior cruciate ligament-injured and -reconstructed knees using quantitative t(1rho) magnetic resonance imaging: 1-year cohort study. Arthroscopy 2011;27(1):65–76.

24. Stahl R, Luke A, Li X, et al. T1rho, T2 and focal knee cartilage abnormalities in physically active and sedentary healthy subjects versus early OA patients—a 3.0-Tesla MRI study. Eur Radiol 2009;19(1):132–43.

25. Regatte RR, Akella SV, Borthaker A, et al. Proteoglycan depletion-induced changes in transverse relaxation maps of cartilage: comparison of T2 and T1rho. Acad Radiol 2002;9(12):1388–94.

26. Peterfy CG, van Dijke CF, Janzen DL, et al. Quantification of articular cartilage in the knee with pulsed saturation transfer subtraction and fat-suppressed MR imaging: optimization and validation. Radiology 1994;192(2):485–91.

27. Rosen MA, Jackson DW, Berger PE. Occult osseous lesions documented by magnetic resonance imaging associated with anterior cruciate ligament ruptures. Arthroscopy 1991;7(1):45–51.

28. Engebretsen L, Arendt E, Fritts HM. Osteochondral lesions and cruciate ligament injuries. MRI in 18 knees. Acta Orthop Scand 1993;64(4):434–6.

29. Graf BK, Cook DA, De Smet AA, et al. Bone bruises" on magnetic resonance imaging evaluation of anterior cruciate ligament injuries. Am J Sports Med 1993;21(2):220–3.

30. Speer KP, Spritzer CE, Basset FH 3rd, et al. Osseous injury associated with acute tears of the anterior cruciate ligament. Am J Sports Med 1992;20(4):382–9.

31. Nakamae A, Engebretsen L, Bahr R, et al. Natural history of bone bruises after acute knee injury: clinical outcome and histopathological findings. Knee Surg Sports Traumatol Arthrosc 2006;14(12):1252–8.

32. Bretlau T, Tuxoe J, Larsen L, et al. Bone bruise in the acutely injured knee. Knee Surg Sports Traumatol Arthrosc 2002;10(2):96–101.

33. Vellet AD, Marks PH, Fowler PJ, et al. Occult posttraumatic osteochondral lesions of the knee: prevalence, classification, and short-term sequelae evaluated with MR imaging. Radiology 1991;178(1):271–6.

34. Johnson DL, Urban WP Jr, Caborn DN, et al. Articular cartilage changes seen with magnetic resonance imaging-detected bone bruises associated with acute anterior cruciate ligament rupture. Am J Sports Med 1998;26(3):409–14.

35. Rangger C, Kathrein A, Freund MC, et al. Bone bruise of the knee: histology and cryosections in 5 cases. Acta Orthop Scand 1998;69(3):291–4.

36. Li X, Ma BC, Bolbos RI, et al. Quantitative assessment of bone marrow edema-like lesion and overlying cartilage in knees with osteoarthritis and anterior cruciate ligament tear using MR imaging and spectroscopic imaging at 3 Tesla. J Magn Reson Imaging 2008;28(2):453–61.

37. Hefti F, Muller W, Jakob RP, et al. Evaluation of knee ligament injuries with the IKDC form. Knee Surg Sports Traumatol Arthrosc 1993;1(3–4):226–34.

38. Scarvell JM, Smith PN, Refshauge KM, et al. Comparison of kinematic analysis by mapping tibiofemoral contact with movement of the femoral condylar centres in healthy and anterior cruciate ligament injured knees. J Orthop Res 2004;22(5): 955–62.

39. Scarvell JM, Smith PN, Refshauge KM, et al. Comparison of kinematics in the healthy and ACL injured knee using MRI. J Biomech 2005;38(2):255–62.

40. Logan M, Dunstan E, Robinson J, et al. Tibiofemoral kinematics of the anterior cruciate ligament (ACL)-deficient weightbearing, living knee employing vertical access open "interventional" multiple resonance imaging. Am J Sports Med 2004;32(3):720–6.

41. von Eisenhart-Rothe R, Bringmann C, Siebert M, et al. Femoro-tibial and menisco-tibial translation patterns in patients with unilateral anterior cruciate ligament deficiency–a potential cause of secondary meniscal tears. J Orthop Res 2004;22(2): 275–82.

42. Shefelbine SJ, Ma CB, Lee KY, et al. MRI analysis of in vivo meniscal and tibiofemoral kinematics in ACL-deficient and normal knees. J Orthop Res 2006;24(6): 1208–17.

43. Barrance PJ, Williams GN, Snyder-Mackler L, et al. Altered knee kinematics in ACL-deficient non-copers: a comparison using dynamic MRI. J Orthop Res 2006;24(2):132–40.

44. Barrance PJ, Williams GN, Snyder-Mackler L, et al. Do ACL-injured copers exhibit differences in knee kinematics?: an MRI study. Clin Orthop Relat Res 2007;454: 74–80.

45. Carpenter RD, Majumdar S, Ma CB. Magnetic resonance imaging of 3-dimensional in vivo tibiofemoral kinematics in anterior cruciate ligament-reconstructed knees. Arthroscopy 2009;25(7):760–6.

46. Logan MC, Williams A, Lavelle J, et al. Tibiofemoral kinematics following successful anterior cruciate ligament reconstruction using dynamic multiple resonance imaging. Am J Sports Med 2004;32(4):984–92.

47. Schairer WW, Haughom BD, Morse LJ, et al. Magnetic resonance imaging evaluation of knee kinematics after anterior cruciate ligament reconstruction with anteromedial and transtibial femoral tunnel drilling techniques. Arthroscopy 2011; 27(12):1663–70.

48. Kothari A, Haughom B, Feely B, et al. Evaluating rotational kinematics of the knee in ACL reconstructed patients using 3.0Tesla magnetic resonance imaging. Knee 2012;19(5):648–51.

49. Haughom BD, Souza R, Shairer WW, et al. Evaluating rotational kinematics of the knee in ACL-ruptured and healthy patients using 3.0 Tesla magnetic resonance imaging. Knee Surg Sports Traumatol Arthrosc 2012;20(4):663–70.

Rotatory Knee Laxity

Mattias Ahldén, MD[a],*, Kristian Samuelsson, MD, PhD[a],
Freddie H. Fu, MD[b], Volker Musahl, MD[b], Jón Karlsson, MD, PhD[a]

KEYWORDS

- Anatomic • Anterior cruciate ligament • Reconstruction • Pivot shift • Rotatory laxity

KEY POINTS

- The interest in rotatory knee laxity has increased with the implementation of anatomic anterior cruciate ligament reconstruction.
- The pivot shift test represents a link between static testing with 1° of freedom and dynamic testing during functional activity such as running.
- The difficulties are how to standardize the performance of the pivot shift test and how to extract measurable and relevant kinematic data. With new technical developments, newer standards are emerging.

INTRODUCTION

Manual clinical examination and the assessment of laxity in the injured knee is one of the foundations for evaluation of the injured knee. It is a key point for enhancement of the optimal treatment selection and clinical follow-up. Most research reports rely on manual clinical examination of laxity as an outcome measure, especially the well-known Lachman test. The Lachman test is considered to be a sensitive manual examination and an important part of the knee investigation when an anterior cruciate ligament (ACL) injury is assessed.[1] Instrumented measurements, such as KT-1000 arthrometer (MEDmetric Corp, San Diego, California), are commonly used to standardize and quantify measurements of anterior-posterior (A-P) knee laxity. However, several studies report that the A-P laxity does not correlate with functional outcome or osteoarthritis, whereas the pivot shift test does.[2,3] The pivot shift test represents dynamic rotatory laxity and entails a complicated motion, which is generally described

The authors did not receive any outside funding or grants directly related to the research presented in this article. The Department of Orthopaedic Surgery from the University of Pittsburgh receives funding from Smith and Nephew to support research related to reconstruction of the ACL. The authors state that this article is an original work submitted only to this journal. All authors contributed to the preparation of this work.
[a] Department of Orthopaedics, Sahlgrenska Academy, University of Gothenburg, Sahlgrenska University Hospital/Mölndal, Mölndal 431 80, Sweden; [b] Department of Orthopaedic Surgery, University of Pittsburgh, 3471 Fifth Avenue, Pittsburgh, PA 15213, USA
* Corresponding author.
E-mail address: mattias.e.ahlden@vgregion.se

as a two-component rotation around the axis of knee flexion and the axis of tibial rotation.[4] However, these rotatory axes are not consistent across patients and subsequently there are interindividual differences.[5] Moreover, the pivot shift represents motion in the extremes of the rotatory laxity envelope and simulates the patient's give-way situation.[6] Rotatory laxity and kinematics during functional activity such as running can be examined using dynamic radiosteremoetry (RSA) or dynamic stereo radiographs (DSX).[7–9] The pivot shift test can be regarded as a link between static laxity testing in 1° of freedom and functional dynamic laxity testing in multiple degrees of freedom. The importance of these different expressions of rotatory laxity, and how they relate to each other, is still not fully understood. DSX is not applicable for office use or in clinical follow-up; the pivot shift test is most likely the most valuable tool in terms of dynamic rotatory laxity evaluation today. Nevertheless, the pivot shift test as an outcome measure needs further improvement and testing in terms of validation and reliability. Important factors to consider when using the pivot shift test are (1) quantification, (2) its subjective nature, and (3) interpretation.[10–12]

In recent years, the interest in evaluating rotatory laxity has markedly increased in parallel with the development and implementation of anatomic ACL reconstruction and double-bundle techniques to improve the outcome of ACL reconstruction. Studies have shown that normal knee kinematics are not restored after traditional nonanatomic ACL reconstruction.[7] The goal of anatomic ACL reconstruction is, therefore, to reproduce the native anatomy of the ACL to improve kinematics and, thereby, long-term prognosis. It seems that anatomic reconstructive techniques better resist rotatory loads than traditional transtibial nonanatomic ACL reconstruction and might, at least theoretically, produce improved long-term outcome.[13–16]

Despite reports on the impact of laxity and the development of osteoarthritis,[17,18] it is still not clear which factors influence the restoration of laxity in the injured knee.[19] Moreover, most studies on rotatory laxity have been conducted on cadavers and little is known about the rotatory laxity in vivo.

The increase in knowledge regarding rotatory laxity has also put emphasis on the development of valid and reliable methods to quantify rotatory laxity and the pivot shift test.

PRIMARY AND SECONDARY RESTRAINTS TO ROTATORY KNEE LAXITY

The contribution of different factors in controlling rotatory laxity in the knee is still poorly understood. The envelope of laxity was described and validated by Bull and colleagues[5] and describes primary restraints (ACL) and secondary restraints (collateral ligaments, menisci, and joint capsule). Thus, the pivot shift grade is not only dependent on the integrity of the ACL. Musahl and colleagues[20] have shown that in a case of grade 1 pivot shift, the ACL injury was more often isolated compared with grade 2 pivot shift. The investigators also reported that the lateral meniscus was more important than the medial meniscus in controlling the pivot shift.

The anterolateral capsule and iliotibial band displays a similar role in controlling rotatory laxity.[21] The anterolateral capsular injury can also be represented by a Segond fracture, a bony avulsion of the insertion site of the anterolateral capsule on the proximal anterolateral tibia. On the other hand, Matsumoto[22] reported a lower pivot shift grade when sectioning the anterolateral secondary restraints. Researchers suggested that sectioning of the iliotibial band produced a less prominent reduction phase of the pivot shift.[23] Furthermore, associated injuries to the medial collateral ligament could reduce the pivot shift, probably because of inability to maintain a distinct pivoting point in the medial compartment.[23]

The influence of bony morphology on the pivot shift is a growing area of interest. Factors reported to influence the rotatory kinematics of the knee and pivot shift are the size and convexity of the lateral tibial plateau,[23,24] tibial slope,[25] and distal femur geometry.[9]

In terms of the ACL as a primary restraint against rotatory laxity, both the anteromedial (AM) and posterolateral (PL) bundle are probably important. It has been implied that the more horizontal orientation of the PL bundle makes it more capable of controlling rotatory loads than the AM bundle.[26] Studies on rotatory laxity in cadavers report differences in rotation of 2° to 3° after cutting the ACL and less when the two bundles are selectively cut.[27–29] Furthermore, the two bundles display a reciprocal behavior and the individual significance in controlling rotatory laxity varies with knee flexion angle.[26] The significance of the PL bundle is greatest in the lower flexion range.[27,30]

METHODS TO MEASURE ROTATORY LAXITY
Static Versus Dynamic Devices

Rotatory laxity measurements are more challenging to perform compared with measurements of A-P laxity. One explanation is that there are large interindividual differences in axial tibial rotation, represented by the individual envelope of laxity.[5] Furthermore, the measured values are usually higher than the actual tibiofemoral motion because skin markers are used in most measurements. Side-to-side differences are preferred to gain relevant data; this is probably even more important for rotatory laxity than for static sagittal laxity. Moreover, important information can be gained from actually analyzing the curves of displacement in response to load.[31] This applies to both static sagittal and rotatory laxity. Devices for measuring rotatory laxity are still undergoing development and differ considerably in terms of patient positioning, knee flexion angle, and applied torques. Static rotatory laxity measurements are more complex than static sagittal measurements and reports on its use are still scarce. Static rotatory laxity measurements have been reported to be able to differentiate between an ACL-deficient and an ACL-intact knee. However, considering the great individual variability in rotatory range, its wider use and validity is still unclear. Bignozzi and colleagues[32] evaluated the relevance of static and dynamic tests after anatomic double-bundle ACL reconstruction using computer-assisted surgery and concluded that static rotatory measurements were inferior in evaluating knee laxity after double-bundle ACL reconstructions. On the other hand, dynamic knee laxity tests are more complex and can be even more difficult to standardize and perform in a reliable way.

The pivot shift is the most specific test of an ACL injury. It is related to ACL function and represents the most common symptom associated with an ACL injury, which is giving-way.[1] The ultimate goal of ACL reconstruction in terms of restoration of laxity is to eliminate the pivot shift and failure to do so is regarded as a failed ACL reconstruction. In certain cases, this is irrespective of the patient's symptoms. The pivot shift represents a comprehensive manifestation of the total joint status and function and correlates to subjective assessments. Pivot shift and dynamic rotatory laxity are obviously more closely correlated with functional deficits and outcome than static laxity; however, they still do not represent a functional movement with weight-bearing. Knee motion during running, for example, is guided by passive structures such as primary and secondary restraints as well as by interaction from gravitational and muscular forces.[7] Kinematic in vivo studies can, therefore, be considered the gold standard when evaluating rotatory laxity. However, kinematic studies, such as DSX, are complex, costly, and labor intensive. On the other hand, the pivot shift test is ideal for use in an office setting in large-scale studies. The main difficulty when performing the pivot shift test is to standardize the force and movement used, especially on patients who are awake. Kinematic recordings of the pivot shift test have shown large rating differences between different examiners.[33] Therefore, a more standardized pivot shift test has been developed that yields more consistent results.[34] A mechanized pivot shifter has also been developed; however, the manually performed pivot shift produces greater rotatory movements than the mechanized procedure.[35] Moreover, the measurements of the anterior tibial translation were more repeatable with the mechanized pivot shifter test than the manual pivot shift. However, the measurement of rotations was less repeatable with the mechanized pivot shifter test. Whether the optimal method consists of recording a standardized manually performed pivot shift or using a mechanized pivot shifter is still not known. If the examiner makes an effort to maximize the pivot shift, the resulting movement could be more consistent and larger than when using a mechanized pivot shifter.[35] The greatest challenge is how to extract measurable and relevant kinematic data from the complex pivot shift movement. Different components of the pivot shift have been reported to correlate with clinical grading, such as posterior tibial acceleration,[36–38] velocity of tibia translation,[39] coupled anterior translation,[36] lateral compartment anterior translation,[40] and the "angle of p."[41] Further studies are needed to evaluate if it is possible to decompose the pivot shift into only one parameter, such as acceleration or lateral compartment translation, or if it is necessary to use several different parameters to best describe a specific pivot shift movement. Ultimately, simple devices that are capable of accurate data acquisition in a noninvasive manner are needed.

Validation of devices

There is a lack of validated measurement devices that can be used to assess rotatory laxity of the knee. Few studies report on external validation of the device and most report internal validation by actually reporting reproducibility.[42] Furthermore, some studies report on validation done when measuring laxity in 1° of freedom in a static or semistatic manner. Such validation cannot be applied when using the same device to measure a quick dynamic motion such as the pivot shift. Moreover, there are obvious differences when using invasive, bone-attached markers as in computer-assisted surgery compared with skin-fixed markers. The skin-fixed markers are less accurate because they allow for motion artifacts from motion between bone and skin and between skin and marker, respectively. Further validation and reliability studies are needed to evaluate the use of skin-fixed markers when assessing dynamic rotatory laxity such as the pivot shift.

Reliable methods to measure rotatory laxity in the clinical setting or operating room are warranted.

Dynamic Rotatory Laxity Devices

There are a variety of techniques reported to measure dynamic rotatory laxity of the knee.[7,36,37,43,44] Comparison of studies is challenging because various methods are used to measure different components of dynamic laxity. Computer-assisted surgery has been used to assess knee kinematics and laxity, which allows for decomposition of the pivot shift as well as direct feedback on laxity testing. Even if the tracking of markers is highly precise, surgeon-specific factors matter greatly because most studies are based on manual examination only. Advantages of manual tests are accuracy and high repeatability due to the direct feedback to the examiner. Disadvantages include its invasiveness and examination confined to the ipsilateral side (**Table 1**).

Bone-attached or skin-fixed electromagnetic sensors can be used to measure rotatory laxity. Electromagnetic sensors can be used in vivo and have been found useful to further define the kinematics of the pivot shift test (**Fig. 1**). Labbe and colleagues[39]

Table 1
Dynamic rotatory laxity devices; advantages and disadvantages

Device	Advantages	Disadvantages
CAS	Accuracy Repeatability of manual tests	Invasive Ipsilateral side only
Electromagnetic tracking	Non invasive	Not wireless Ferromagnetic influence
RSA	Accuracy	Invasive Cost Labor intensive Radiation
DSX	Accuracy Non invasive	Cost Labor intensive Radiation
MRI open	Display of soft tissues No radiation	Low frame rate Restricted space for exam
Accelerometer	Non invasive Wireless Small	Skin motion Only acceleration

used an electromagnetic device to study different components of the pivot shift and found that velocity and acceleration of the pivot shift test accounted for many of the differences and were more closely correlated to clinical grade than other features of the pivot shift test, such as A-P translation.

RSA is a highly precise system with reported accuracy of 0.2 mm in translation and 0.3° in rotation when evaluating in vivo joint motion.[7] The procedure involves insertion of multiple tantalum markers with the diameters of 0.8 to 1.6 mm in the bone of femur and tibia. Imaging is done with biplane radiographs with a sample rate of up to 300 Hz. To capture significant events during running or jumping, a sample rate of at least 100 to 300 Hz and an exposure time of 1 millisecond or less are required.[45]

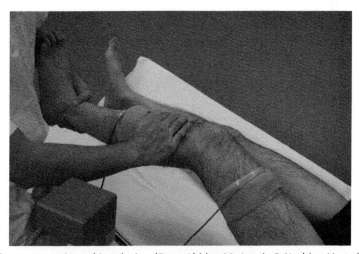

Fig. 1. Electromagnetic tracking device. (*From* Ahlden M, Araujo P, Hoshino Y, et al. Clinical grading of the pivot shift test correlates best with tibial acceleration. Knee Surg Sports Traumatol Arthrosc 2012;20(4):708–12; with kind permission from Springer Science and Business Media.)

DSX is a similar but noninvasive technique that evolved from RSA. A model-based tracking technique is used to align three-dimensional CT scans with the radiographic image pairs (**Fig. 2**). Precision when measuring joint motion during running was less than 1.0° for rotation and less than 1.0 mm for translation.[46] Disadvantages for the DSX and RSA include high costs, exposure to radiation, and the need for manual labor-intensive analysis.

Open MRI has been introduced for in vivo analysis of knee joint kinematics that can be correlated to meniscal kinematics and joint contact areas.[47] Disadvantages are low frame rates and restricted space for functional weight-bearing movements. With new technical developments, the ability to monitor high-speed activities will most probably improve.

The accelerometer is a fairly new device that can be used in a noninvasive setting.[37,44] The tibial sensor is mounted on the anterolateral tibia between the lateral aspect of the tibial tuberosity and the Gerdy tubercle (**Fig. 3**). A second sensor can be mounted on the femur for reference. The limited size and wireless connection favors an office-based use and the accelerometer has shown promising results in quantification of the pivot shift test. The sensor can also be packed into a sterile envelope that allows intraoperative testing. However, further validation and reliability testing are still warranted.[37,44]

QUANTITATIVE MEASUREMENT OF THE PIVOT SHIFT

During the Panther summit meeting (August 2011 in Pittsburgh, PA, USA), a multi-center pivot shift study was performed. The purpose of the study was to demonstrate several different techniques for the pivot shift examination and to correlate a surgeon-specific clinical grading to objective measurements of the pivot shift using three different measurement devices.[33,34,38,48]

Twelve expert surgeons from around the world performed the pivot shift test on a whole lower-extremity cadaver. The ACL and anterior horn of the lateral meniscus of the right knee were transected to produce a high-grade pivot shift. Surgeons performed the pivot shift test using their preferred technique and used International Knee Documentation Committee (IKDC) guidelines for clinical grading. Video motion analysis was used to capture each individual surgeon's technique. For analysis, the pivot shift was broken down into fixed rotation versus motion-allowing, high force versus low force, and reduction versus dislocation maneuver. Simultaneous data samplings were performed using three different measurement devices: bone-attached and skin-fixed

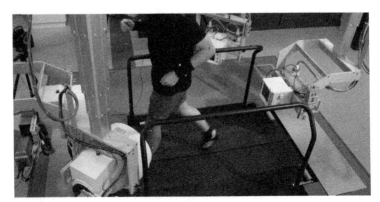

Fig. 2. DSX. (*From* Ahlden M, Araujo P, Hoshino Y, et al. Clinical grading of the pivot shift test correlates best with tibial acceleration. Knee Surg Sports Traumatol Arthrosc 2012;20(4):708–12; with kind permission from Springer Science and Business Media.)

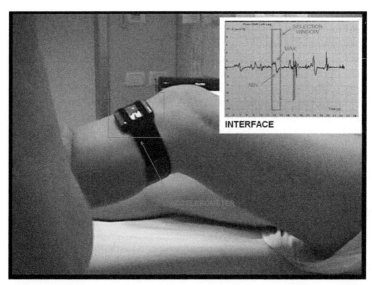

Fig. 3. Accelerometer. (*From* Ahlden M, Araujo P, Hoshino Y, et al. Clinical grading of the pivot shift test correlates best with tibial acceleration. Knee Surg Sports Traumatol Arthrosc 2012;20(4):708–12; with kind permission from Springer Science and Business Media.)

electromagnetic tracking system, triaxial accelerometer system, and video image analysis. The expert surgeons' average clinical grading was 2.3 ± 0.5. Five genuinely different pivot shift test maneuvers were observed. The most common type of pivot shift test used was a fixed internal rotation-type. There was no difference in average clinical grading when using high force during the pivot shift test (2.5 ± 0.6) versus low force (2.3 ± 0.5), or when using fixed rotation (2.2 ± 0.5) versus motion-allowing (2.3 ± 0.6) tests. Clinical grading displayed the best correlation to the acceleration of reduction as measured by the electromagnetic tracking system with bone-attached sensors ($r = 0.674$, $P<.05$). A similar correlation coefficient was found for acceleration of reduction ($r = 0.575$, $P = .05$) and the "jerk" component of acceleration ($r = 0.609$, $P<.05$) measured by means of the triaxial accelerometer system.

The conclusion were: (1) clinical grading varies among surgeons but not between different techniques, (2) tibial acceleration parameters during the pivot shift most closely correlate with the clinical grading assessed by 12 expert surgeons, and (3) a standardized pivot shift test improved measurement accuracy.[33,34,38,48]

A standardized technique based on the original technique of Galway and MacIntosh[49] was introduced to the surgeons by manual instruction and by watching a 2-minute instructional video. The standardized technique resulted in significantly less variation in the acceleration between different surgeons.[34] Therefore, the standardized technique for the pivot shift test may standardize tibial acceleration and, thereby, clinical grading of the pivot shift. Standardization of the pivot shift test itself, and its quantifiable measurement, may enable multicenter clinical outcome research to improve outcome for patients following ACL reconstruction.

SUMMARY

The standard of knee laxity testing is changing toward improved understanding of the significance and importance of rotatory laxity, especially dynamic testing. The quantification of rotatory laxity presents a challenge in terms of validation and reliability testing. The pivot shift test represents a link between static testing and functional dynamic testing of rotatory laxity. With new technical development, newer standards are emerging and noninvasive methods based on electromagnetic or acceleration sensors have been shown to evaluate the pivot shift in a quantitative manner. Kinematic parameters can be recorded during functional activity with weight bearing, such as when using high-frequency biplane radiographs (RSA or DSX).

The goal of ACL reconstruction should be to eliminate the pivot shift and normalize kinematics in the knee. In the future, individual treatment plans can be made for each patient based on information from preoperative imaging, contralateral native knee anatomy, and examinations on rotatory laxity. Ultimately, accurate assessment of rotatory knee laxity preoperatively will enable individualized and functional restoration of native ACL anatomy.

REFERENCES

1. Prins M. The Lachman test is the most sensitive and the pivot shift the most specific test for the diagnosis of ACL rupture. Aust J Physiother 2006;52(1):66.
2. Kocher MS, Steadman JR, Briggs KK, et al. Relationships between objective assessment of ligament stability and subjective assessment of symptoms and function after anterior cruciate ligament reconstruction. Am J Sports Med 2004; 32(3):629–34.
3. Jonsson H, Riklund-Ahlström K, Lind J. Positive pivot shift after ACL reconstruction predicts later osteoarthrosis: 63 Patients followed 5–9 years after surgery. Acta Orthop Scand 2004;75(5):594–9.
4. Bull AM, Amis AA. The pivot-shift phenomenon: a clinical and biomechanical perspective. Knee 1998;5(3):141–58.
5. Bull AM, Earnshaw PH, Smith A, et al. Intraoperative measurement of knee kinematics in reconstruction of the anterior cruciate ligament. J Bone Joint Surg Br 2002;84(7):1075–81.
6. Losee RE, Johnson TR, Southwick WO. Anterior subluxation of the lateral tibial plateau. A diagnostic test and operative repair. J Bone Joint Surg Am 1978; 60(8):1015–30.
7. Tashman S, Collon D, Anderson K, et al. Abnormal rotational knee motion during running after anterior cruciate ligament reconstruction. Am J Sports Med 2004; 32(4):975–83.
8. Tashman S, Kolowich P, Collon D, et al. Dynamic function of the ACL-reconstructed knee during running. Clin Orthop Relat Res 2007;454:66–73.
9. Hoshino Y, Wang JH, Lorenz S, et al. The effect of distal femur bony morphology on in vivo knee translational and rotational kinematics. Knee Surg Sports Traumatol Arthrosc 2011. http://dx.doi.org/10.1007/s00167-011-1661-3.
10. Bach BR Jr, Warren RF, Wickiewicz TL. The pivot shift phenomenon: results and description of a modified clinical test for anterior cruciate ligament insufficiency. Am J Sports Med 1988;16(6):571–6.
11. Noyes FR, Grood ES, Cummings JF, et al. An analysis of the pivot shift phenomenon. The knee motions and subluxations induced by different examiners. Am J Sports Med 1991;19(2):148–55.
12. Kuroda R, Hoshino Y, Kubo S, et al. Similarities and differences of diagnostic manual tests for anterior cruciate ligament insufficiency: a global survey and kinematics assessment. Am J Sports Med 2011. http://dx.doi.org/10.1177/0363546511423634.
13. Yagi M, Wong EK, Kanamori A, et al. Biomechanical analysis of an anatomic anterior cruciate ligament reconstruction. Am J Sports Med 2002;30(5):660–6.

14. Fu FH, Shen W, Starman JS, et al. Primary anatomic double-bundle anterior cruciate ligament reconstruction: a preliminary 2-year prospective study. Am J Sports Med 2008;36(7):1263–74.

15. Hussein M, van Eck CF, Cretnik A, et al. Prospective randomized clinical evaluation of conventional single-bundle, anatomic single-bundle, and anatomic double-bundle anterior cruciate ligament reconstruction: 281 cases with 3- to 5-year follow-up. Am J Sports Med 2011. http://dx.doi.org/10.1177/0363546511426416.

16. Samuelsson K, Andersson D, Karlsson J. Treatment of anterior cruciate ligament injuries with special reference to graft type and surgical technique: an assessment of randomized controlled trials. Arthroscopy 2009;25(10):1139–74.

17. Anderst WJ, Tashman S. The association between velocity of the center of closest proximity on subchondral bones and osteoarthritis progression. J Orthop Res 2009;27(1):71–7.

18. Andriacchi TP, Mundermann A, Smith RL, et al. A framework for the in vivo pathomechanics of osteoarthritis at the knee. Ann Biomed Eng 2004;32(3):447–57.

19. Tanaka M, Vyas D, Moloney G, et al. What does it take to have a high-grade pivot shift? Knee Surg Sports Traumatol Arthrosc 2012;20(4):737–42.

20. Musahl V, Citak M, O'Loughlin PF, et al. The effect of medial versus lateral meniscectomy on the stability of the anterior cruciate ligament-deficient knee. Am J Sports Med 2010;38(8):1591–7.

21. Hughston JC, Andrews JR, Cross MJ, et al. Classification of knee ligament instabilities. Part II. The lateral compartment. J Bone Joint Surg Am 1976;58(2):173–9.

22. Goldman AB, Pavlov H, Rubenstein D. The Segond fracture of the proximal tibia: a small avulsion that reflects major ligamentous damage. AJR Am J Roentgenol 1988;151(6):1163–7.

23. Matsumoto H. Mechanism of the pivot shift. J Bone Joint Surg Br 1990;72(5):816–21.

24. Musahl V, Ayeni OR, Citak M, et al. The influence of bony morphology on the magnitude of the pivot shift. Knee Surg Sports Traumatol Arthrosc 2010;18(9):1232–8.

25. Brandon ML, Haynes PT, Bonamo JR, et al. The association between posterior-inferior tibial slope and anterior cruciate ligament insufficiency. Arthroscopy 2006;22(8):894–9.

26. Yasuda K, van Eck CF, Hoshino Y, et al. Anatomic single- and double bundle anterior cruciate ligament reconstruction, part 1: basic science. Am J Sports Med 2011;39(8):1789–99.

27. Amis AA. The functions of the fibre bundles of the anterior cruciate ligament in anterior drawer, rotational laxity and the pivot shift. Knee Surg Sports Traumatol Arthrosc 2012;20(4):613–20.

28. Lorbach O, Pape D, Maas S, et al. Influence of the anteromedial and posterolateral bundles of the anterior cruciate ligament on external and internal tibiofemoral rotation. Am J Sports Med 2010;38(4):721–7.

29. Diermann N, Schumacher T, Schanz S, et al. Rotational instability of the knee: internal tibial rotation under a simulated pivot shift test. Arch Orthop Trauma Surg 2009;129(3):353–8.

30. Gabriel MT, Wong EK, Woo SL, et al. Distribution of in situ forces in the anterior cruciate ligament in response to rotatory loads. J Orthop Res 2004;22(1):85–9.

31. Musahl V, Seil R, Zaffagnini S, et al. The role of static and dynamic rotatory laxity testing in evaluating ACL injury. Knee Surg Sports Traumatol Arthrosc 2012;20(4):603–12.

32. Bignozzi S, Zaffagnini S, Lopomo N, et al. Clinical relevance of static and dynamic tests after anatomical double-bundle ACL reconstruction. Knee Surg Sports Traumatol Arthrosc 2010;18(1):37–42.
33. Araujo PH, Ahldén M, Hoshino Y, et al. Comparison of three non-invasive quantitative measurement systems for the pivot shift test. Knee Surg Sports Traumatol Arthrosc 2012;20(4):692–7.
34. Hoshino Y, Araujo P, Ahldén M, et al. Standardized pivot shift test improves measurement accuracy. Knee Surg Sports Traumatol Arthrosc 2012;20(4):732–6.
35. Musahl V, Voos J, O'Loughlin PF, et al. Mechanized pivot shift test achieves greater accuracy than manual pivot shift test. Knee Surg Sports Traumatol Arthrosc 2010;18(9):1208–13.
36. Hoshino Y, Kuroda R, Nagamune K, et al. In vivo measurement of the pivot-shift test in the anterior cruciate ligament-deficient knee using an electromagnetic device. Am J Sports Med 2007;35(7):1098–104.
37. Lopomo N, Zaffagnini S, Signorelli C, et al. An original clinical methodology for non-invasive assessment of pivot-shift test. Comput Methods Biomech Biomed Engin 2011. http://dx.doi.org/10.1080/10255842.2011.591788.
38. Ahldén M, Araujo P, Hoshino Y, et al. Clinical grading of the pivot shift test correlates best with tibial acceleration. Knee Surg Sports Traumatol Arthrosc 2012; 20(4):708–12.
39. Labbe DR, de Guise JA, Mezghani N, et al. Feature selection using a principal component analysis of the kinematics of the pivot shift phenomenon. J Biomech 2010;43(16):3080–4.
40. Bedi A, Musahl V, Lane C, et al. Lateral compartment translation predicts the grade of pivot shift: a cadaveric and clinical analysis. Knee Surg Sports Traumatol Arthrosc 2010;18(9):1269–76.
41. Lane CG, Warren RF, Stanford FC, et al. In vivo analysis of the pivot shift phenomenon during computer navigated ACL reconstruction. Knee Surg Sports Traumatol Arthrosc 2008;16(5):487–92.
42. Ahldén M, Hoshino Y, Samuelsson K, et al. Dynamic knee laxity measurement devices. Knee Surg Sports Traumatol Arthrosc 2012;20(4):621–32.
43. Zaffagnini S, Klos TV, Bignozzi S. Computer-assisted anterior cruciate ligament reconstruction: an evidence-based approach of the first 15 years. Arthroscopy 2010;26(4):546–54.
44. Kopf S, Kauert R, Halfpaap J, et al. A new quantitative method for pivot shift grading. Knee Surg Sports Traumatol Arthrosc 2012;20(4):718–23.
45. Tashman S. Comments on "validation of a non-invasive fluoroscopic imaging technique for the measurement of dynamic knee joint motion." J Biomech 2008;41(15):3290–1.
46. Anderst W, Zauel R, Bishop J, et al. Validation of three-dimensional model-based tibio-femoral tracking during running. Med Eng Phys 2009;31(1):10–6.
47. Haughom B, Schairer W, Souza RB, et al. Abnormal tibiofemoral kinematics following ACL reconstruction are associated with early cartilage matrix degeneration measured by MRI T1rho. Knee 2012;19(4):482–7.
48. Musahl V, Hoshino Y, Ahldén M, et al. The pivot shift: a global user guide. Knee Surg Sports Traumatol Arthrosc 2012;20(4):724–31.
49. Galway HR, MacIntosh DL. The lateral pivot shift: a symptom and sign of anterior cruciate ligament insufficiency. Clin Orthop Relat Res 1980;147:45–50.

Effects of Anterior Cruciate Ligament Reconstruction on In Vivo, Dynamic Knee Function

Scott Tashman, PhD[a,b,]*, Daisuke Araki, MD, PhD[c,d]

KEYWORDS

- Anterior cruciate ligament • In vivo knee kinematics • Dynamic stereo X-ray system
- Knee • Anatomic • Double-bundle • Single-bundle

KEY POINTS

- Current treatment approaches are moderately successful for restoring function, with most individuals able to return to their preinjury level of sports activity.
- Although there are many factors that may contribute to joint degeneration, persistent abnormal knee mechanics are often implicated in the initiation and progression of osteoarthritis in the anterior cruciate ligament–injured/reconstructed knee.
- Concerns about the high rates of osteoarthritis are largely responsible for the increased interest during the past several years on more anatomic approaches to anterior cruciate ligament repair and reconstruction.

INTRODUCTION

The goals of anterior cruciate ligament (ACL) reconstruction are to restore stability and enable return to unrestricted function during the short term and ideally to protect joint health during the long term. Current treatment approaches are moderately successful for restoring function, with most individuals able to return to their preinjury level of sports activity.[1,2] However, surgical ligament reconstruction does not seem to prevent the development of osteoarthritis after ACL injury.[3–5] Although there are many factors that may contribute to joint degeneration, persistent abnormal knee mechanics are

Funding sources: Dr Tashman: NIH, Arthritis Foundation. Dr Araki: None.
Conflict of interest: None.
[a] Orthopaedic Biodynamics Laboratory, Department of Orthopaedic Surgery, School of Medicine, University of Pittsburgh, 3820 South Water Street, Pittsburgh, PA 15203, USA; [b] Department of Bioengineering, School of Engineering, University of Pittsburgh, South Water Street, 15203 Pittsburgh, PA, USA; [c] Department of Orthopaedic Surgery, School of Medicine, University of Pittsburgh, 3471 Fifth Avenue, Pittsburgh, PA 15213, USA; [d] Department of Orthopaedic Surgery, Graduate School of Medicine, Kobe University, Kobe, Japan
* Corresponding author. Orthopaedic Biodynamics Laboratory, Department of Orthopaedic Surgery, School of Medicine, University of Pittsburgh, 3820 South Water Street, Pittsburgh, PA 15203.
E-mail address: tashman@pitt.edu

often implicated in the initiation and progression of osteoarthritis (OA) in the ACL-injured/reconstructed knee.[6,7] Concerns about the high rates of OA are largely responsible for the increased interest during the last several years on more anatomic approaches to ACL repair and reconstruction. Although no current techniques can restore the true insertion site anatomy or physiology of the native ACL, procedures that attempt to improve tunnel placement and graft geometry to more closely resemble the original ligament are gaining in popularity. The premise for these newer procedures is that better restoration of native anatomy will lead to more normalized joint mechanics and improved long-term joint health.

Ultimately, determining the efficacy of these procedures for reducing OA risk after ACL injury will require large, well-designed clinical studies with long-term follow-up to directly evaluate joint degeneration. However, considerable insights about the relative merits of different ACL reconstruction techniques can be obtained during the short term by investigating their effectiveness for restoring normal joint function. The goals of this narrative review are to discuss key factors for assessing joint function, present some recent findings, and propose future directions for evaluating the function of the ACL-injured/reconstructed knee.

METHODOLOGIC CONSIDERATIONS FOR ASSESSING KNEE FUNCTION
The Case for In Vivo, Human Studies

Definitive conclusions on the relative efficacy of different ACL reconstruction techniques can only be drawn from in vivo, human studies. Cadaveric studies have contributed a wealth of information on the basic biomechanics and passive structural properties of the knee and can be beneficial for development and initial evaluation of surgical techniques. However, cadaver studies cannot reproduce the complex combination of gravitational, inertial, and active muscular forces that influence knee mechanics during functional activities. Cadaver studies also represent only "time zero" conditions and cannot account for biologic responses (such as healing, remodeling, tunnel enlargement, etc) that can have a significant influence on knee and ligament function. Conversely, animal models are well suited for studying biologic tissue response, but they differ too extensively in joint morphology and function for direct transfer of kinematic findings to humans (with the possible exception of large primates, which are rarely used for orthopedic studies because of cost and ethical considerations).

Laxity Versus Stability

In vivo knee function can be evaluated under a wide range of conditions. Which measures are most relevant to outcomes after ACL reconstruction? With the progression from laxity testing to static weight-bearing to dynamic, functional activities, assessment becomes more technically demanding but also potentially more relevant to joint health. Central to most theories relating joint mechanics to OA development is the idea that altered joint contact patterns and joint loads, encountered during routine activities, can be detrimental to long-term cartilage health.[6,8] These theories would suggest that the most relevant measures of joint function are those that reflect the behavior of the knee during common, functional activities. It is especially important to distinguish between evaluations of laxity versus assessments of dynamic knee function and functional stability. In a recent review, Musahl and colleagues[9] stated, "In biomechanical terms, laxity is the passive response of a joint to an externally applied force or torque. Stability, on the other hand, is a functional measure; that is, a knee, regardless of laxity, is only unstable if it 'gives way' during functional activities." Laxity tests are typically performed without the compressive joint forces required to properly engage the conforming condylar surfaces, which play an important role in joint stabilization. Thus, although laxity tests may be effective for identifying structural deficits, the results cannot predict joint behavior during dynamic, functional activities. In fact, many studies relating static laxity and clinical/functional outcomes have reported correlations that are at best weak.[10–14]

Knee Function Is Task Dependent

In vivo studies incorporating body-weight loading and active muscular control provide a much more comprehensive and realistic picture of the natural function of the knee joint as a complex neuromusculoskeletal system. However, the knee has a wide envelope of possible motions, and joint function is highly activity dependent. Patterns of joint motion and articular contact vary considerably with loading and activity, even during similar ranges of knee flexion.[15,16] Knee tissues are highly viscoelastic and respond nonlinearly to load magnitude and loading rate,[17,18] so the behavior of the knee under low-demand conditions cannot be simply "scaled up" to predict behavior during functional activities. Thus, studies incorporating body-weight loading during quasi-static activities (eg, sequential fixed knee angles[19]) or low-effort movements (eg, half-speed gait[20]) may not predict knee behavior during more complex, demanding tasks. This may be especially important for ACL-injured athletes, who will routinely expose their joints to high-magnitude, rapidly changing loads after returning to sports.

Measurement Options for Dynamic, In Vivo Studies

Meaningful characterization of dynamic joint function during common activities poses unique challenges, especially for measurements directly relevant to soft tissue behavior. Peak ACL strains during activities of daily living are on the order of 4% or less[21]; for a typical ACL size, this represents a length change of only 1.2 mm. Assessing articular contact kinematics (arthrokinematics) requires a measurement error substantially smaller than the thickness of the cartilage layer (typically 2–4 mm thick for the tibiofemoral joint). The most widely used technology for studying knee function after ACL reconstruction is video-motion analysis, which tracks motion of multiple skin-mounted markers placed on the thigh and shank to determine limb movement. This technology is noninvasive, widely available, and reliable and has been effective for identifying differences in knee kinematics between ACL-intact, ACL-deficient, and ACL-reconstructed joints (as described later). But, conventional motion analysis cannot achieve the submillimeter accuracy required for tissue-relevant measurements, because of the displacement of skin-mounted markers relative to underlying bone.[22–24] Magnetic resonance (MR) imaging can achieve submillimeter accuracy and enables direct visualization of soft tissue, but sample rates are too slow and the imaging environment is too restrictive for most functional movement tasks.

Dynamic radiographic imaging enables direct visualization and 3-dimensional tracking of bone motion and has been gaining in popularity during the past decade. Although some measurements have been performed using a single imaging plane, dual or biplane imaging systems are generally required to obtain submillimeter resolution in all 3 movement planes. Many systems are now in use across the United States, with capabilities that vary based on the specific equipment and analysis techniques used. Conventional "C-arm" fluoroscopy systems are limited by low frame rates (≤30 Hz) and long exposure times (≥8 ms) but are adequate for quasi-static and low-speed activities.[25,26] Custom-built systems can achieve much higher sample rates and have validated submillimeter accuracy for more physically demanding tasks, such as running.[27–29]

DYNAMIC KNEE FUNCTION: TRADITIONAL ACL RECONSTRUCTION

The ACL is often described as consisting of 2 functional bundles, the anteromedial (AM) and the posterolateral (PL) bundles, named in relation to their typical orientation and insertion on the tibia and femur (**Fig. 1**).[30,31] The AM and PL bundles function synergistically to provide both anterior and rotational stability of the knee. Cadaver studies suggest that the AM bundle is taut throughout the range of motion of the knee, reaching a maximum tension between 45° and 60°, whereas the PL bundle is tight primarily in extension.[32–35]

Traditional ACL reconstruction procedures have been performed using a single graft bundle, without attempting to recreate the native double-bundle ACL anatomy. The tunnel placement techniques commonly used (eg, transtibial drilling of the femoral tunnels and/or the "o'clock" method for drill orientation) also failed to reliably place the graft within the native ACL footprint.[36,37] These single-bundle, nonanatomic procedures may eliminate anteroposterior (AP) laxity and successfully restore normal AP translation but fail to restore rotational stability.[38,39] Numerous in vivo kinematic studies using a variety of loading conditions have confirmed that these procedures fail to restore normal dynamic knee function. Logan and colleagues,[40] using open-access MR imaging, reported that ACL reconstruction reduced sagittal laxity to within normal limits but did not restore normal tibiofemoral kinematics during static weight-bearing. Georgoulis and colleagues[41] examined ACL-deficient individuals before and after bone–patellar tendon–bone ACL reconstruction during walking using video-motion analysis. The ACL-deficient patients demonstrated greater tibial internal rotation, which decreased closer to normal levels after ACL reconstruction. In a subsequent investigation with higher-demand activities (stair descent and pivoting), tibial rotation was significantly larger in the ACL reconstructed knees compared with the contralateral, intact legs.[42] Kinematics after ACL reconstruction have also been investigated using radiographic techniques to analyze in vivo knee kinematics without errors from skin motion artifacts. Brandsson and colleagues[43] found that tibial rotation and AP translation were not restored by ACL reconstruction (using bone–patella tendon–bone autografts) in 9 unilateral ACL patients 1 year after surgery using continuous radiostereometric analysis. Papannagari and colleagues[44] reported that although anterior laxity was restored

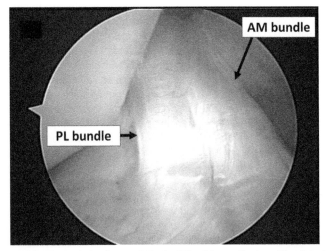

Fig. 1. Arthroscopic view of the intact ACL, in 90° of knee flexion. The intact native ACL consists of 2 instinct bundles; AM and PL bundles can been seen, separated by a septum.

according to KT-1000 arthrometer (Medmetric Inc, San Diego, CA) testing, ACL reconstruction did not restore normal knee kinematics under weight-bearing conditions when measured using a dual-orthogonal fluoroscopic system. Studies of more physically demanding tests require specialized high-speed radiographic imaging systems. Further evidence of rotational instability following ACL reconstruction was provided by Tashman and colleagues[45,46] who used a 250 frame/s dynamic stereo x-ray system to evaluate in vivo kinematics of the knee during downhill running for patients who underwent traditional, nonanatomic single-bundle reconstruction. This traditional single-bundle ACL reconstruction restored normal AP translation, but the reconstructed knees were more externally rotated (mean 4°) and more adducted (mean 3°) relative to the contralateral, uninjured knees. These rotational changes were associated with shifts in the areas of joint contact and a reduction in medial-compartment joint space under dynamic loading. Thus, there is substantial and growing evidence from in vivo knee kinematics studies that nonanatomic single-bundle ACL reconstruction fails to restore preinjury knee function under functional loading conditions.

This evidence, along with increasing knowledge of ACL anatomy, led to greater interest in double-bundle ACL reconstruction techniques. Several in vitro biomechanical studies have suggested that double-bundle ACL reconstruction might improve anterior tibial translational and rotational stability.[47,48] Conversely, other studies have reported no significant differences in clinical outcome between single-bundle and double-bundle ACL reconstruction procedures.[49,50] Yasuda and colleagues[51] performed a prospective comparative cohort study of 72 patients evaluated 2 years after surgery to compare the clinical outcomes of anatomic double-bundle ACL reconstruction with those of nonanatomic single- and double-bundle reconstructions. They observed no significant differences in the range of motion, the muscle torque and International Knee Documentation Committee evaluation scores. However, side-to-side laxity measurements (KT2000 arthrometer, Medmetric Inc, San Diego, CA) and pivot shift examination of anatomic double-bundle ACL reconstruction showed significantly better results than in the single-bundle procedure. Because "double bundle" does not necessarily imply "anatomic," interpretation of these findings is complicated by uncertainty as to whether the double-bundle procedures in some studies were actually performed anatomically (ie, with tunnels drilled in the footprints of the native ACL bundles). Nonanatomic and anatomic tunnel placements are shown in **Fig. 2**. There is insufficient high-quality data in the literature to adequately assess whether nonanatomic double-bundle ACL reconstruction is kinematically superior to nonanatomic single-bundle procedures.

DYNAMIC KNEE FUNCTION: ANATOMIC ACL RECONSTRUCTION

In the past decade, anatomic placement of ACL grafts has become a more widely accepted principle for ligament reconstruction. Anatomic ACL reconstruction techniques aim to better restore the normal anatomy and biomechanics of the knee and are hypothesized to potentially decrease the incidence of OA after ACL reconstruction. Cadaver studies have shown mixed results comparing anatomic single-bundle ACL reconstruction procedures to anatomic double-bundle procedures, with some reporting superior stability for double-bundle[52] and others reporting little difference for anatomic double-bundle compared with centrally placed single-bundle reconstructions.[53] Although differences in the outcomes of single-bundle and double-bundle ACL reconstruction comprise a topic of ongoing discussion, it is generally believed that both methods benefit from anatomic tunnel placement.[38,54,55]

Controversy regarding the possible merits of both anatomic and double-bundle techniques for restoring knee function has motivated several in vivo kinematics

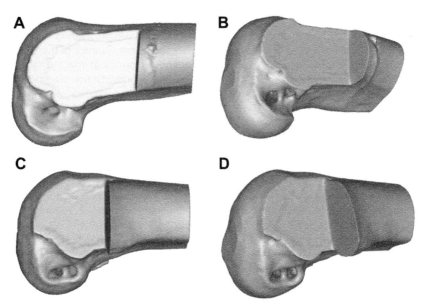

Fig. 2. Nonanatomic tunnel placement in double-bundle ACL reconstruction (*A, B*). Anatomic tunnel placement in double-bundle ACL reconstruction (*C, D*).

studies during the past several years. Abebe and colleagues,[56] using biplanar fluoroscopy and MR imaging, reported that anatomic femoral placement of the graft in single-bundle reconstruction resulted in a more stable knee (see **Fig. 2**). Although subjects with nonanatomic graft placement had up to 3.4 mm more anterior tibial translation, 1.1 mm more medial tibial translation, and 3.7° more internal tibial rotation compared with the contralateral side, subjects with anatomic graft placement had motion that more closely replicated that of the intact knee (**Fig. 3**). The additional benefit of double-bundle (versus single-bundle) anatomic reconstruction for restoring kinematics has, however, yet to be established. Several video-motion analysis studies have found no differences in knee kinematics and rotational stability between double-bundle and single-bundle ACL-reconstructed knees during gait, high-demand pivoting activities, and other dynamic movement tasks (**Figs. 4** and **5**).[57–60] These studies concluded that both techniques were able to restore tibial rotational excursion compared with the contralateral knees and/or with control knees from uninjured subjects. However, these studies cannot definitively address differences between single- and double-bundle anatomic ACL reconstruction, as a result of concerns regarding the ability of surface marker–based techniques for assessing small (but potentially important) differences in transverse and coronal-plane rotations or assessing shifts in tibiofemoral contact locations.

Radiographic studies reporting dynamic knee function during high-demand activities after anatomic reconstruction (single-bundle or double-bundle) have yet to appear in the peer-reviewed literature. A pilot study was performed at the University of Pittsburgh Biodynamics Laboratory to evaluate the effectiveness of anatomic double-bundle ACL reconstruction for restoring normal knee kinematics. Eight subjects with isolated ACL ruptures were tested during downhill running approximately 6 months after ACL reconstruction, using methods similar to those used for previous studies.[46] An anatomic double-bundle surgical procedure was used to place graft tunnels within

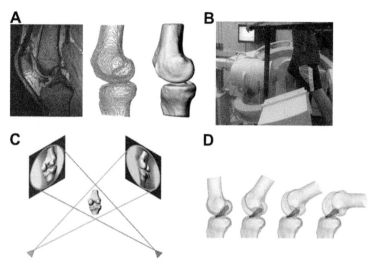

Fig. 3. Multiplanar, high-resolution MR imaging was used to create 3-dimensional models of the knee, including the attachment sites of the ACL and graft (*A*). Biplanar fluoroscopy was used to record each subject's knee motion during a single leg lunge (*B*). Fluoroscopic images and 3-dimensional models were used to reproduce the motion of the each subject's knees during the lunge (*C*). From these models, the length and orientation of the ACL and graft were measured (*D*). (*Reprinted from* Abebe ES, Utturkar GM, Taylor DC, et al. The effects of femoral graft placement on in vivo knee kinematics after anterior cruciate ligament reconstruction. J Biomech 2011;44(5):924–9; with permission.)

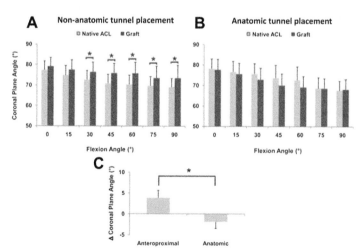

Fig. 4. In the sagittal plane, anteroproximal grafts were more vertical than the native ACL (*A*), whereas the anatomic grafts (*B*) more closely restored the sagittal plane orientation of the native ACL. When their respective differences from native were averaged across all flexion angles, anteroproximal grafts were more vertical compared with the anatomic grafts (*C*) (*$P<.05$). (*Reprinted from* Abebe ES, Utturkar GM, Taylor DC, et al. The effects of femoral graft placement on in vivo knee kinematics after anterior cruciate ligament reconstruction. J Biomech 2011;44(5):924–9; with permission.)

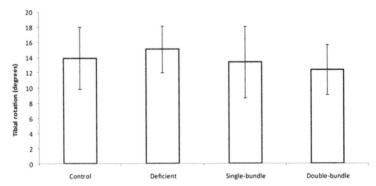

Fig. 5. Tibial rotation (mean ± SD) of examined groups. There was no significant difference in tibial rotation either between the 4 groups or between sides. The mean knee rotation for the single- and double-bundle groups was lower than the control group. (*Reprinted from* Tsarouhas A, Iosifidis M, Kotzamitelos D, et al. Three-dimensional kinematic and kinetic analysis of knee rotational stability after single- and double-bundle anterior cruciate ligament reconstruction. Arthroscopy 2010;26(7):885–93; with permission.)

the native footprints of the AM and PL bundles. Biplane radiograph images were collected at 150 frames/s during the early to mid-stance phase of running, and a model-based tracking method was used to determine tibiofemoral kinematics.[28] Tibiofemoral rotations and translations were determined and compared for the reconstructed and uninvolved limbs. No statistically (or clinically) significant differences were found between reconstructed and contralateral limbs for any kinematic variables after anatomic double-bundle reconstruction; mean between-limb differences were 0.4° for external rotation, 0.1° for abduction, and 0.7 mm for A/P translation. These preliminary results suggest that anatomic double-bundle reconstruction may be more effective in restoring preinjury knee function than more traditional techniques (**Fig. 6**). A larger, randomized study is currently under way to rigorously evaluate this hypothesis.[61]

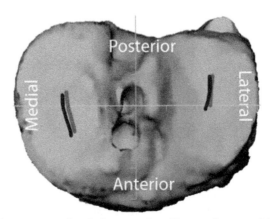

Fig. 6. Estimated contact paths during running (foot strike to mid-stance) for ACL-reconstructed (anatomic double-bundle, *red traces*) versus contralateral, uninjured joints (*blue traces*). There were no significant differences.

DISCUSSION

Several methods for the objective assessment of in vivo motion have been developed. The most common methods use high-speed cameras or skin marker based video-motion capture systems.[62] The advantages of these systems are their ease of application, safety and quick data processing. However, the accuracy of these methods is limited (to several millimeters at best) by the relative motion between the markers and the skin[63] and may be inadequate to detect meaningful differences between similar procedures. Dual fluoroscopy (for relatively low-demand tasks)[25] and dynamic stereo-radiography (providing short imaging times and high frames rates for more strenuous activities)[27] are more complex, expensive, and invasive (because of radiation exposure) but provide reliable, high-precision assessment of tibiofemoral kinematics (typically ±0.1–0.3 mm accuracy, an order of magnitude or more better than surface-marker techniques, even when using artifact reduction approaches). These radiographic methods are becoming more widely available and are likely during the next few years to provide definitive answers regarding the relative merits of different surgical procedures for restoring dynamic joint function and stability.

In vitro biomechanics studies can focus on very specific aspects of ligament properties and behavior but are insufficient to establish clinical efficacy. For example, the mechanical properties of different graft materials have been well characterized using tensile testing machines. However, the relationship between preimplantation graft properties and actual graft function after months of healing, loading, and remodeling has not been established. Conversely, in vivo human studies have direct clinical relevance but may be confounded by uncontrolled factors that can cloud interpretation of results. Thus, basic/cadaver research studies are well suited for establishing a scientific basis for developing improved ACL reconstruction procedures. However, these studies must be followed by carefully designed and controlled clinical investigations with appropriate outcome measures.

Most ACL-reconstructed knees are clinically stable, regardless of surgical technique. Differences in functional stability have been identified between ACL-reconstructed and contralateral knees, but these differences are subtle and require sensitive outcome measures to detect. Rotational instability has been discussed as a potentially important indicator of surgical outcome, although there are no standardized approaches for assessing rotational laxity. A measurement of tibial rotation in response to an applied torque was insufficient to detect the difference between single- and double-bundle reconstructions,[53,64] whereas the dynamic evaluation of the clinically performed pivot shift test found that double-bundle reconstruction led to improved rotational stability.[39,65,66] Because simple load-displacement types of laxity measurement seem to be relatively insensitive to surgical procedure and do not reliably correlate with clinical outcomes, tests that better replicate functional knee loading are necessary to evaluate knee function after reconstruction. Previous in vivo dynamic studies demonstrated residual rotational instability in ACL-reconstructed patients with normal anterior stability but nonanatomically placed grafts.[41,45,67] Similar studies are under way and required to evaluate the potential benefits of anatomic reconstruction techniques.

SUMMARY

Concerns about the high rates of OA after ACL reconstruction, along with recent evidence of inadequate restoration of joint kinematics in reconstructed knees, have lead to a reevaluation of surgical procedures with the goals of better restoring both native ACL anatomy and dynamic knee function. Although consensus is growing concerning the benefits of more anatomic graft placement, the merits of double-bundle reconstruction for further improving knee function have yet to be firmly established. Well-designed studies, using state-of-the art tools to assess knee kinematics under in vivo, dynamic, high-loading conditions, are necessary to evaluate the relative performance of different procedures for restoring normal joint motion. Additionally, long-term studies are required to establish whether better restoration of knee kinematics is associated with superior clinical results and reduced incidence of OA after ACL injury.

REFERENCES

1. Biau DJ, Tournoux C, Katsahian S, et al. ACL reconstruction: a meta-analysis of functional scores. Clin Orthop Relat Res 2007;458:180–7.
2. Freedman KB, D'Amato MJ, Nedeff DD, et al. Arthroscopic anterior cruciate ligament reconstruction: a metaanalysis comparing patellar tendon and hamstring tendon autografts. Am J Sports Med 2003;31(1):2–11.
3. Daniel DM, Stone ML, Dobson BE, et al. Fate of the ACL-injured patient: a prospective outcome study. Am J Sports Med 1994;22(5):632–44.
4. Kessler MA, Behrend H, Henz S, et al. Function, osteoarthritis and activity after ACL-rupture: 11 years follow-up results of conservative versus reconstructive treatment. Knee Surg Sports Traumatol Arthrosc 2008;16(5):442–8.
5. Lohmander LS, Ostenberg A, Englund M, et al. High prevalence of knee osteoarthritis, pain, and functional limitations in female soccer players twelve years after anterior cruciate ligament injury. Arthritis Rheum 2004;50(10):3145–52.
6. Andriacchi TP, Mundermann A, Smith RL, et al. A framework for the in vivo pathomechanics of osteoarthritis at the knee. Ann Biomed Eng 2004;32(3):447–57.
7. Tochigi Y, Vaseenon T, Heiner AD, et al. Instability dependency of osteoarthritis development in a rabbit model of graded anterior cruciate ligament transection. J Bone Joint Surg Am 2011;93(7):640–7.
8. Dye SF. The knee as a biologic transmission with an envelope of function: a theory. Clin Orthop Relat Res 1996;(325):10–8.
9. Musahl V, Hoshino Y, Becker R, et al. Rotatory knee laxity and the pivot shift. Knee Surg Sports Traumatol Arthrosc 2012;20(4):601.
10. Snyder-Mackler L, Fitzgerald GK, Bartolozzi AR, et al. The relationship between passive joint laxity and functional outcome after anterior cruciate ligament injury. Am J Sports Med 1997;25(2):191–5.
11. Harter RA, Osternig LR, Singer KM. Long-term evaluation of knee stability and function following surgical reconstruction for anterior cruciate ligament insufficiency. Am J Sports Med 1988;16:434–43.
12. Barber SD, Noyes FR, Mangine RE, et al. Quantitative assessment of functional limitations in normal and anterior cruciate ligament-deficient knees. Clin Orthop Relat Res 1990;255:204–14.
13. Seto JL, Orofino AS, Morrissey MC. Assessment of quadriceps/hamstring strength, knee ligament stability, functional and sports activity levels five years after anterior cruciate ligament reconstruction. Am J Sports Med 1988;16:170–80.
14. Cross MJ, Wootton JR, Bokor DJ. Acute repair of injury to the anterior cruciate ligament: a long-term followup. Am J Sports Med 1993;21:128–31.
15. Andriacchi TP, Dyrby CO. Interactions between kinematics and loading during walking for the normal and ACL deficient knee. J Biomech 2005;38(2):293–8.
16. Moro-oka TA, Hamai S, Miura H, et al. Dynamic activity dependence of in vivo normal knee kinematics. J Orthop Res 2008;26(4):428–34.

17. van Dommelen JA, Jolandan MM, Ivarsson BJ, et al. Nonlinear viscoelastic behavior of human knee ligaments subjected to complex loading histories. Ann Biomed Eng 2006;34(6):1008–18.
18. Dortmans L, Jans H, Sauren A, et al. Nonlinear dynamic behavior of the human knee joint. Part II: time-domain analyses: effects of structural damage in post-mortem experiments. J Biomech Eng 1991;113(4):392–6.
19. Hosseini A, Gill TJ, Li G. In vivo anterior cruciate ligament elongation in response to axial tibial loads. J Orthop Sci 2009;14(3):298–306.
20. Wu JL, Hosseini A, Kozanek M, et al. Kinematics of the anterior cruciate ligament during gait. Am J Sports Med 2010;38(7):1475–82.
21. Beynnon BD, Fleming BC. Anterior cruciate ligament strain in-vivo: a review of previous work. J Biomech 1998;31(6):519–25.
22. Gao B, Zheng NN. Investigation of soft tissue movement during level walking: translations and rotations of skin markers. J Biomech 2008;41(15):3189–95.
23. Holden JP, Orsini JA, Siegel KL, et al. Surface movement errors in shank kinematics and knee kinetics during gait. Gait Posture 1997;5:217–27.
24. Manal K, Davis IM, Galinat B, et al. The accuracy of estimating proximal tibial translation during natural cadence walking: bone vs. skin mounted targets. Clin Biomech 2003;18(2):126–31.
25. Li G, Van de Velde SK, Bingham JT. Validation of a non-invasive fluoroscopic imaging technique for the measurement of dynamic knee joint motion. J Biomech 2008;41(7):1616–22.
26. Tashman S. Comments on "validation of a non-invasive fluoroscopic imaging technique for the measurement of dynamic knee joint motion". J Biomech 2008;41(15):3290–1 [author reply: 3292–3].
27. Tashman S, Bey M, Anderst WJ, et al. Model-based tracking of knee kinematics from biplane radiographs: in-vivo validation. Chicago: Orthopaedic Research Society; 2006.
28. Anderst W, Zauel R, Bishop J, et al. Validation of three-dimensional model-based tibio-femoral tracking during running. Med Eng Phys 2009;31(1):10–6.
29. Miranda DL, Schwartz JB, Loomis AC, et al. Static and dynamic error of a biplanar videoradiography system using marker-based and markerless tracking techniques. J Biomech Eng 2011;133(12):121002.
30. Girgis FG, Marshall JL, Monajem A. The cruciate ligaments of the knee joint. anatomical, functional and experimental analysis. Clin Orthop Relat Res 1975;(106):216–31.
31. Odensten M, Hamberg P, Nordin M, et al. Surgical or conservative treatment of the acutely torn anterior cruciate ligament. Clin Orthop Relat Res 1985;198:87–93.
32. Chhabra A, Starman JS, Ferretti M, et al. Anatomic, radiographic, biomechanical, and kinematic evaluation of the anterior cruciate ligament and its two functional bundles. J Bone Joint Surg Am 2006;88(Suppl 4):2–10.
33. Ferretti A, Monaco E, Labianca L, et al. Double bundle or single bundle plus extra-articular tenodesis in ACL reconstruction? A CAOS Study. Knee Surg Sports Traumatol Arthrosc 2008;16(1):98.
34. Gabriel MT, Wong EK, Woo SL, et al. Distribution of in situ forces in the anterior cruciate ligament in response to rotatory loads. J Orthop Res 2004;22(1):85–9.
35. Tischer T, Ronga M, Tsai A, et al. Biomechanics of the goat three bundle anterior cruciate ligament. Knee Surg Sports Traumatol Arthrosc 2009;17(8):935–40.
36. Abebe ES, Moorman CT 3rd, Dziedzic TS, et al. Femoral tunnel placement during anterior cruciate ligament reconstruction: an in vivo imaging analysis comparing

transtibial and 2-incision tibial tunnel-independent techniques. Am J Sports Med 2009;37(10):1904–11.

37. Kopf S, Forsythe B, Wong AK, et al. Nonanatomic tunnel position in traditional transtibial single-bundle anterior cruciate ligament reconstruction evaluated by three-dimensional computed tomography. J Bone Joint Surg Am 2010;92(6): 1427–31.

38. Araki D, Kuroda R, Kubo S, et al. A prospective randomised study of anatomical single-bundle versus double-bundle anterior cruciate ligament reconstruction: quantitative evaluation using an electromagnetic measurement system. Int Orthop 2011;35(3):439–46.

39. Yagi M, Kuroda R, Nagamune K, et al. Double-bundle ACL reconstruction can improve rotational stability. Clin Orthop Relat Res 2007;454:100–7.

40. Logan M, Dunstan E, Robinson J, et al. Tibiofemoral kinematics of the anterior cruciate ligament (ACL)-deficient weightbearing, living knee employing vertical access open "interventional" multiple resonance imaging. Am J Sports Med 2004;32(3):720–6.

41. Georgoulis AD, Papadonikolakis A, Papageorgiou CD, et al. Three-dimensional tibiofemoral kinematics of the anterior cruciate ligament-deficient and recon-structed knee during walking. Am J Sports Med 2003;31(1):75–9.

42. Ristanis S, Giakas G, Papageorgiou CD, et al. The effects of anterior cruciate liga-ment reconstruction on tibial rotation during pivoting after descending stairs. Knee Surg Sports Traumatol Arthrosc 2003;11(6):360–5.

43. Brandsson S, Karlsson J, Sward L, et al. Kinematics and laxity of the knee joint after anterior cruciate ligament reconstruction: pre- and postoperative radioster-eometric studies. Am J Sports Med 2002;30(3):361–7.

44. Papannagari R, Gill TJ, Defrate LE, et al. In vivo kinematics of the knee after ante-rior cruciate ligament reconstruction: a clinical and functional evaluation. Am J Sports Med 2006;34(12):2006–12.

45. Tashman S. Abnormal rotational knee motion during running after anterior cruciate ligament reconstruction. Am J Sports Med 2004;32(4):975–83.

46. Tashman S, Kolowich P, Collon D, et al. Dynamic function of the ACL-reconstructed knee during running. Clin Orthop Relat Res 2007;454:66–73.

47. Mae T, Shino K, Miyama T, et al. Single- versus two-femoral socket anterior cru-ciate ligament reconstruction technique: biomechanical analysis using a robotic simulator. Arthroscopy 2001;17(7):708–16.

48. Yagi M, Wong EK, Kanamori A, et al. Biomechanical analysis of an anatomic ante-rior cruciate ligament reconstruction. Am J Sports Med 2002;30(5):660–6.

49. Hamada M, Shino K, Horibe S, et al. Single- versus bi-socket anterior cruciate ligament reconstruction using autogenous multiple-stranded hamstring tendons with endobutton femoral fixation: a prospective study. Arthroscopy 2001;17(8): 801–7.

50. Adachi N, Ochi M, Uchio Y, et al. Reconstruction of the anterior cruciate ligament. single- versus double-bundle multistranded hamstring tendons. J Bone Joint Surg Br 2004;86(4):515–20.

51. Yasuda K, Kondo E, Ichiyama H, et al. Clinical evaluation of anatomic double-bundle anterior cruciate ligament reconstruction procedure using hamstring tendon grafts: comparisons among 3 different procedures. Arthroscopy 2006; 22(3):240–51.

52. Yamamoto Y, Hsu WH, Woo SL, et al. Knee stability and graft function after ante-rior cruciate ligament reconstruction: a comparison of a lateral and an anatomical femoral tunnel placement. Am J Sports Med 2004;32(8):1825–32.

53. Ho JY, Gardiner A, Shah V, et al. Equal kinematics between central anatomic single-bundle and double-bundle anterior cruciate ligament reconstructions. Arthroscopy 2009;25(5):464–72.
54. Irrgang JJ, Bost JE, Fu FH. Re: Outcome of single-bundle versus double-bundle reconstruction of the anterior cruciate ligament: a meta-analysis. Am J Sports Med 2009;37(2):421–2 [author reply: 422].
55. Meredick RB, Vance KJ, Appleby D, et al. Outcome of single-bundle versus double-bundle reconstruction of the anterior cruciate ligament: a meta-analysis. Am J Sports Med 2008;36(7):1414–21.
56. Abebe ES, Utturkar GM, Taylor DC, et al. The effects of femoral graft placement on in vivo knee kinematics after anterior cruciate ligament reconstruction. J Biomech 2011;44(5):924–9.
57. Claes S, Neven E, Callewaert B, et al. Tibial rotation in single- and double-bundle ACL reconstruction: a kinematic 3-D in vivo analysis. Knee Surg Sports Traumatol Arthrosc 2011;19(Suppl 1):S115–21.
58. Ristanis S, Stergiou N, Siarava E, et al. Effect of femoral tunnel placement for reconstruction of the anterior cruciate ligament on tibial rotation. J Bone Joint Surg Am 2009;91(9):2151–8.
59. Tsarouhas A, Iosifidis M, Kotzamitelos D, et al. Three-dimensional kinematic and kinetic analysis of knee rotational stability after single- and double-bundle anterior cruciate ligament reconstruction. Arthroscopy 2010;26(7):885–93.
60. Misonoo G, Kanamori A, Ida H, et al. Evaluation of tibial rotational stability of single-bundle vs. anatomical double-bundle anterior cruciate ligament reconstruction during a high-demand activity - a quasi-randomized trial. Knee 2012;19(2):87–93.
61. Irrgang JJ, Tashman S, Moore C, Fu FH. Challenge accepted: description of an ongoing NIH-funded randomized clinical trial to compare anatomic single-bundle versus anatomic double-bundle ACL reconstruction. Arthroscopy 2012;28(6):747–8.
62. Pappas E, Zampeli F, Xergia SA, et al. Lessons learned from the last 20 years of ACL-related in vivo-biomechanics research of the knee joint. Knee Surg Sports Traumatol Arthrosc 2012. [Epub ahead of print].
63. Garling EH, Kaptein BL, Mertens B, et al. Soft-tissue artefact assessment during step-up using fluoroscopy and skin-mounted markers. J Biomech 2007;40(Suppl 1):S18–24.
64. Lorenz S, Tashman S, Fu FH. Failed exploration of rotational instability in single- and double-bundle ACL reconstruction. Arthroscopy 2009;25(9):949 [author reply: 949–50].
65. Hoshino Y, Kuroda R, Nagamune K, et al. In vivo measurement of the pivot-shift test in the anterior cruciate ligament-deficient knee using an electromagnetic device. Am J Sports Med 2007;35(7):1098–104.
66. Araki D, Kuroda R, Kubo S, et al. The use of an electromagnetic measurement system for anterior tibial displacement during the Lachman test. Arthroscopy 2011;27(6):792–802.
67. Georgoulis AD, Ristanis S, Chouliaras V, et al. Tibial rotation is not restored after ACL reconstruction with a hamstring graft. Clin Orthop Relat Res 2007;454:89–94.

Innovative Technology for Knee Laxity Evaluation

Clinical Applicability and Reliability of Inertial Sensors for Quantitative Analysis of the Pivot-Shift Test

Stefano Zaffagnini, MD[a,*], Nicola Lopomo, PhD[a,b],
Cecilia Signorelli[a,c], Giulio Maria Marcheggiani Muccioli, MD[a],
Tommaso Bonanzinga, MD[a], Alberto Grassi, MD[a],
Andrea Visani, MD[a], Maurilio Marcacci, MD[a]

KEYWORDS

- Knee kinematics • Anterior cruciate ligament injury • Dynamic instability
- Pivot-shift test • Acceleration

KEY POINTS

- There has been an increased interest in the quantification of the knee laxity secondary to anterior cruciate ligament (ACL) injury. In clinical practice, the diagnosis is performed by clinical examination and magnetic resonance imaging analysis and confirmed arthroscopically under anesthesia.
- The pivot-shift (PS) phenomenon has been identified as one of the essential signs of functional ACL insufficiency.
- During the preoperative phase, the importance of the PS test for a complete evaluation of the injury is well acknowledged. Moreover, PS is the test that correlates with functional instability and patient outcomes better than does any other physical examination test. Thus, a reliable system to adequately assess patients with ACL injury, quantifying the PS test outcome, is needed to determine the efficacy of such reconstructions and aid in managing patient recovery.
- Several studies have been conducted in this regard using navigation systems, electromagnetic sensors, or other devices. Unfortunately, because of various problems, the proposed methods remain confined to a research area.
- The goal of this article is to summarize the actual knowledge and current concepts with respect to the use of acceleration as a quantitative parameter in the assessment of the dynamic knee movement during the PS test.

Conflict of Interest Statement: The authors declare they have no conflict of interest.
[a] Laboratorio di Biomeccanica e Innovazione Tecnologica, Istituto Ortopedico Rizzoli, Via di Barbiano 1/10, 40136 Bologna, Italy; [b] Laboratorio di NanoBiotecnologie - NaBi, Istituto Ortopedico Rizzoli, Via Di Barbiano 1/10, 40136 Bologna, Italy; [c] Dipartimento di Bioingegneria, Politecnico di Milano, Via Golgi 39, 20133 Milano, Italy
* Corresponding author.
E-mail address: s.zaffagnini@biomec.ior.it

INTRODUCTION

Instability of the tibiofemoral joint secondary to an anterior cruciate ligament (ACL) injury is considered a critical issue and relates to the concept of joint *laxity*.[1] By definition, laxity is the displacement, or the rotation, produced in response to an applied load or moment. Moreover, it is defined as *static* laxity when only one degree of freedom is involved and *dynamic* when more than two are considered.[2]

Because the ACL represents the primary restraint to tibia anteroposterior (AP) displacement,[3] historically, the first approach to the evaluation of the tibiofemoral joint laxity involved the measurement of joint AP translation. From this point of view, Lachman and drawer tests are still the most commonly used tests to quantify the static laxity of the knee joint.

Although the previous tests are useful in the detection of a large part of ACL injuries, they do not provide information about rotational and dynamic laxity of the joint. Moreover, analyzing solely static laxity makes it difficult to isolate the injured ligament because of the different structures involved in the restraining phenomenon.[4] Thus, additional stress tests have been introduced.

The pivot-shift (PS) phenomenon is commonly described as the anterior subluxation of the lateral tibial plateau followed by its sudden reduction during combined stresses.[2,5] This pathway has been widely identified to be one of the essential signs of functional ACL insufficiency[6,7]; thus, clinicians have been trying to mimic it by means of a combination of valgus stress and tibial internal rotation during limb flexion.[5,7]

Lachman and PS are the two clinical tests most commonly used to assess knee laxity.[8] Although the PS test could be considered the most specific test in detecting ACL injury,[4,9,10] the Lachman test, involving only one knee grade of freedom, remains more easily quantifiable and sensitive.

Moreover, literature reported that PS grade more closely correlates with instability symptoms,[11] reduced sport activity,[12] articular cartilage damage, and meniscal damage[13] with respect to the standard clinical examinations addressing only static joint laxity (ie, Lachman and drawer tests).[14]

The major problem using PS test lays in the complexity of the maneuver itself, which provokes a large variability both between testers and patients and making it a highly surgeon-subjective clinical examination.[15–17] Furthermore, given that the test itself is a combined stress, PS test lacks a generally recognized quantitative and overall measurement.

In the past years, several studies proposed a quantification of this phenomenon, promoting different kinematic parameters.

The goal of this article is to summarize the actual knowledge and current concepts about the quantification of PS test and, above all, about the use of acceleration as a quantitative parameter in the assessment of the dynamic knee movement during the test. The authors specifically reported the performed in vitro and in vivo validations in the use of an inertial sensor (ie, accelerometer) to quantify PS test.

QUANTITATIVE EVALUATION OF THE PS TEST

During the past decade, several systems and methods have been developed and proposed to quantify knee dynamic laxity level because of ligament injuries, providing a standardized approach as a basis for the clinical examination. The importance of any grading system lies in how helpful it can be in making decisions concerning diagnosis, treatment and recovery phase after surgery. A quantification of knee laxity can be valuable during the course of the diagnosis assessment and preoperative planning to determine *if* and *what* surgery is required, as well as during the postoperative evaluation to quantify the laxity reduction after surgery. Moreover, it would enable results from different centers and different studies to be compared more accurately.

Thus, rather complex systems have been developed, using skin markers, force footplates, robotic technology, or image-based systems in dynamic condition, such as magnetic resonance imaging.[18–21]

Navigation Systems

Among the most commonly used systems, more recently, navigation systems have enabled surgeons to analyze the dynamic motion of the components associated with the PS phenomenon.[4,10,22–28] Colombet and colleagues,[29] Pearle and colleagues,[30] and Lopomo and colleagues[4] measured in in vivo and in vitro setups, respectively, the kinematic tests using a commercial navigation system, with an accuracy of within 1° and 1 mm. Lane and colleagues[27] reported on correlations between clinical grading of PS and navigation data, defining the "p-angle," described by the movement of the pathologic limb during PS test compared with a reference movement, finding a good correlation between this parameter and the clinical grade of the PS. As recently reported by Bignozzi and colleagues,[10] the use of Computer Aided Surgery (CAS) system has been increased parallel to the development of double-bundle ACL reconstructions. Specifically, Lopomo and colleagues[4] and Bignozzi and colleagues[31] reported the use of navigation system in assessing dynamic laxity during anatomic double-bundle reconstruction, analyzing the kinematic behavior of the limb during the maneuver before and after surgery, and thus identifying specific parameters enabling the assessment of PS grade.

Despite the fact that the PS analysis obtained using navigation system provides a reliable and quantitative description of the test correlated with the clinical laxity classification,[4] its application, because of the invasiveness, is however limited to the surgical site, preventing a side-to-side comparison. The only exception is the work of Miura and colleagues,[32] in which knee-laxity between ACL-reconstructed knees and controlateral stable knees was compared intraoperatively by the use of a navigation system.

Toward Noninvasive Methodologies

In recent years, less invasive methodologies of quantifying the PS test noninvasively in an in-office setup have been developed.

Several studies reported the use of electromagnetic sensors[15,33–36] to quantitatively analyze the PS test. Bull and colleagues[2] were the first to use electromagnetic systems with skin-mounted sensors. Similarly, Kubo and colleagues[37] developed a noninvasive measurement system using commercial electromagnetic tracking system, finding a good correlation with bone-fixed measurements and identifying the velocity as a good parameter to grade PS test. Analogously, Hoshino and colleagues[16,33,36] used a noninvasive electromagnetic measurement system, finding positive correlations between anterior tibial translation and posterior tibial acceleration during the PS test and clinical grading of the PS test itself. Acceleration was also analyzed by Araki and colleagues[38] in a comparison between anatomic single-bundle versus double-bundle ACL reconstruction using an electromagnetic device. Lopomo and colleagues,[39] using an electromagnetic tracking system, identified the 3-dimensional acceleration as the parameter most correlated to the clinical grade. Electromagnetic tracking devices can be used in vivo with an optimal accuracy, but the wired sensors and possible disturbance from ferromagnetic material limit their clinical utility.

More recently, Hoshino and colleagues[40] proposed a noninvasive method based on image analysis for capturing the lateral PS movement, identifying specific landmarks by means of ring-shaped stickers. However, the measured accuracy of the digital analysis requires further validation, including the influence of skin artifacts.

THE USE OF ACCELERATION SENSORS

As reported earlier, acceleration has been used as a parameter to evaluate the dynamic condition of the knee joint during the PS maneuver, using either intraoperative methods to analyze the lateral compartment kinematics[41] or electromagnetic systems.[16,33,36]

Recently, Lopomo and colleagues,[39] Maeyama and colleagues,[42] and Debandi and colleagues[43] proposed in 2 different setups (in vivo and in animal model) a novel procedure that uses a single triaxial accelerometer in the evaluation of dynamic knee laxity during the PS maneuver. One single accelerometer able to detect ACL injury is in fact easy to use in the office setting as well.

Lopomo and colleagues,[39] applying a single triaxial acceleration sensor on the lateral side of the tibia, specifically tried to analyze the dynamic behavior of the joint, including the 3-dimensional amount of acceleration measured by the sensor during execution of the clinical maneuver. The acquisition system (KiRA, Orthokey LLC, Lewes, DE, USA) consisted of a sensor embedded in a triaxial accelerometer wirelessly connected to a common laptop. The sensor was skin-affixed to the tibia, between the lateral aspect of the anterior tuberosity and the Gerdy tubercle. A sterile drape was used to reduce the movement between the box and the tibia. The main axis of the sensor was aligned with the tibial mechanical axis (**Fig. 1**). The localization of the

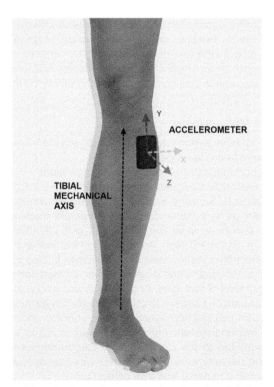

Fig. 1. In vivo setup with a single accelerometer placed on the tibia in a stable and reliable position.

sensor has been defined according to the outcomes of Lopomo and colleagues[4] and Bedi and colleagues.[44] They stated that the acceleration reached during the reduction of the lateral compartment is most influenced by the presence of PS phenomenon.

Their method afforded a simple setup and the definition of few parameters on the 3-dimensional acceleration signal (**Fig. 2**). Moreover, they were able to automatically detect the PS event by evaluating in a sample-by-sample manner the Pearson correlation coefficient between a specific window-template–previously defined on a set of trial patients–and the corresponding part of the analyzed signal.[45]

Reliability of the Acceleration in PS Quantification

Recent articles on the same in vitro setup analyzed the reliability of the use of a single accelerometer in discriminating the grade of the PS, compared with an electromagnetic system used as a gold standard and involving 12 expert surgeons performing a preferred and a standardized technique (**Fig. 3**).

In particular, Ahlden and colleagues[46] reported a good correlation between the maximum acceleration measured by the sensor and between the jerk and the average PS grade. Moreover, Araujo and colleagues[47] found that the triaxial accelerometer system demonstrated from moderate to good correlation with the reference measurement for the acceleration parameter, depending on the use of a standardized or a preferred technique.

Again, preliminary in vivo analyses have been performed. In a cohort study, Lopomo and colleagues[48] compared the results obtained with a navigation system to the acceleration simultaneously measured with an acceleration sensor. They reported an average root-mean-square displacement because of soft tissue artifacts of 4.9 ± 2.6 mm, good repeatability of the obtained parameters, an optimal interpatient and intrapatient similarity in acceleration curves (**Fig. 4**) and a good positive correlation with the anteroposterior acceleration measured with the navigation system.

Clinical Validation of the Methodology

Lopomo and colleagues[49–51] and Zaffagnini and colleagues[52–54] reported in different in vivo studies the clinical validation of the use of a single accelerometer in quantification of the PS test. Specifically in analysis of their novel procedure[39] performed on 66 consecutive patients after anesthesia, they reported a fair/good intratester reliability of the analyzed parameters, finding a high effect size between the injured and the contralateral knee, thus reporting a probability of about 70% to 80% of whether a knee is in the injured group, only analyzing the acceleration parameters.

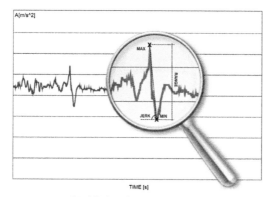

Fig. 2. Acceleration parameters highlighted on a typical acquisition signal.

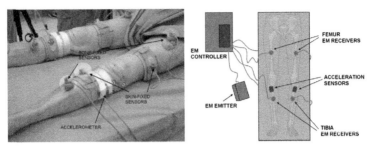

Fig. 3. In vitro setup. The acceleration and the electromagnetic system as used by Ahlden and colleagues[46] and Araujo and colelagues[47] is highlighted.

This clinical validation represented a great pace for clinical practice, especially for the ambulatory assessment. Indeed, a noninvasive tool able to quantify the knee dynamic laxity always represents a challenge.

Current Limitations of the Methodology

An excellent review by Kuroda and colleagues[55] highlighted how muscular resistance could suppress the PS phenomenon, and therefore, most of the studies were conducted under anesthesia to eliminate the effect of muscular resistance. However, the PS test is primarily performed when the patients are awake, so the appropriate muscle relaxation might not be achieved. Without properly eliciting the PS test, any quantitative measurement would not work. Patient guarding during performance of PS should be considered. A preliminary analysis[51,54] reported no differences between preanesthesia and postanesthesia tests with the use of a single acceleration sensor, if considering the patient's guarding strategy and trying to perform the PS maneuver in the most relaxing way.

Moreover, as highlighted by Noyes and colleagues,[56] Hoshino and colleagues,[36,40] Ahlden and colleagues,[57] and Kuroda and colleagues,[15,55] the variability among examiners remains an important issue. In fact, as clearly reported by Kuroda and colleagues,[55] the speed of PS test procedure, the angle of hip abduction, and the force applied to the knee could negatively affect test outcome, above all considering only one sensor and measuring a parameter (ie, acceleration) that is more sensitive to motion variability. It is possible to accomplish better consistency and accuracy of the measurement by standardizing the testing procedure.[16]

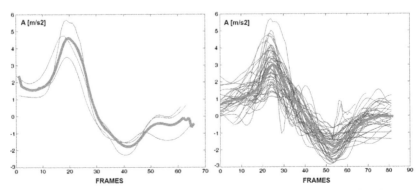

Fig. 4. Intratester (*left*) and intertester similarity of acceleration curves for the in vivo acquisitions.

SUMMARY

In this article, the authors reported that the acceleration of the tibial reduction during the PS test could be detected using a single noninvasive acceleration sensor. This in vivo measurement methodology can be applied to quantitative evaluation of dynamic laxity of the knee joint during the PS test. All the reported articles highlighted how the use of the acceleration as a parameter able to discriminate the ACL injury can be easily applicable under in vivo conditions; a quantitative description of the dynamic instability of the PS test, which could not be easily and noninvasively detected by the conventional devices, is thus possible. This is also confirmed by the reliability of the analyzed PS quantitative parameters. A fair/good intraclass correlation value was obtained[39] even when compared with the reliability results of system that are considered the state of the art for the static laxity tests.[58] Moreover, in vitro biomechanical evidence demonstrates the usefulness of this methodology and system in the quantitative analysis of the PS test. A further application is the use of accelerometers as a teaching tool to instruct young surgeons to perform the PS test in a more standardized way, ultimately enabling comparison of clinical outcome following ACL reconstruction surgery.

REFERENCES

1. Bonnet A. Traité des maladies des articulations. Paris: Avec Atlas Balliére; 1845.
2. Bull AM, Andersen HN, Basso O, et al. Incidence and mechanism of the pivot shift. An in vitro study. Clin Orthop Relat Res 1999;363:219–31.
3. Butler DL, Noyes FR, Grood ES, et al. Ligamentous restraints to anterior-posterior drawer in the human knee. A biomechanical study. J Bone Joint Surg Am 1980; 62(2):259–70.
4. Lopomo N, Zaffagnini S, Bignozzi S, et al. Pivot-shift test: analysis and quantification of knee laxity parameters using a navigation system. J Orthop Res 2010;28(2):164–9.
5. Galway HR, MacIntosh DL. The lateral pivot shift: a symptom and sign of anterior cruciate ligament insufficiency. Clin Orthop Relat Res 1980;147:45–50.
6. Slocum DB, James SL, Larson RL, et al. Clinical test for anterolateral rotary instability of the knee. Clin Orthop Relat Res 1976;118:63–9.
7. Jakob RP, Stäubli HU, Deland JT. Grading the pivot shift. Objective tests with implications for treatment. J Bone Joint Surg Br 1987;69:294–9.
8. Oberlander M, Shalvoy R, Hughston J. The accuracy of the clinical knee examination documented by arthroscopy: a prospective study. Am J Sports Med 1993; 21:773–8.
9. Prins M. The Lachman test is the most sensitive and the pivot shift the most specific test for the diagnosis of ACL rupture. Aust J Physiother 2006;52:66.
10. Bignozzi S, Zaffagnini S, Lopomo N. Clinical relevance of static and dynamic tests after anatomical double-bundle ACL reconstruction. Knee Surg Sports Traumatol Arthrosc 2010;18:37–42.
11. Kujala UM, Nelimarkka O, Koskinen KS. Relationship between the pivot shift and the configuration of the lateral tibial plateau. Arch Orthop Trauma Surg 1992; 111(4):228–9. http://dx.doi.org/10.1007/BF00571483.
12. Kaplan N, Wickiewicz TL, Warren RF. Primary surgical treatment of anterior cruciate ligament ruptures. A long-term follow-up study. Am J Sports Med 1990;18(4):354–8.
13. Noyes FR, Mooar PA, Matthews DS. The symptomatic anterior cruciate-deficient knee. Part I: the long-term functional disability in athletically active individuals. J Bone Joint Surg Am 1983;65(2):154–62.

14. Kocher MS, Steadman JR, Briggs KK, et al. Relationships between objective assessment of ligament stability and subjective assessment of symptoms and function after anterior cruciate ligament reconstruction. Am J Sports Med 2004; 32:629–34.

15. Kuroda R, Hoshino Y, Kubo S, et al. Similarities and differences of diagnostic manual tests for anterior cruciate ligament insufficiency: a global survy and kinematics assessment. Am J Sports Med 2012;40(1):91–9.

16. Hoshino Y, Araujo P, Ahlden M, et al. Standardized pivot shift test improves measurement accuracy. Knee Surg Sports Traumatol Arthrosc 2012. http://dx.doi.org/10.1007/s00167-011-1850-0.

17. Musahl V, Hoshino Y, Ahlden M, et al. The pivot shift: a global user guide. Knee Surg Sports Traumatol Arthrosc 2012. http://dx.doi.org/10.1007/s00167-011-1859-4.

18. Csintalan RP, Ehsan A, McGarry MH, et al. Biomechanical and anatomical effects of an external rotational torque applied to the knee: a cadaveric study. Am J Sports Med 2006;34:1623–9.

19. Amis A, Bull A, Lie D. Biomechanics of rotational instability and anatomic anterior cruciate ligament reconstruction. Oper Tech Orthop 2005;15:29–35.

20. Diermann N, Schumacher T, Schanz S, et al. Rotational instability of the knee: internal tibial rotation under a simulated pivot shift test. Arch Orthop Trauma Surg 2009;129:353–8.

21. Tashiro Y, Okazaki K, Miura H. Quantitative assessment of rotatory instability after anterior cruciate ligament reconstruction. Am J Sports Med 2009;37:909–16.

22. Kuroda R, Hoshino Y, Nagamune K, et al. Intraoperative measurement of pivot shift by electromagnetic sensors. Oper Tech Orthop 2008;18:190–5.

23. Lopomo N, Bignozzi S, Zaffagnini S, et al. Quantitative correlation between IKDC score, static laxity, and pivot-shift test: a kinematic analysis of knee stability in anatomic double-bundle anterior cruciate ligament reconstruction. Oper Tech Orthop 2008;18:185–9.

24. Pearle AD, Kendoff D, Musahl V, et al. The pivot-shift phenomenon during computer-assisted anterior cruciate ligament reconstruction. J Bone Joint Surg Am 2009;91(Suppl 1):115–8.

25. Kendoff D, Citak M, Voos J, et al. Surgical navigation in knee ligament reconstruction. Clin Sports Med 2009;28:41–50.

26. Colombet PD, Robinson JR. Computer-assisted, anatomic, double-bundle anterior cruciate ligament reconstruction. Arthroscopy 2008;24:1152–60.

27. Lane CG, Warren RF, Stanford FC, et al. In vivo analysis of the pivot shift phenomenon during computer navigated ACL reconstruction. Knee Surg Sports Traumatol Arthrosc 2008;16:487–92.

28. Ishibashi Y, Tsuda E, Yamamoto Y, et al. Navigation evaluation of the pivot-shift phenomenon during double-bundle anterior cruciate ligament reconstruction: is the posterolateral bundle more important? Arthroscopy 2009;25:488–95.

29. Colombet P, Robinson J, Christel P, et al. Using navigation to measure rotation kinematics during ACL reconstruction. Clin Orthop Relat Res 2007;454:59–65.

30. Pearle AD, Solomon DJ, Wanich T, et al. Reliability of navigated knee stability examination: a cadaveric evaluation. Am J Sports Med 2007;35(8):1315–20.

31. Bignozzi S, Zaffagnini S, Lopomo N, et al. Does a lateral plasty control coupled translation during antero-posterior stress in single-bundle ACL reconstruction? An in vivo study. Knee Surg Sports Traumatol Arthrosc 2009;17(1):65–70.

32. Miura K, Ishibashi Y, Tsuda E, et al. Intraoperative comparison of knee laxity between anterior cruciate ligament-reconstructed knee and contralateral stable knee using navigation system. Arthroscopy 2010;26(9):1203–11.

33. Hoshino Y, Kuroda R, Nagamune K. In vivo measurement of the pivot-shift test in the anterior cruciate ligament-deficient knee using an electromagnetic device. Am J Sports Med 2007;35:1098–104.

34. Amis AA, Cuomo P, Rama RB, et al. Measurement of knee laxity and pivot-shift kinematics with magnetic sensors. Oper Tech Orthop 2008;18:196–203.

35. Labbe D, Deguise J, Godbout V, et al. Development of an objective measurement tool for the pivot shift phenomenon of the knee. J Biomech 2008;41:S207–S207.

36. Hoshino Y, Kuroda R, Nagamune K, et al. Optimal measurement of clinical rotational test for evaluating anterior cruciate ligament insufficiency. Knee Surg Sports Traumatol Arthrosc 2011. http://dx.doi.org/10.1007/s00167-011-1643-5.

37. Kubo S, Muratsu H, Yoshiya S, et al. Reliability and usefulness of a new in vivo measurement system of the pivot shift. Clin Orthop Relat Res 2007;454:54–8.

38. Araki D, Kuroda R, Kubo S, et al. A prospective randomised study of anatomical single-bundle versus double-bundle anterior cruciate ligament reconstruction: quantitative evaluation using an electromagnetic measurement system. Int Orthop 2011;35(3):439–46.

39. Lopomo N, Zaffagnini S, Signorelli C, et al. An original clinical methodology for noninvasive assessment of pivot-shift test. Comput Methods Biomech Biomed Engin 2011. http://dx.doi.org/10.1080/10 255842.2011.591788.

40. Hoshino Y, Araujo P, Irrgang JJ, et al. An image analysis method to quantify the lateral pivot shift test. Knee Surg Sports Traumatol Arthrosc 2012;20(4):703–7.

41. Zaffagnini S, Marcheggiani Muccioli GM, Lopomo N, et al. Can the pivot-shift be eliminated by anatomic double-bundle anterior cruciate ligament reconstruction? Knee Surg Sports Traumatol Arthrosc 2012;20(4):743–51.

42. Maeyama A, Hoshino Y, Debandi A, et al. Evaluation of rotational instability in the anterior cruciate ligament deficient knee using triaxial accelerometer: a biomechanical model in porcine knees. Knee Surg Sports Traumatol Arthrosc 2011; 19(8):1233–8.

43. Debandi A, Maeyama A, Hoshino Y, et al. The effect of tunnel placement on rotational stability after ACL reconstruction: evaluation with use of triaxial accelerometry in a porcine model. Knee Surg Sports Traumatol Arthrosc 2012. http://dx.doi.org/10.1007/s00167-012-1961-2.

44. Bedi A, Musahl V, O'Loughlin P, et al. A comparison of the effect of central anatomical single-bundle anterior cruciate ligament reconstruction and double-bundle anterior cruciate ligament reconstruction on pivot-shift kinematics. Am J Sports Med 2010;38(9):1788–94.

45. Signorelli C, Lopomo N, Bignozzi S, et al. Automatic screening of acceleration signal during pivot-shift test based on Pearson's correlation coefficient. Paper presented at: BIOSTEC, BIOSIGNALS 2010, International Conference on Bio-inspired Systems and Signal. Valencia, January 20–23, 2010.

46. Ahlden M, Araujo P, Hoshino Y, et al. Clinical grading of the pivot shift test correlates best with tibial acceleration. Knee Surg Sports Traumatol Arthrosc 2012; 20(4):708–12.

47. Araujo P, Ahlden M, Hoshino Y, et al. Comparison of three noninvasive quantitative measurement systems for the pivot shift test. Knee Surg Sports Traumatol Arthrosc 2012;20(4):692–7.

48. Lopomo N, Signorelli C, Bonanzinga T, et al. Quantitative assessment of pivot-shift using inertial sensors. Knee Surg Sports Traumatol Arthrosc 2012;20(4): 713–7.

49. Lopomo N, Signorelli C, Visani A, et al. Intra-operative validation of a novel method dedicated to quantify pivot-shift phenomenon. 24th International Society

for Technology in Arthroplasty – Annual Congress. Bruges, September 20–23, 2011.

50. Lopomo N, Signorelli C, Bignozzi S, et al. A new tool for quantifying knee dynamic instability based on automatic classification of acceleration signal during pivot-shift test. 17th European Society of Biomechanics – ESB Congress. Edinburgh, July 4–8, 2010.

51. Signorelli C, Lopomo N, Bignozzi S, et al. Clinical validation of a novel method dedicated to quantify knee joint dynamic instability. 17th European Society of Biomechanics – ESB Congress. Edinburgh, July 4–8, 2010.

52. Zaffagnini S, Lopomo N, Signorelli C, et al. Clinical validation of a non-invasive system dedicated to quantify pivot-shift. American Accademy of Orthopaedic Surgeons. San Diego, February 15–19, 2011.

53. Zaffagnini S, Signorelli C, Lopomo N, et al. Clinical validation and preliminary results of a system for knee joint dynamic instability quantification. 56th Annual Meeting of the Orthopaedic Research Society-ORS. New Orleans, March 6–9, 2010.

54. Zaffagnini S, Signorelli C, Lopomo N, et al. Clinical validation and preliminary results of a new tool used to quantify pivot-shift test. 14th European Society of Sports Traumatology, Knee Surgery and Arthroscopy- ESSKA Congress. Oslo, June 9–12, 2010.

55. Kuroda R, Hoshino Y, Araki D, et al. Quantitative measurement of the pivot shift, reliability, and clinical applications. Knee Surg Sports Traumatol Arthrosc 2012; 20(4):686–91.

56. Noyes FR, Grood ES, Cummings JF, et al. An analysis of the pivot shift phenomenon. The knee motions and subluxations induced by different examiners. Am J Sports Med 1991;19(2):148–55.

57. Ahlden M, Hoshino Y, Samuelsson K, et al. Dynamic knee laxity measurement devices. Knee Surg Sports Traumatol Arthrosc 2012;20(4):621–32.

58. Muellner T, Bugge W, Johansen S. Inter- and intratester comparison of the Rolimeter knee tester: effect of tester's experience and the examination technique. Knee Surg Sports Traumatol Arthrosc 2001;9(5):302–6.

Evidence-Based Practice to Improve Outcomes of Anterior Cruciate Ligament Reconstruction

O.R. Ayeni, MD, MSc, FRCSC[a],*, N. Evaniew, MD[a],
R. Ogilvie, MD, FRCSC[b], D.C. Peterson, MD, FRCSC[c],
M.R. Denkers, MD, FRCSC[d], M. Bhandari, MD, PhD, FRCSC[e]

KEYWORDS

- Anterior cruciate ligament • Evidence-based medicine • Knee surgery
- Expertise-based trails • Anatomic reconstruction • Narrative review

KEY POINTS

- An evidence-based approach to anterior cruciate ligament (ACL) reconstruction integrates best available research with clinical expertise and patient values.
- Appropriately powered expertise-based trials should be emphasized to minimize bias, enhance validity, and reduce crossover.
- Best-practice rehabilitation protocols can guide postoperative care while minimizing heterogeneity within studies.
- Functional outcome scores should be sensitive, responsive, and able to reliably detect small changes.
- Tunnel position should be measured accurately, reported, and scrutinized if the benefits of anatomic ACL reconstruction are to be verified.

INTRODUCTION

The earliest attempts to salvage the anterior cruciate ligament (ACL)-deficient knee were described by Battle in 1900 and Mayo Robson in 1903.[1,2] In 1917, Groves was among the first to advocate reconstruction with graft tissue rather than primary

Conflicts of Interest: None declared.
[a] Division of Orthopaedic Surgery, McMaster University Medical Center, McMaster University, 1200 Main Street West, Room 4E17, Hamilton, Ontario L8N3Z5, Canada; [b] Division of Orthopaedic Surgery, McMaster University, 203-323 Wilson Street East, Ancaster, Ontario L9G4A8, Canada; [c] Division of Orthopaedic Surgery, Department of Surgery, McMaster University Medical Center, McMaster University, 1200 Main Street West Hamilton, Ontario L8N3Z5, Canada; [d] Division of Orthopaedic Surgery, Hamilton General Hospital, McMaster University, 237 Barton Street East, 5North - Room 532, Hamilton, Ontario L8L2X2, Canada; [e] Division of Orthopaedic Surgery, McMaster University, 293 Wellington Street North, Suite 110, Hamilton, Ontario L8L8E7, Canada
* Corresponding author.
E-mail address: ayenif@mcmaster.ca

Clin Sports Med 32 (2013) 71–80
http://dx.doi.org/10.1016/j.csm.2012.08.008
0278-5919/13/$ – see front matter © 2013 Elsevier Inc. All rights reserved.
sportsmed.theclinics.com

repair.[3] Many advances have taken place, and ACL surgery is among the most successful operations in orthopedic surgery. In the last 30 years, techniques in ACL reconstruction have evolved from open and extra-articular reconstruction techniques, to arthroscopic and more anatomic techniques. Considerable research has focused on graft selection, graft fixation, and tunnel placement.[4] Modern techniques allow for minimal tissue trauma, accelerated recovery, and reproducible outcomes. For example, the use of an accessory medial portal for femoral tunnel drilling, based on an improved understanding of tunnel positioning, has led to an emphasis on anatomic ACL reconstruction.[5]

As described by Karlsson and colleagues,[5] anatomic ACL reconstruction involves 4 key principles: the restoration of native insertion-site anatomy, the restoration of the 2 functional bundles of the native ACL, the restoration of native tensioning behavior between these 2 bundles, and the individualization of surgical techniques to each patient. However, anatomic ACL reconstruction is not synonymous with double-bundle ACL reconstruction. Just as the principles may be applied to single-bundle anatomic ACL reconstruction, they may likewise be discounted in nonanatomic double-bundle ACL reconstruction. A recent report has identified that while many studies have evaluated anatomic ACL reconstruction techniques, few provide enough surgical description to substantiate such claims.[6]

Whereas the immediate surgical goal of anatomic ACL reconstruction is to replicate native knee anatomy and biomechanical function, the long-term clinical goal is to stabilize the knee and minimize the development of symptomatic ACL-deficient degenerative arthrosis.[5] Several cadaveric and in vivo kinematic studies have demonstrated improved biomechanical function and stability when anatomic ACL reconstruction techniques are compared with traditional nonanatomic techniques.[7] Although early clinical results appear promising, long-term outcome data are lacking.[8,9] Well-designed prospective studies with detailed technical descriptions and appropriate patient-centered outcomes will accurately investigate the benefits of this technique.

Evidence-based medicine (EBM) is the integration of best available research with clinical expertise and patient values to facilitate clinical decision making.[10] Introduced by Sackett in the early 1980s and coined by Guyatt in the 1990s, both at McMaster University, EBM has been identified by the *BMJ* as one of the top 15 medical breakthroughs in the last 160 years.[11,12]

The purpose of this article is to describe how EBM must be applied to future research on the ACL-deficient knee to optimize short- and long-term clinical outcomes. Pitfalls in current understanding and identification of areas of deficiency will illustrate the necessity of proper protocols for future research.

DIAGNOSTIC CHALLENGES: ASSESSMENT OF THE ACL-DEFICIENT KNEE
Evidence for Clinical Maneuvers

Study of anatomic ACL reconstruction begins with clinical assessment of the ACL-deficient knee. Validated and reproducible examination maneuvers are essential to ensure accurate diagnosis and to appraise the success of surgical interventions.

The Lachman and instrumented Lachman tests have shown excellent sensitivity, specificity, and reproducibility in describing anterior–posterior laxity, but current literature suggests that a measure of rotatory laxity may be more meaningful.

Benjaminise and colleagues[13] performed a meta-analysis of 28 studies to evaluate the accuracy of clinical tests for ACL tears. The included reports displayed some heterogeneity, but the Lachman test was identified as the most valid for ACL deficiency, with a pooled sensitivity of 85% and a pooled specificity of 94%. The pivot–shift test had a higher specificity, 98%, but a much lower sensitivity, 24%. The anterior drawer test had poor validity in acute tears, but good sensitivity and specificity in chronic cases. Despite these findings, preferential use of the Lachman test has been criticized due to its poor correlation with subjective and objective functional outcomes after ACL reconstruction surgery.[14] Further, residual rotational laxity has been correlated with decreased patient satisfaction, functional instability, and the development of osteoarthritis.[15–17]

Role of the Pivot–Shift Test

Whereas reconstruction of the posterolateral bundle of the ACL during anatomic ACL reconstruction specifically aims to restore rotatory laxity, the pivot–shift test has received significant recent attention. Elimination of the pivot–shift phenomenon is a well-regarded goal of ACL reconstruction,[18] and a recent systematic review identified an 85% correlation between reported pivot–shift test results and functional outcomes.[19]

Nonetheless, performance and grading of the pivot–shift test remain subjective and poorly standardized. Applied forces and rotational moments, resulting tibial translation and tibial acceleration, and clinical grading all vary significantly between expert examiners.[18] In a recent cadaveric study, Hoshino and colleagues[20] demonstrated that standardization of the manual pivot–shift test might be possible. Variations in tibial acceleration were minimized after simple training, but the validity and reliability of this effect on clinical grading have not yet been investigated.

Other reports have described increasingly precise techniques to quantify the pathologic movements of the pivot–shift phenomenon. Noninvasive techniques include electromagnetic tracking of skin sensors, triaxial accelerometers, and digital image analysis.[21] Even more precise, but also invasive, expensive, and complex, are intraoperative kinematic analysis with computer-assisted surgery, fixed electromagnetic tracking devices, fixed accelerometers, dynamic roentgen sterometric analysis (RSA), and open magnetic resonance imaging (MRI).[22] Although these techniques demonstrate excellent promise, investigations of validity, reliability, and feasibility are required.

MRI continues to provide an important adjunct in the evaluation of ACL-deficient knees. Historical and recent reports have confirmed the high accuracy of conventional MRI in diagnosing ACL tears. Van Dyck and colleagues[23] demonstrated accuracies of 97% and 95% for complete and partial ACL tears, respectively. MRI also identifies associated pathology, such as mensical injuries, that aid in preoperative planning.[24]

SURGICAL TECHNIQUES: CLINICAL STUDIES AND TRIAL DESIGN
Expertise-Based Trials

Sackett and colleagues described that "Evidence based medicine is the conscientious, explicit, and judicious use of current best evidence in making decisions about the care of individual patients."[25] Importance is placed on high-quality research including well-designed randomized controlled trials (RCTs), rigorous systematic reviews, and meta-analyses. Due in part to some unique challenges when designing surgical RCTs, surgical decision making has long relied on nonsystematic clinical observations, expert opinion, and eminence-based decision-making.[26]

To conduct high-quality RCTs of surgical techniques, the following challenges must be overcome: a general lack of pre-existing EBM knowledge, difficulty with proper blinding, ethical considerations, and a tendency to defend historical procedures. Likewise, the effect of the learning curve effect, whereby seniority and experience often result in superior outcomes, must be considered.[25] The latter can be overcome by well-designed expertise-based clinical trials.

Devereaux and colleagues[26] describe differential expertise bias as being inherent to many RCTs of surgical procedures. A surgeon's training and experience necessarily lead to the refinement of limited particular techniques to solve a given surgical problem. This creates restricted expertise. Subsequently, if surgeons with expertise in the novel intervention treat a majority of the patients in both treatment arms, and surgeons with expertise in the comparison intervention treat a minority of those in both arms, results could be biased toward the novel intervention. The inverse is also possible. Practically, the greater the disparity in distribution of expertise among the 2 groups, the greater risk of expertise bias to be present in a trial.

Many studies either fail to ensure or fail to report that the number of surgeons with expertise in each procedure is equal. Some studies stipulate surgeons complete a requisite number of cases with the novel procedure before entering the study, but bias may persist, because outcomes often continue to improve with extensive experience.[26] That is, surgeons are unlikely to reach the plateau of the learning curve by simply completing the minimum number of cases required to enter the trial. This has been demonstrated in large observational studies.[27,28] Most recently, Marx and colleagues[29] demonstrated that 60 or more ACL reconstructions are needed to reduce the risk of a patient requiring revision ACL surgery.

In an expertise-based clinical trial, 1 surgeon with specific expertise in the new technique performs the novel procedure, while another surgeon with specific expertise in the standard technique performs the comparison procedure. This obviates the need for surgeons to be skilled in both techniques and eliminates the learning curve effect.[26] It also addresses criticism that either a surgeon's lack of technical expertise or an unblinded surgeon's belief in 1 of the procedures compromises the validity or applicability of the results.[26] Finally, it also minimizes differential crossover, a well-described phenomenon in which procedural crossovers are initiated by surgeons with limited experience in the novel procedure.[26]

Graft Selection

At present, primary ACL-reconstruction is most commonly performed with either a central third bone–patellar tendon–bone (PT) or hamstrings–tendon (HT) autograft construct.[30] Despite prolific investigation, graft selection remains controversial. Purported advantages of PT constructs include secure fixation, increased graft incorporation, relative ease of harvest, and excellent graft strength. Possible disadvantages include risks of patellar tendonitis, patellar tendon rupture, patellar fracture, and anterior knee pain. Purported advantages of HT constructs include reduced donor site morbidity, multiple-bundled structure to increase strength, and larger graft size to increase incorporation, while disadvantages include hamstring weakness and prominent hardware.[30]

Several recent systematic reviews and meta-analyses have examined outcomes of ACL reconstruction using PT versus HT autografts. Mohtadi and colleagues[31] performed a Cochrane Review of 19 randomized and quasi-randomized controlled trials. Pooled analysis demonstrated no significant differences in primary outcomes of return to activity, Tegner and Lysholm knee scores, International Knee Documentation Committee (IKDC) scores, rerupture, or single-leg hop test. Analysis of secondary outcomes revealed improved Lachman results, pivot–shift results, and knee flexion strength in the PT constructs, and reduced anterior knee pain and improved knee extension range-of-motion in HT constructs. Important methodological limitations include the heterogeneity of surgical techniques, rehabilitation protocols, and presentation of results in each of the included studies. Among both PT and HT groups, various fixation methods including screws and washers, suture posts, staples, buttons, and interference screws were used. Among the HT groups, various combinations of semitendinosus and gracilis tendons, and various doubling, tripling, and quadrupling of strands were used.

Poolman and colleagues[32] summarized 11 recent overlapping systematic reviews and found variable success in quality of reporting, internal validity, use of formal sensitivity analysis, and citation of prior reviews in all relevant studies. Based on the most methodologically sound meta-analyses, HT constructs were favored for reduced anterior knee pain, while limited evidence favored PT constructs for stability. Ultimately, they concluded that a large, appropriately powered, ideally multicentered and expertise-based, randomized trial using a validated patient-oriented outcome instrument to measure a clinically relevant treatment effect remains necessary to resolve the issue of graft selection.

Tunnel Position

Given that anatomic ACL reconstruction aims to place graft tunnels in the native insertion sites of the anteromedial and posterolateral bundles of the ACL, an important feature of future trials will include assessment of whether this has been accomplished. Such data will reveal technical challenges while validating outcomes as truly reflecting anatomic reconstruction. Kopf and colleagues[33] and Forstyth and colleagues[34] recently used 3-dimensional computed tomography (CT) analysis to evaluate tunnel position in actual patient and cadaver knees. They showed that transtibial drilling frequently placed the tunnels outside of the anatomic insertions, but that meticulous arthroscopic dissection and double-bundle techniques accurately led to anatomic tunnel placement. Their postoperative 3-dimensional CT data correlated well with existing anatomic literature, providing an important reference set for future studies.

Recent reports have emphasized anatomic drilling of the femoral tunnel via an anteromedial portal.[35] In a cadaveric study, Bedi and colleagues[36] demonstrated improved coronal obliquity, but increased risks of posterior blowout and critically short tunnel lengths with a standard anteromedial portal and a conventional 6 mm offset guide. In a 3-dimensional model analysis, however, Hensler and colleagues[37] suggested excellent control of tunnel position and length by considering the combined effects of drill bit start position, drill bit diameter, transverse drill angle, and knee flexion angle. Femoral tunnel geometry most closely matched native ACL anatomy when a 9 mm drill bit was positioned in the anatomic femoral origin with the knee in 102° of flexion and drilled at a transverse angle of 40°. Positioning of the tunnel using anatomic landmarks rather than relying on offset guides,[38] and use of a central viewing portal to enhance visualization of the lateral wall may further minimize complications.[39] To clarify the benefits of the anteromedial portal, future prospective clinical trials should include precise descriptions of surgical techniques and intraoperative complications.[6]

Rehabilitation Protocols

To achieve optimal outcomes after ACL reconstruction, an evidence-based approach to rehabilitation is critical. Wright and colleagues[40] performed a detailed systematic review and meta-analysis of 54 RCTs investigating multiple aspects of ACL rehabilitation. Analysis was limited by methodological heterogeneity and potential bias within studies, but some conclusions were possible. Based on 6 RCTs, no significant clinical benefit has been shown to support the use of continuous passive motion (CPM). Based on 4 RCTs, minimally supervised home physiotherapy programs have been shown to be safe and adequate for selected highly motivated patients when compared with traditional intensively supervised clinic-based programs. Selection and performance bias were possible in 3 of the 4 studies, and particular therapeutic protocols were varied. A single RCT demonstrated no complications and improved anterior knee pain with early weight bearing and range of motion.[41]

In a systematic review of 11 RCTs, there were no associated increases in injury rates, postoperative pain, knee laxity, or reduced range of motion when patients were not braced with stabilizing hinged rehabilitation braces postoperatively.[42] The authors concluded that postoperative bracing is not necessary following routine primary ACL reconstruction. This conclusion is limited by potential selection bias due to poor description of randomization and blinding methods.

Multiple reports have examined the role of accelerated rehabilitation after ACL reconstruction surgery. Ekstrand found no significant differences at 12 months follow-up in a group of 20 soccer players randomized to either a 6- or 8-month postoperative return to sport, but both groups underwent otherwise very similar protocols, including a 3-month period of delayed full weight bearing. Randomization method, power analysis, and confidence intervals were not described.[43] Beynnon and colleagues[44] described 42 patients randomized to either a 19- or 32-week rehabilitation program and followed them prospectively with double binding to 2 years. Patients in the accelerated group demonstrated improved thigh muscle strength at 3 months after surgery, but there were otherwise no differences in clinical assessment, patient satisfaction, function, and proprioception. Roentgen Stereophotogrammetric Analysis (RSA) was used to demonstrate no significant differences in either anterior-posterior (A-P) or rotational laxity between the groups.

Van Grinsven and colleagues[45] recently published a best evidence therapy protocol after their own systematic review of 32 RCTs. They describe an accelerated program of rehabilitation without postoperative bracing. Early goals include reduction of pain, swelling, and inflammation, and emphasis is placed on regaining range of motion, strength, and neuromuscular control. Preoperative educational sessions, clear time points, and interim objective and subjective tests are also included. Nonetheless, prospective evaluation and widespread consensus are lacking. Continued study and critical review remain essential for an evidence-based approach to rehabilitation after ACL reconstruction.

OUTCOMES ASSESSMENT: EVIDENCE-BASED EVALUATION

An essential requirement for future trials is the use of sensitive, responsive, reliable, and validated outcome measures.[10] Improvement in surgical outcomes can only be determined when those outcomes can be measured, repeated, and compared with other reports. With regard to anatomic ACL reconstruction, short- and long-term patient-focused scoring instruments and objective measures of laxity are essential. Long-term studies will provide the gold standard measure of postreconstruction radiologic and symptomatic osteoarthritis, but postoperative 3-dimensional CT analysis of tunnel position may provide important prognostic information.

Knee Scores

Commonly used knee scores in ACL reconstruction include the IKDC subjective and objective forms, the modified Lysholm score, the Knee Injury and Osteoarthritis Outcome Score, the Cincinnati Knee Rating System, the Tegner Activity Score, and the Marx Activity Score.[10] Most have demonstrated validity and reliability in evaluative studies, but some key criticisms must be highlighted.

Irrgang and colleagues[46] described a potentially significant limitation of conventionally reported IKDC scores for the pivot–shift test. Grouping the nearly normal and normal groups allows dichotomous contrast to the abnormal and severely abnormal groups, which may minimize any subjective bias of the IKDC instrument. However, it also suggests that nearly normal is good enough.[46] When the data from the meta-analysis of RCT comparing single- and double-bundle ACL reconstruction by Meredick and colleagues[46] were reanalyzed with the nearly normal and normal groups separated, statistically significant differences favoring double-bundle ACL reconstruction were revealed. Irrgang and colleagues[46] hypothesized that such small differences may be clinically meaningful at long-term follow-up.

In multiple systematic review and meta-analyses, many knee scores have demonstrated only minor functional outcomes during comparisons of technique, graft type, and tunnel positions.[31] Karlsson and colleagues[5] discuss that the relatively poor ability of current knee scores to detect small differences in function may be responsible. Improvements in outcome instruments that allow detection of smaller but potentially very meaningful differences may be of paramount importance. Future well-designed trials should include a general health outcome measure, an activity level scale, and a disease-specific scale that considers patients' sensation of stability while participating in strenuous activities.[10,46] To date, the Anterior Cruciate Ligament Quality of Life (ACL-QOL) is the only validated, disease-specific measure of health-related quality of life for ACL deficiency.[31,47] In their prospective cohort trial, Tanner and colleagues[48] demonstrated superiority of this instrument to detect symptoms and disabilities important to patients with ACL tears.

Long-term Data

The long-term clinical goal of anatomic ACL reconstruction is to stabilize the knee and in turn protect knee health and minimize the development of symptomatic ACL-deficient degenerative arthrosis.[5] In their retrospective review of 103 patients who underwent traditional ACL reconstruction, Ait si Selmi and colleagues[49] demonstrated up to 22% prevalence of radiographic osteoarthritis at 17 years of follow-up. Lohmander and colleagues[50] showed up to 46% prevalence of symptomatic radiographic osteoarthritis in ACL-reconstructed knees at 12 years of follow-up. More recently, Li and colleagues[40] reported a 38.6% incidence of radiographic knee Osteoarthritis (OA) at 7.8 years of follow-up. Although early clinical results of anatomic ACL reconstruction appear promising, long-term data investigating the onset of OA are lacking.[8,9,51] Ultimately, prospective studies of anatomic ACL reconstruction with extensive follow-up and detailed evaluation of knee health will demonstrate the benefits of this technique.

SUMMARY

Recent studies of anatomic ACL reconstruction have considered native knee anatomy and biomechanical function, and emphasized the long-term clinical goals of protecting knee health and preventing the development of symptomatic ACL-deficient degenerative arthrosis. Ultimately, extensive follow-up will be required to possibly demonstrate the benefits of this technique. An evidence-based approach integrates best available research with clinical expertise and patient values.

Validated and reproducible examination maneuvers are necessary for accurate diagnosis and for appraisal of surgical interventions. Appropriately powered expertise-based trials should be emphasized to minimize bias, enhance validity, and reduce crossover. Best practice rehabilitation protocols can guide postoperative care while minimizing heterogeneity within studies. Functional outcome scores should be sensitive, responsive, and able to reliably detect small changes. Tunnel position should be measured accurately, reported, and scrutinized if the benefits of anatomic ACL reconstruction are to be verified.

REFERENCES

1. Battle WH. A case of open section of the knee joint for irreducible traumatic dislocation. Clinical Society of London Transactions 1900;33:232–3.
2. Mayo Robson AW. Ruptured crucial ligaments and their repair by operation. Ann Surg 1903;37:716–8.
3. Hey Groves EW. The crucial ligaments of the knee joint: their function, rupture and the operative treatment of the same. Br J Surg 1919;7:505–15.
4. McCulloch PC, Lattermann C, Boland AL, et al. An illustrated history of anterior cruciate ligament surgery. J Knee Surg 2007;20(2):95–104.
5. Karlsson J, Irrgang JJ, van Eck CF, et al. Anatomic single- and double-bundle anterior cruciate ligament reconstruction, part 2: clinical application of surgical technique. Am J Sports Med 2011;39:2016.
6. van Eck CF, Schreiber VM, Mejia HA, et al. "Anatomic" anterior cruciate ligament reconstruction: a systematic review of surgical techniques and reporting of surgical data. Arthroscopy 2010;26(Suppl 9):S2–12.
7. Yasuda K, van Eck CF, Hoshino Y, et al. Anatomic single- and double-bundle anterior cruciate ligament reconstruction, part 1: basic science. Am J Sports Med 2011;39(8):1789–99.
8. Fu FH, Shen W, Starman JS, et al. Primary anatomic double-bundle anterior cruciate ligament reconstruction: a preliminary 2-year prospective study. Am J Sports Med 2008;36(7):1263–74.
9. Siebold R, Dehler C, Ellert T. Prospective randomized comparison of double-bundle versus single-bundle anterior cruciate ligament reconstruction. Arthroscopy 2008;24:137–45.
10. Audigé L, Ayeni OR, Bhandari M, et al. A practical guide to research: design, execution, and publication [erratum in Arthroscopy 2011;27(6):878]. Arthroscopy 2011;27(Suppl 4):S1–112.
11. Sackett D, Rosenberg W, Gray J, et al. Evidence-based medicine: what it is and what it isn't. BMJ 1996;312:71–2.
12. Watts G. Let's pension off the "major breakthrough." BMJ 2007;334:4.
13. Benjaminse A, Gokeler A, van der Schans CP. Clinical diagnosis of an anterior cruciate ligament rupture: a meta-analysis. J Orthop Sports Phys Ther 2006;36:267–88.
14. Kocher MS, Steadman JR, Briggs KK, et al. Determinants of patient satisfaction with outcome after anterior cruciate ligament reconstruction. J Bone Joint Surg 2002;84(9):1560–72.
15. Leitze Z, Losee RE, Jokl P, et al. Implications of the pivot shift in the ACL: deficient knee. Clin Orthop Relat Res 2005;436:229–36.
16. Kocher MS, Steadman JR, Briggs KK, et al. Relationships between objective assessment of ligament stability and subjective assessment of symptoms and function after anterior cruciate ligament reconstruction. Am J Sports Med 2004; 32:629–34.
17. Jonsson H, Riklund-Ahlström K, Lind J. Positive pivot shift after ACL reconstruction predicts later osteoarthrosis: 63 patients followed 5–9 years after surgery. Acta Orthop Scand 2004;75:594–9.
18. Musahl V, Hoshino Y, Ahlden M, et al. The pivot shift: a global user guide. Knee Surg Sports Traumatol Arthrosc 2012;20(4):724–31.
19. Ayeni OR, Chahal M, Tran MN, et al. Pivot shift as an outcome measure for ACL reconstruction: a systematic review. Knee Surg Sports Traumatol Arthrosc 2012; 20(4):767–77.

20. Hoshino Y, Araujo P, Ahlden M, et al. Standardized pivot shift test improves measurement accuracy. Knee Surg Sports Traumatol Arthrosc 2011;20(4): 732–6.
21. Araujo PH, Ahlden M, Hoshino Y, et al. Comparison of three non-invasive quantitative measurement systems for the pivot shift test. Knee Surg Sports Traumatol Arthrosc 2012;20(4):692–7.
22. Ahldén M, Hoshino Y, Samuelsson K, et al. Dynamic knee laxity measurement devices. Knee Surg Sports Traumatol Arthrosc 2011;20(4):621–32.
23. Van Dyck P, Vanhoenacker FM, Gielen JL, et al. Three tesla magnetic resonance imaging of the anterior cruciate ligament of the knee: can we differentiate complete from partial tears? Skeletal Radiol 2011;40(6):701–7.
24. Sampson MJ, Jackson MP, Moran CJ, et al. Three tesla MRI for the diagnosis of meniscal and anterior cruciate ligament pathology: a comparison to arthroscopic findings. Clin Radiol 2008;63:1106–11.
25. Panesar SS, Philippon MJ, Bhandari M. Principles of evidence-based medicine. Orthop Clin North Am 2010;41(2):131–8.
26. Devereaux PJ, Bhandari M, Clarke M, et al. Need for expertise based randomised controlled trials. BMJ 2005;330(7482):88.
27. Prystowsky JB, Bordage G, Feinglass JM. Patient outcomes for segmental colon resection according to surgeon's training, certification, and experience. Surgery 2002;132:663–70.
28. Bridgewater B, Grayson AD, Au J, et al. Improving mortality of coronary surgery over first four years of independent practice: retrospective examination of prospectively collected data from 15 surgeons. BMJ 2004;329:421.
29. Marx RG, Ghomrawi H, Do H, et al. "Practice makes perfect" in ACL reconstruction. Presented at the AAOS Sessions, The 2012 American Academy of Orthopaedic Surgeons/Orthopaedic Research Society Annual Meeting. San Francisco, February 7, 2012.
30. Freedman KB, D'Amato MJ, Nedeff DD, et al. Arthroscopic anterior cruciate ligament reconstruction: a meta-analysis comparing patellar tendon and hamstring tendon autografts. Am J Sports Med 2003;31(1):2–11.
31. Mohtadi NG, Chan DS, Dainty KN, et al. Patellar tendon versus hamstring tendon autograft for anterior cruciate ligament rupture in adults. Cochrane Database Syst Rev 2011;(9):CD005960.
32. Poolman RW, Abouali JA, Conter HJ, et al. Overlapping systematic reviews of anterior cruciate ligament reconstruction comparing hamstring autograft with bone-patellar tendon-bone autograft: why are they different? J Bone Joint Surg Am 2007;89(7):1542–52.
33. Kopf S, Forsythe B, Wong AK, et al. Nonanatomic tunnel position in traditional transtibial single-bundle anterior cruciate ligament reconstruction evaluated by three-dimensional computed tomography. J Bone Joint Surg Am 2010;92(6): 1427–31.
34. Forsythe B, Kopf S, Wong AK, et al. The location of femoral and tibial tunnels in anatomic double-bundle anterior cruciate ligament reconstruction analyzed by three-dimensional computed tomography models. J Bone Joint Surg Am 2010; 92(6):1418–26.
35. Lubowitz JH. Anteromedial portal technique for the anterior cruciate ligament femoral socket: pitfalls and solutions. Arthroscopy 2009;25(1):95–101.
36. Bedi A, Raphael B, Maderazo A, et al. Transtibial versus anteromedial portal drilling for anterior cruciate ligament reconstruction: a cadaveric study of femoral tunnel length and obliquity. Arthroscopy 2010;26(3):342–50.

37. Hensler D, Working ZM, Illingworth KD, et al. Medial portal drilling: effects on the femoral tunnel aperture morphology during anterior cruciate ligament reconstruction. J Bone Joint Surg Am 2011;93(22):2063–71.

38. Ferretti M, Ekdahl M, Shen W, et al. Osseous landmarks of the femoral attachment of the anterior cruciate ligament: an anatomic study. Arthroscopy 2007;23: 1218–25.

39. Araujo PH, van Eck CF, Macalena JA, et al. Advances in the three-portal technique for anatomical single- or double-bundle ACL reconstruction. Knee Surg Sports Traumatol Arthrosc 2011;19(8):1239–42.

40. Wright RW, Preston E, Fleming BC, et al. A systematic review of anterior cruciate ligament reconstruction rehabilitation: part I: continuous passive motion, early weight bearing, postoperative bracing, and home-based rehabilitation. J Knee Surg 2008;21(3):217–24.

41. Li RT, Lorenz S, Xu Y, et al. Predictors of radiographic knee osteoarthritis after anterior cruciate ligament reconstruction. Am J Sports Med 2011;39:2595.

42. Wright RW, Fetzer GB. Bracing after ACL reconstruction: a systematic review. Clin Orthop 2007;455:162–8.

43. Ekstrand J. Six versus eight months of rehabilitation after reconstruction of the anterior cruciate ligament: a prospective randomized study on soccer players. Science and Football 1990;3:31–6.

44. Beynnon BD, Johnson RJ, Naud S, et al. Accelerated versus nonaccelerated rehabilitation after anterior cruciate ligament reconstruction: a prospective, randomized, double-blind investigation evaluating knee joint laxity using roentgen stereophotogrammetric analysis. Am J Sports Med 2011;39(12):2536–48.

45. van Grinsven S, van Cingel RE, Holla CJ, et al. Evidence-based rehabilitation following anterior cruciate ligament reconstruction. Knee Surg Sports Traumatol Arthrosc 2010;18(8):1128–44.

46. Irrgang JJ, Bost JE, Fu FH. Re: outcome of single-bundle versus double-bundle reconstruction of the anterior cruciate ligament: a meta-analysis. Am J Sports Med 2009;37(2):421–2.

47. Mohtadi N. Development and validation of the quality of life outcome measure (questionnaire) for chronic anterior cruciate ligament deficiency. Am J Sports Med 1998;26(3):350–9.

48. Tanner SM, Dainty KN, Marx RG, et al. Knee-specific quality-of-life instruments: which ones measure symptoms and disabilities most important to patients? Am J Sports Med 2007;35(9):1450–8.

49. Aït Si Selmi T, Fithian D, Neyret P. The evolution of osteoarthritis in 103 patients with ACL reconstruction at 17 years follow-up. Knee 2006;13:353–8.

50. Lohmander LS, Ostenberg A, Englund M, et al. High prevalence of knee osteoarthritis, pain, and functional limitations in female soccer players twelve years after anterior cruciate ligament injury. Arthritis Rheum 2004;50(10):3145–52.

51. Hussein M, van Eck CF, Cretnik A, et al. Prospective randomized clinical evaluation of conventional single-bundle, anatomic single-bundle, and anatomic double-bundle anterior cruciate ligament reconstruction: 281 cases with 3- to 5-year follow-up. Am J Sports Med 2011;40(3):512–20.

Double-Bundle Versus Single-Bundle Anterior Cruciate Ligament Reconstruction

Timo Järvelä, MD, PhD[a,b,]*, Sally Järvelä, MD, PhD[c]

KEYWORDS

- Anterior cruciate ligament reconstruction • ACL • Reconstruction • Double-bundle
- Single-bundle

KEY POINTS

- Anatomic and biomechanical studies have shown that the anterior cruciate ligament (ACL) mainly consists of 2 distinct bundles, the anteromedial (AM) bundle and the posterolateral (PL) bundle, which act separately during the knee's range of motion.
- Conventional ACL reconstruction techniques have focused on restoration of the AM bundle only, while giving limited attention to the PL bundle.
- In recent years, following the desire to better replicate ACL anatomy and its 2 bundles, many orthopedic surgeons developed double-bundle ACL reconstruction techniques.

INTRODUCTION

Anatomic and biomechanical studies have shown that the anterior cruciate ligament (ACL) mainly consists of 2 distinct bundles, the anteromedial (AM) bundle and the posterolateral (PL) bundle, which act separately during the knee's range of motion.[1–7] Conventional ACL reconstruction techniques have focused on restoration of the AM bundle only, while giving limited attention to the PL bundle. The outcomes of these single-bundle techniques have been relatively good in ACL reconstructive surgery. In recent years, following the desire to better replicate ACL anatomy and its 2 bundles, many orthopedic surgeons developed double-bundle ACL reconstruction techniques.

The purpose of this review was to analyze the clinical results of the double-bundle versus single-bundle ACL reconstruction according to the current literature. The main focus in reviewing these clinical studies is on the randomized controlled trials.

a Sports Clinic, Hospital Mehiläinen, Itäinenkatu 3, FIN-33210 Tampere, Finland; b Tampere University, Teiskontie 35, Tampere 33210, Finland; c Department of Orthopaedics and Traumatology, Tampere University Hospital, Teiskontie 35, Tampere 33210, Finland
* Corresponding author. Sports Clinic, Hospital Mehiläinen, Itäinenkatu 3, FIN-33210 Tampere, Finland.
E-mail address: timo.jarvela@sci.fi

Clin Sports Med 32 (2013) 81–91
http://dx.doi.org/10.1016/j.csm.2012.08.009
0278-5919/13/$ – see front matter © 2013 Elsevier Inc. All rights reserved.

RANDOMIZED CONTROLLED TRIALS

The first prospective, randomized study comparing single-bundle and double-bundle techniques in ACL reconstruction was published by Adachi and colleagues[8] in 2004; however, the investigators used only 1 tunnel on the tibial side and 2 tunnels on the femoral side, so the double-bundle technique used in their study was not an anatomic double-bundle ACL reconstruction. They did not find any significant differences concerning knee stability, knee scores, and subjective evaluations between their single-bundle and double-bundle groups at an average of 32-months of follow-up.

Aglietti and colleagues[9] randomized 75 patients into 3 groups of ACL reconstruction: a single-bundle technique, a double-bundle with transtibial technique, and a double-bundle with a double-incision technique. They found significantly better rotational and anterior stability at the 2-year follow-up using the double-bundle with double-incision technique compared with the transtibial double-bundle or single-bundle techniques.

In the other prospective, randomized study of Aglietti and colleagues[10] published in 2010, they compared single-bundle and double-bundle ACL reconstruction with a double-incision technique in both groups with 70 patients. At a minimum of 2-year follow-up, the double-bundle group had significantly better visual analog scale for pain, anterior knee stability, and knee scores than the single-bundle group.

Järvelä[11] compared his anatomic double-bundle technique with hamstring grafts and bioabsorbable screw fixation with his single-bundle ACL reconstruction using similar fixation and graft material in a prospective, randomized study of 65 patients (**Figs. 1** and **2**). The anteromedial portal and freehand technique were used in both groups to create the femoral tunnels as anatomically as possible. At a minimum of 1-year follow-up, the rotational stability, as evaluated by the pivot shift, was significantly better in the double-bundle group than in the single-bundle group. However, the anterior stability and the International Knee Documentation Committee (IKDC) and Lysholm knee scores were equally good in both groups.

In another prospective, randomized study of Järvelä and colleagues,[12] 77 patients were divided into 3 groups: single-bundle with metallic screw fixation, single-bundle with bioabsorbable screw fixation, and double-bundle with bioabsorbable screw fixation. At a minimum of 2-year follow-up, the rotational stability was best in the double-bundle group. In addition, the patients in the single-bundle groups had 6 graft failures leading to revision ACL surgery, whereas only 1 patient in the double-bundle group had a graft failure. These differences were significant.

In the third prospective, randomized study of Järvelä and colleagues,[13] 60 patients were divided into either double-bundle or single-bundle ACL reconstruction using

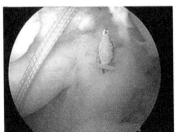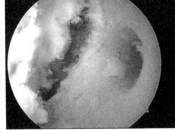

Fig. 1. Arthroscopic view of the left knee showing tunnel placements of the single-bundle ACL reconstruction on the tibial side (*left*) and on the femoral side (*right*).

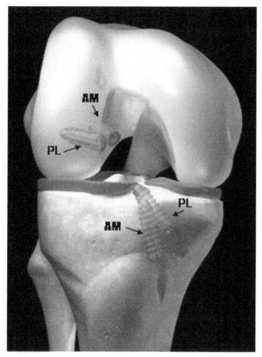

Fig. 2. Schematic view of the right knee showing the tunnel and screw placements of the double-bundle ACL reconstruction.

hamstring autografts and bioabsorbable screw fixation in both groups. At the minimum of 2-year follow-up, the double-bundle group had significantly less tunnel enlargement in the tibial side evaluated by magnetic resonance imaging (MRI) than the single-bundle group; however, there were no differences in the stability evaluations or the IKDC and Lysholm knee scores between the groups.

Yagi and colleagues[14] randomized 60 patients into 3 groups: an anteromedial bundle reconstruction group, a posterolateral bundle reconstruction group, and a double-bundle reconstruction group. All the patients were examined 1 year after surgery. Anterior stability and the IKDC knee scores were equal in each group; however, rotational stability, as evaluated by the pivot shift and by 3-dimensional electromagnetic sensors, was best in the double-bundle group.

Muneta and colleagues[15] randomized 68 patients into double-bundle or single-bundle ACL reconstruction groups. At the 2-year follow-up, the double-bundle group had significantly better rotational and anterior stability than the single-bundle group, although no differences were found in the subjective knee scores.

Streich and colleagues[16] randomized 50 male athletes into anatomic double-bundle or anatomic single-bundle (low femoral tunnel) ACL reconstruction. At the 2-year follow-up, no significant differences were found between the groups concerning rotational and anterior stability of the knee. Also, the objective and subjective knee scores were equal in both groups. The investigators concluded that ACL reconstruction with a single-bundle technique and more horizontal femoral tunnel placement obtained comparable clinical results than those with a double-bundle technique in high-demand athletes.

Siebold and colleagues[17] randomized 70 patients into double-bundle or single-bundle ACL reconstruction. At an average of 19 months of follow-up, the double-bundle group had significantly better rotational and anterior stability than the single-bundle group. Also, the objective IKDC score was significantly better in the double-bundle group, although no differences were found in the subjective knee scores.

Sastre and colleagues[18] randomized 40 patients into double-bundle or single-bundle ACL reconstruction with an anatomic low femoral tunnel position in both techniques. At the 2-year follow-up, no differences were found between the groups in anterior or rotational stability or in the IKDC knee scores.

Zaffagnini and colleagues[19] randomized 100 patients into double-bundle or single-bundle ACL reconstruction with extra-articular augmentation on the lateral side of the knee. Seventy-two patients were available for 3-year follow-up. The double-bundle group showed significantly better results in terms of subjective, objective, and functional evaluations of the knee. Also, anterior stability was significantly better in the double-bundle group compared with the single-bundle group.

Zaffagnini and colleagues[20] have published another prospective randomized study. In that study, 79 patients were evaluated with a minimum of 8-year follow-up; however, the double-bundle technique they used was nonanatomic with only one tunnel on the femoral and tibial side combined with one "over-the-top" passage of the graft. The investigators concluded that although both the single-bundle and the nonanatomic double-bundle techniques provided satisfactory results, the nonanatomic double-bundle reconstruction showed significantly better functional results with a faster return to sports activity, a lower reoperation rate, and lower degenerative knee changes determined radiographically than the single-bundle technique.

Wang and colleagues[21] randomized 64 patients into double-bundle or single-bundle ACL reconstruction using hamstring grafts and cortical fixation on the femoral side. At the 10-month follow-up, no differences were found between the groups in anterior or rotational stability or in the IKDC knee scores.

Ibrahim and colleagues[22] randomized 218 patients with unilateral ACL deficiency into 4 groups: one group was performed with an anatomic double-bundle technique and the 3 other groups with single-bundle techniques using different fixation methods in each group on the femoral side (Endobutton [Smith & Nephew, USA], RigidFix [DePuy Mitek, USA], TransFix [Arthrex, USA]). For tibial fixation, a bioabsorbable screw fixation was used in all patients. Also, hamstring autografts were used in all patients. At a mean of 29-month follow-up, the double-bundle method showed significantly better rotational and anterior stability, as evaluated by the pivot shift test and by KT-1000 (San Diego, CA, USA), measurements, compared with the single-bundle methods. However, no differences were found in the IKDC knee scores between the groups.

Suomalainen and colleagues[23] compared the double-bundle technique with hamstring autografts and aperture screw fixation with single-bundle ACL reconstruction using similar fixation and graft material in a prospective, randomized study of 153 patients. At a minimum of 2-year follow-up, the revision rate was significantly lower with the double-bundle technique than that with the single-bundle technique (7 revision ACL reconstructions in the single-bundle group, and 1 revision in the double-bundle group). In addition, 7 patients (5 in the single-bundle group and 2 in the double-bundle group) had an invisible graft on the MRI assessment at the 2-year follow-up; however, no differences were found in the IKDC or Lysholm knee scores between the groups. Also, the stability evaluations did not show any significant differences between these 2 techniques at the follow-up.

Araki and colleagues[24] randomized 20 patients into anatomic single-bundle or double-bundle ACL reconstruction. At the 1-year follow-up, there were no significant differences between the groups in the clinical stability evaluations or Lysholm knee scores. According to the 6-degrees-of-freedom of knee kinematic measurement system using an electromagnetic device, however, the double-bundle technique tended to have biomechanically better results than the anatomic single-bundle technique.

Fujita and colleagues[25] randomized 55 patients into 3 groups of ACL reconstruction: an anteromedial bundle reconstruction, a posterolateral bundle reconstruction, and a double-bundle reconstruction. At the minimum of 2-year follow-up, the patients undergoing double-bundle ACL reconstruction had significantly better anterior stability than the patients having a single-bundle posterolateral reconstruction, whereas in the pivot shift test, the posterolateral reconstruction group had fewer negative results than the double-bundle reconstruction group; however, the anteromedial bundle reconstruction group (conventional single-bundle reconstruction) had results similar to the double-bundle reconstruction group concerning both the anterior and rotatory stability of the knee. The investigators concluded that, overall, the clinical outcome, as measured by Lysholm and Tegner scores, was not different among the groups.

Hussein and colleagues[26] randomized 281 patients into 3 groups of ACL reconstruction: a conventional single-bundle group, an anatomic single-bundle group, and an anatomic double-bundle ACL reconstruction group. At 3-year to 5-year follow-up, the anatomic double-bundle technique resulted in significantly better anterior stability measured by KT-1000 arthrometer, and significantly better rotational stability as evaluated by pivot shift test than the conventional and anatomic single-bundle techniques. Also, the Lysholm knee score was significantly better with the anatomic double-bundle technique than with the conventional single-bundle technique. The investigators concluded that the anatomic double-bundle ACL reconstruction was significantly superior to conventional single-bundle ACL reconstruction and better than anatomic single-bundle reconstruction, although the differences were small and might not be clinically relevant.

Lee and colleagues[27] randomized 42 patients into single-bundle or double-bundle ACL reconstruction. They used a navigation system to measure anterior and rotatory laxity of the knee before and after the fixation of the graft during reconstruction, and found that the double-bundle ACL reconstruction improved rotatory laxity significantly better than the single-bundle technique. However, at the 2-year follow-up, there was no group-difference in functional outcome.

All of the randomized, controlled trials comparing double-bundle and single-bundle ACL reconstruction are summarized in **Table 1**.

PREVIOUS SYSTEMATIC REVIEWS

In 2008, Meredick and colleagues[28] published a meta-analysis of randomized controlled trials comparing single-bundle versus double-bundle ACL reconstruction. According to their meta-analysis of the 4 level I studies published in the literature, double-bundle reconstruction did not result in clinically significant differences in KT-1000 measurements for anterior stability or in pivot-shift testing for rotational stability. They concluded that the results do not support the theory that double-bundle reconstruction better controls knee rotation; however, the investigators grouped "normal" and "nearly normal" outcome together, which was criticized and discussed later in the literature.[29]

Yasuda and colleagues[30] published a current concepts review of the anatomic double-bundle ACL reconstruction. They reported the results of 10 prospective, randomized studies comparing single-bundle and double-bundle ACL reconstruction.

Table 1
Randomized controlled trials comparing double-bundle (DB) and single-bundle (SB) anterior cruciate ligament reconstruction

Authors	Year Published	Number of Patients	Follow-up Time	Results
Adachi et al[8]	2004	108	32 mo	No difference
Aglietti et al[9]	2007	75	2 y	Better rotational and anterior stability in DB-group
Aglietti et al[10]	2010	70	2 y	Better anterior stability and subjective and objective knee scores in DB-group
Järvelä[11]	2007	65	14 mo	Better rotational stability in DB-group
Järvelä et al[12]	2008	77	2 y	Better rotational stability and fewer graft failures in DB group
Järvelä et al[13]	2008	60	2 y	Less tunnel enlargement in DB group
Yagi et al[14]	2007	60	1 y	Better rotational stability in DB group
Muneta et al[15]	2007	68	2 y	Better rotational and anterior stability in DB group
Streich et al[16]	2008	50	2 y	No difference
Siebold et al[17]	2008	70	19 mo	Better rotational and anterior stability and objective knee scores in DB group
Sastre et al[18]	2010	40	2 y	No difference
Zaffagnini et al[19]	2008	100	3 y	Better anterior stability and objective and subjective knee scores in DB group
Zaffagnini et al[20]	2010	79	8 y	Better functional scores and fewer graft failures and less degenerative changes in DB group
Wang et al[21]	2009	64	10 mo	No difference
Ibrahim et al[22]	2009	218	29 mo	Better rotational and anterior stability in DB group
Suomalainen et al[23]	2011	153	2 y	Fewer graft failures in DB group
Araki et al[24]	2011	20	1 y	No difference
Fujita et al[25]	2011	55	2 y	No difference
Hussein et al[26]	2011	281	51 mo	Better rotational and anterior stability in DB group
Lee et al[27]	2012	42	2 y	Better rotational stability in DB group

In 8 of the 10 studies, the anterior and/or rotational stability of the knee was significantly better with the anatomic double-bundle ACL reconstruction than with the conventional single-bundle reconstruction; however, many controversies concerning the surgical techniques remain in the field of anatomic double-bundle ACL reconstruction. There were many differences in procedures for creating anatomic tunnels, graft preparation, tensioning, and fixation among the clinical trials included in the review.

Yasuda and colleagues[30] concluded that the utility of the anatomic double-bundle reconstruction has not yet been established.

Boyer and Meislin[31] published a review of double-bundle versus single-bundle ACL reconstruction in 2010. They included both retrospective nonrandomized studies and prospective randomized studies comparing double-bundle and single-bundle ACL reconstruction. They criticized a large variability of the methodology of these studies. Also, several different surgical techniques were represented, which made pooling the data difficult. They concluded that there is a need for more standardization of measuring parameters and the future application of advanced technologies that would inform more correct models how to improve the techniques of ACL reconstruction.

Järvelä and Suomalainen[32] published a review comparing the clinical results between double-bundle and single-bundle ACL reconstruction. They reported 14 randomized controlled trials found from the literature comparing the clinical results of these 2 techniques. According to their review, 4 trials (29%) did not find any significant differences in the results between double-bundle and single-bundle ACL reconstruction. Ten trials (71%) reported significantly better results with the double-bundle technique than with the single-bundle technique, of which 7 reported better rotational stability, 6 reported better anterior stability, 3 reported better objective knee scores, 3 reported better subjective knee scores, 2 reported fewer graft failures, and 1 reported fewer degenerative changes of the knee. In addition, none of the trials found the single-bundle technique to have better results in any of these evaluations than the double-bundle technique; however, 13 of the 14 trials had only a short-term follow-up (1–3 years), and only 1 trial had a long-term follow-up (8–10 years). They concluded that only through long-term follow-up studies will we be able to determine whether the double-bundle reconstruction is really better than the single-bundle technique.

Longo and colleagues[33] published a systematic review comparing single-bundle and double-bundle ACL reconstruction. They found that double-bundle ACL reconstruction could provide better outcome for patients in terms of closer restoration of normal knee biomechanics and improving the rotatory laxity of the knee; however, they did not recommend the systematic use of double-bundle ACL reconstruction for patients, because even though biomechanical results are encouraging, subjective patient evaluation is similar for single-bundle and double-bundle ACL reconstruction. They concluded that with the current evidence available, a simple single-bundle ACL reconstruction is a suitable technique, and it should not be abandoned until stronger scientific evidence in favor of double-bundle ACL reconstruction is produced.

Kongtharvonskul and colleagues[34] published a systematic review of randomized controlled trials comparing clinical outcomes of double-bundle versus single-bundle ACL reconstruction. They included 13 studies in their review. They reported that the double-bundle technique was approximately 4 times more likely to show a normal pivot shift than the single-bundle technique. Also, the IKDC grading was 2 times better with the double-bundle technique. They concluded that the double-bundle ACL reconstruction may be better than the single-bundle technique in rotational stability but not for function, translation, and complications.

DISCUSSION

According to the 20 prospective, randomized studies found from the English literature and included into this review, 6 studies (30%) did not find any significant differences in the clinical results between double-bundle and single-bundle ACL reconstructions; however, 14 studies (70%) reported significantly better results with the double-bundle technique than with the single-bundle technique. Nine of these trials reported better rotational stability, 7 trials noted better anterior-posterior stability, 3 trials showed better objective knee scores, 3 trials had better subjective knee scores, 3 trials had fewer graft failures, 1 trial had less tunnel enlargement, and 1 trial was found to have fewer degenerative changes in the knee joint with the double-bundle technique compared with the single-bundle technique. In addition, none of the studies found that the single-bundle technique had better results in any of these evaluations than the double-bundle technique.

Although the current scoring systems may not be very sensitive in finding differences between double-bundle and single-bundle techniques, and there is a large variation between the techniques and terminology used in the ACL double-bundle surgery (nonanatomic vs anatomic), it appears that the double-bundle ACL reconstruction is either equal to or significantly better than the single-bundle ACL reconstruction.

There are some risks associated with the double-bundle technique, however. Because there are more tunnels to be created, and more grafts to be fixed, the double-bundle technique provides more opportunity to have some technical difficulties or failures during the operation than the traditional single-bundle technique. The double-bundle ACL reconstruction can be a very demanding procedure with increased costs associated with a need for more fixation material, grafts, and a longer operation time, as well as potential complications related to the steep learning curve for the surgeon. That is why the double-bundle technique is not recommended for every ACL surgeon but only for the hands of the most experienced ACL surgeons.

Also, the size of the knee is important when making the decision as to whether to use the double-bundle or single-bundle technique in ACL reconstruction. If the knee is very small, there is no room to perform a good double-bundle ACL reconstruction. Then, it is better to make an anatomic single-bundle ACL reconstruction. In addition, if the hamstring autografts, especially the gracilis tendon graft, are very thin, and allograft is not available, it is better to make 1 good graft than 2 very thin grafts. The minimum diameter for the PL-bundle graft should be 5 to 6 mm, and for the AM-bundle 6 to 7 mm, respectively.

The activity level of the patient may have some importance in deciding which technique to use in ACL reconstruction. Patients with a high activity level may have some benefit from the double-bundle ACL reconstruction, because almost half of the prospective randomized studies included in this review reported that the double-bundle technique resulted in significantly better stability of the knee than the single-bundle technique. Especially athletes who perform demanding pivoting sports (eg, ball games, skiing, gymnastics) could have a more stable knee with the double-bundle technique compared with the single-bundle technique.

Also, the injury model of the knee plays a role in the decision of which technique to use. Musahl and colleagues[35] showed in their cadaveric study that the double-bundle

| Table 2 |
| Suggested indications for anatomic single-bundle versus double-bundle ACL reconstruction |

Single-bundle ACL Reconstruction	Double-bundle ACL Reconstruction
Small knee (not room for the DB technique)	Large enough knee
Thin hamstring tendons	Good quality of the hamstring tendons
Nonathlete or	High-level athlete
Recreational athlete	Pivoting sports
Isolated ACL injury	ACL injury combined with meniscal injury

ACL reconstruction was able to restore intact knee kinematics during the pivot shift testing significantly better than the anatomic single-bundle or nonanatomic single-bundle technique in the setting of ACL injury and concomitant medial and lateral meniscus deficiency.

SUMMARY

According to this systematic review of prospective, randomized studies comparing double-bundle and single-bundle ACL reconstruction, 6 studies (30%) did not find any significant differences in the clinical results between these techniques. However, 14 studies (70%) reported significantly better results with the double-bundle technique than with the single-bundle technique. In addition, none of the studies showed the single-bundle technique to have better results than the double-bundle technique. However, double-bundle surgery may not yet be a standard procedure for every surgeon or for every patient until stronger scientific evidence with longer follow-ups in favor of double-bundle ACL reconstruction is produced. The suggested indications for the anatomic double-bundle and single-bundle ACL reconstruction are presented in **Table 2**.

REFERENCES

1. Palmer I. On the injuries to the ligaments of the knee joint. Acta Chir Scand 1938; 91:282.
2. Girgis FG, Marshall JL, Monajem A. The cruciate ligaments of the knee joint. Anatomical, functional, and experimental analysis. Clin Orthop 1975;106:216–31.
3. Ferretti M, Levicoff EA, Macpherson TA, et al. The fetal anterior cruciate ligament: an anatomic and histologic study. Arthroscopy 2007;23:278–83.
4. Amis AA, Dawkins GP. Functional anatomy of the anterior cruciate ligament. Fiber bundle actions related to ligament replacements and injuries. J Bone Joint Surg Br 1991;73:260–7.
5. Ishibashi Y, Tsuda E, Fukuda A, et al. Stability evaluation of single-bundle and double-bundle reconstruction during navigated ACL reconstruction. Sports Med Arthrosc 2008;16:77–83.
6. Ishibashi Y, Tsuda E, Yamamoto Y, et al. Navigation evaluation of the pivot-shift phenomenon during double-bundle anterior cruciate ligament reconstruction: is the posterolateral bundle more important? Arthroscopy 2009;25:488–95.
7. Wu J, Seon J, Gadikota H, et al. In situ forces in the anteromedial and posterolateral bundles of the anterior cruciate ligament under simulated functional loading conditions. Am J Sports Med 2010;38:558–63.
8. Adachi N, Ochi M, Uchio Y, et al. Reconstruction of the anterior cruciate ligament: single- versus double-bundle multistranded hamstring tendons. J Bone Joint Surg Br 2004;86:515–20.
9. Aglietti P, Giron F, Cuomo P, et al. Single- and double-incision double-bundle ACL reconstruction. Clin Orthop Relat Res 2007;454:108–13.
10. Aglietti P, Giron F, Losco M, et al. Comparison between single-and double-bundle anterior cruciate ligament reconstruction: a prospective, randomized, single-blinded clinical trial. Am J Sports Med 2010;38(1):25–34.
11. Järvelä T. Double-bundle versus single-bundle anterior cruciate ligament reconstruction: a prospective, randomized clinical study. Knee Surg Sports Traumatol Arthrosc 2007;15:500–7.
12. Järvelä T, Moisala AS, Sihvonen R, et al. Double-bundle anterior cruciate ligament reconstruction using hamstring autografts and bioabsorbable interference screw

fixation: prospective, randomized, clinical study with 2-year results. Am J Sports Med 2008;36:290–7.

13. Järvelä T, Moisala AS, Paakkala T, et al. Tunnel enlargement after double-bundle anterior cruciate ligament reconstruction: a prospective, randomized study. Arthroscopy 2008;24:1349–57.

14. Yagi M, Kuroda R, Nagamune K, et al. Double-bundle ACL reconstruction can improve rotational stability. Clin Orthop Relat Res 2007;454:100–7.

15. Muneta T, Koga H, Mochizuki T, et al. A prospective randomized study of 4-strand semitendinosus tendon anterior cruciate ligament reconstruction comparing single-bundle and double-bundle techniques. Arthroscopy 2007;23: 618–28.

16. Streich NA, Friedrich K, Gotterbarm T, et al. Reconstruction of the ACL with a semitendinosus tendon graft: a prospective randomized single blinded comparison of double-bundle versus single-bundle technique in male athletes. Knee Surg Sports Traumatol Arthrosc 2008;16:232–8.

17. Siebold R, Dehler C, Ellert T. Prospective randomized comparison of double-bundle versus single-bundle anterior cruciate ligament reconstruction. Arthroscopy 2008;24:137–45.

18. Sastre S, Popescu D, Nunez M, et al. Double-bundle versus single-bundle ACL reconstruction using the horizontal femoral position: a prospective, randomized study. Knee Surg Sports Traumatol Arthrosc 2010;18:32–6.

19. Zaffagnini S, Bruni D, Russo A, et al. ST/G ACL reconstruction: double strand plus extra-articular sling vs double bundle, randomized study at 3-year follow-up. Scand J Med Sci Sports 2008;18:573–81.

20. Zaffagnini S, Bruni D, Marcheggiani Muccioli GM, et al. Single-bundle patellar tendon versus non-anatomical double-bundle hamstrings ACL reconstruction: a prospective randomized study at 8-year minimum follow-up. Knee Surg Sports Traumatol Arthrosc 2011;19:740–6.

21. Wang JQ, Ao YF, Yu CL, et al. Clinical evaluation of double-bundle anterior cruciate ligament reconstruction procedure using hamstring tendon grafts: a prospective, randomized and controlled study. Chin Med J (Engl) 2009;122: 706–11.

22. Ibrahim SA, Hamido F, Al Misfer AK, et al. Anterior cruciate ligament reconstruction using autologous hamstring double bundle graft compared with single bundle procedures. J Bone Joint Surg Br 2009;91:1310–5.

23. Suomalainen P, Moisala AS, Paakkala A, et al. Double-bundle versus single-bundle anterior cruciate ligament reconstruction: randomized clinical and magnetic resonance imaging study with 2-year follow-up. Am J Sports Med 2011;39:1615–22.

24. Araki D, Kuroda R, Kubo S, et al. A prospective randomized study of anatomical single-bundle versus double-bundle anterior cruciate ligament reconstruction: quantitative evaluation using an electromagnetic measurement system. Int Orthop 2011;35:439–46.

25. Fujita N, Kuroda R, Matsumoto T, et al. Comparison of the clinical outcome of double-bundle, anteromedial single-bundle, and posterolateral single-bundle anterior cruciate ligament reconstruction using hamstring tendon graft with minimum 2-year follow-up. Arthroscopy 2011;27:906–13.

26. Hussein M, van Eck CF, Cretnik A, et al. Prospective randomized clinical evaluation of conventional single-bundle, anatomic single-bundle, and anatomic double-bundle anterior cruciate ligament reconstruction: 281 cases with 3- to 5-year follow-up. Am J Sports Med 2012;40(3):512–20.

27. Lee S, Kim H, Jang J, et al. Comparison of anterior and rotatory laxity using navigation between single- and double-bundle ACL reconstruction: prospective randomized trial. Knee Surg Sports Traumatol Arthrosc 2012;20(4):752–61.
28. Meredick RB, Vance KJ, Appleby D, et al. Outcome of single-bundle versus double-bundle reconstruction of the anterior cruciate ligament: a meta-analysis. Am J Sports Med 2008;36:1414–21.
29. Irrgang JJ, Bost JE, Fu FH. Re: outcome of single-bundle versus double-bundle reconstruction of the anterior cruciate ligament: a meta-analysis. Am J Sports Med 2009;37:421–2.
30. Yasuda K, Tanabe Y, Kondo E, et al. Anatomic double-bundle anterior cruciate ligament reconstruction. Arthroscopy 2010;26(Suppl 9):S21–34.
31. Boyer J, Meislin RJ. Double-bundle versus single-bundle ACL reconstruction. Bull NYU Hosp Jt Dis 2010;68:119–26.
32. Järvelä T, Suomalainen P. ACL reconstruction with double-bundle technique: a review of clinical results. Phys Sportsmed 2011;39:85–92.
33. Longo UG, Buchmann S, Franceschetti E, et al. A systematic review of single-bundle versus double-bundle anterior cruciate ligament reconstruction. Br Med Bull 2012;103:147–68.
34. Kongtharvonskul J, Attia J, Thamakalson S, et al. Clinical outcomes of double- vs single-bundle anterior cruciate ligament reconstruction: a systematic review of randomized control trials. Scand J Med Sci Sports 2012. http://dx.doi.org/10.1111/j.1600–0838.2011.01439.x.
35. Musahl V, Bedi A, Citak M, et al. Effect of single-bundle and double-bundle anterior cruciate ligament reconstructions on pivot-shift kinematics in anterior cruciate ligament- and meniscus-deficient knees. Am J Sports Med 2011;39:289–95.

ACL Graft Healing and Biologics

Bart Muller, MD[a,b], Karl F. Bowman Jr, MD[a], Asheesh Bedi, MD[c,*]

KEYWORDS

• Tendon-bone healing • Autograft • Allograft • Cytokine • ACL reconstruction

KEY POINTS

• Operative reconstruction of a torn anterior cruciate ligament (ACL) has become the most broadly accepted treatment, aiming to restore native anatomy and a complete return to functional demands.
• Although the reported success rates of ACL reconstruction vary between 69% and 95%, return to previous activity level has recently been reported to be less than 50%.
• The mechanism of graft failure is multifactorial in nature and may be attributed to either traumatic or nontraumatic causes.

INTRODUCTION

Operative reconstruction of a torn anterior cruciate ligament (ACL) has become the most broadly accepted treatment, aiming to restore native anatomy and a complete return to functional demands.[1] Although the reported success rates of ACL reconstruction vary between 69% and 95%, return to previous activity level has recently been reported to be less than 50%.[1–6] In addition, current surgical techniques have not been shown to prevent the development of late osteoarthritis after ACL injury.

An important, but underreported, outcome of ACL reconstruction is graft failure. Although this is a devastating outcome for the patient, treatment of failed primary ACL reconstructions also poses a challenge for the orthopedic surgeon. Basic science studies have shown that an anatomically placed graft sees forces that are similar to those of the native ACL and are substantially greater than the forces on a nonanatomically placed graft.[7,8] The successful restoration of native knee kinematics through ACL reconstruction relies on the assumption that there is adequate healing of the graft/bone tunnel interface and reconstructed tissues to withstand the forces transmitted to the native ACL with athletic activity. With the well-established, inferior functional

[a] Department of Orthopaedic Surgery, UPMC Center for Sports Medicine, University of Pittsburgh, 3200 South Water Street, Pittsburgh, PA 15213, USA; [b] Department of Orthopaedic Surgery, Orthopaedic Research Center Amsterdam, Meibergdreef 9, 1105AZ Amsterdam, The Netherlands; [c] Department of Orthopaedic Surgery, University of Michigan, 24 Frank Lloyd Wright Drive, PO Box 0391, Ann Arbor, MI 48106-0391, USA
* Corresponding author. Department of Orthopaedic Surgery, University of Michigan, 24 Frank Lloyd Wright Drive, PO Box 0391, Ann Arbor, MI 48106-0391, USA.
E-mail address: abedi@umich.edu

Clin Sports Med 32 (2013) 93–109
http://dx.doi.org/10.1016/j.csm.2012.08.010   **sportsmed.theclinics.com**

outcomes of revision ACL reconstruction compared with primary ACL reconstruction, prevention of graft failure should be the focus of early after-treatment.[9,10] Recent efforts at advancing the clinical success of ACL reconstruction have focused on strategies to enhance and optimize the biologic environment of the graft-bone interface, promoting and potentially improving the healing rate and strength of the reconstruction.

The mechanism of graft failure is multifactorial in nature and may be attributed to either traumatic or nontraumatic causes. Recurrent trauma, resulting from early aggressive rehabilitation, a premature return to play, or reinjury of a well-healed graft can lead to graft failure. In addition, nontraumatic causes may include technical error in tunnel placement, occult limb malalignment or ligamentous laxity, failure of fixation, or poor biological incorporation.[10] Often, multiple factors may be present to variable degrees. Biomechanical testing has shown that the time-zero strength of the most common graft choices is greater than the native ACL.[11,12] Rather, the weakest link after ACL reconstruction is not the graft but the fixation points on the tibial and femoral side until the graft has adequately healed in the bone tunnel.[13–16] The gradual healing at the enthesis and the intra-articular ligamentization process together make up the 2 main sites of biological incorporation after ACL reconstruction.[17] An understanding of the tendon-bone healing and the intra-articular ligamentization process is crucial for orthopedic surgeons to make appropriate graft choices and to be able to initiate optimal rehabilitation protocols after surgical ACL reconstruction.

Graft-tunnel healing is influenced by many different factors, including surgical technical variables such as graft placement, graft length within the bone tunnel, graft fixation, graft tensioning, and graft-tunnel micromotion. These variables may even vary for different regions of the bone tunnels.[18,19] However, the principal form of healing that occurs in the bone tunnels is primarily dependent on the graft used. Grafts with a bone plug (eg, bone-patellar tendon-bone graft, bone-quadriceps tendon graft) rely on bone-to-bone healing, whereas soft tissue grafts rely on tendon-bone healing, a slow process that does not recapitulate the native anatomy of the ACL insertion with regard to morphology or mechanical strength.[20,21] However, all grafts depend on tendon-to-bone healing at the intra-articular tunnel apertures.[22] Tissue engineering and biomechanical stimulation approaches to enhance this healing process have shown promising results in animal studies and include, but are not limited to, the use of a fibrin clot, platelet rich plasma, growth factors, stem cells, scaffolds, periosteum graft augmentation, bisphosphonates, autologous ruptured tissue, and mechanical loading.

This article focuses on the current understanding of the tendon-to-bone healing process for both autografts and allografts and discusses strategies to biologically augment healing.

TENDON-BONE HEALING: AUTOGRAFT

Healing of a tendon graft inside a bone tunnel is particularly challenged by the complex transition site, which must allow for load transfer between the 2 distinct, inhomogeneous tissues: tendon and bone.[23] Moreover, this transition site is markedly different from the load-transferring architecture of the insertion site of the native ACL.

The native ACL inserts into the bone through an insertion site that changes from ligament to bone directly and functions to transmit complex mechanical loads. This insertion site is made up of highly specialized tissue that gradually changes from ligament to bone through 4 zones: ligament, unmineralized fibrocartilage, mineralized fibrocartilage, and bone (**Fig. 1**).[24] The increase of tissue stiffness along the insertion site from

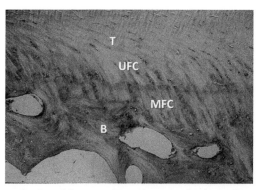

Fig. 1. Native direct enthesis architecture. Note the organized transition from tendon (T) to unmineralized fibrocartilage (UFC) to mineralized fibrocartilage (MFC) and bone (B). This organization is optimized for load transmission and is not recapitulated after ACL reconstruction.

tendon to bone is likely controlled by collagen fiber alignment and a gradual increase of mineralization.[25] A direct insertion from ligament to bone as the ACL has different from other ligaments and tendons, such as the medial collateral ligament (MCL), that run parallel to the bone and insert through an indirect insertion site. Indirect insertion sites do not gradually change from ligament to bone, but rather consist of specialized collagen fibers, called Sharpey fibers, which are oriented obliquely to the long axis of the bone and ligament and provide anchorage between the 2 tissues.

With anatomic ACL reconstruction, the native insertion sites are restored with respect to the insertion site locations on the femur and tibia.[26,27] However, because the grafts are placed in bone tunnels, the structure and composition of the direct insertion site are not reproduced. Instead, the graft heals with a fibrovascular scar at the graft-tunnel interface and forms perpendicular collagen bundles to counteract the shear stresses, attaching the tendon to the bone.[13,15,28] These perpendicular bundles resemble the Sharpey fibers of an indirect insertion site.[13,15] The formation of these fibers begins at 3 to 4 weeks after graft placement and their size and number are positively correlated with the graft pull-out strength.[13,15,28] Sharpey-like fibers continue to be present at 1 year after surgery while gradual osseointegration occurs, improving the graft attachment and incorporating the graft into the surrounding bone.[13]

The earliest phase of healing comprises an inflammatory response characterized by the presence of distinct subpopulations of macrophages. Around 4 days after surgery, macrophages recruited from the circulation and neutrophils are present in the healing tendon-bone interface and are involved in phagocytizing cellular debris, recruiting additional inflammatory cells, and assisting in proinflammatory cytokine release. After 10 days, resident, progenerative macrophages can be identified.[29] These inflammatory cells repopulate the graft and produce numerous cytokines, like transforming growth factor β (TGF-β), which contribute to the formation of the fibrovascular scar tissue interface between the graft and the bone tunnel (**Fig. 2**).[29] However, the formation of this scar tissue results in a mechanically inferior tendon-bone interface, with less organized collagen deposition and decreased pull-out strength than when this scar formation is diminished by macrophage depletion in animal models (**Fig. 3**).[30] Macrophages, TGF-β, and the cyclooxygenase 2 (COX-2) pathway have a complex interplay, and although a depletion of macrophages may be accomplished by inhibiting the COX-2 pathway,[31] different studies have shown that selectively inhibiting the COX-2 pathway delays healing with significantly decreased load to failure.[32,33]

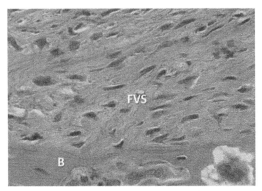

Fig. 2. Healing tendon-bone interface after rotator cuff repair surgery. Note the interposed fibrovascular scar (FVS) tissue and lack of an organized architecture at the healing enthesis. Sharpey-like fibers begin to form at the interface over time with narrowing and maturation of the fibrovascular tissue.

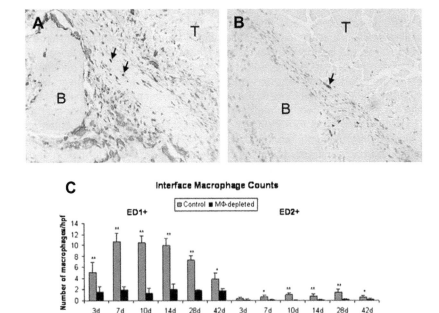

Fig. 3. The effect of macrophage depletion on tendon-bone healing after ACL reconstruction in a rat model. Immunostaining for the ED1 antigen at the tendon-bone interface of control (A) and macrophage-depleted (B) specimens 7 days after ACL reconstruction (original magnification x160). Specimens from animals that had been administered liposomal clodronate showed significantly fewer positively staining macrophages (*arrows*) than control specimens at all time points (C). Macrophage depletion after ACL reconstruction resulted in significantly improved morphologic and biomechanical properties at the healing tendon-bone interface. *$P<.05$. **$P<.01$. B, bone; T, tendon. (*From* Hays PL, Kawamura S, Deng XH, et al. The role of macrophages in early healing of a tendon graft in a bone tunnel. J Bone Joint Surg Am 2008;90(3):568; with permission.)

During the first 8 weeks postoperatively, the tendon-bone interface undergoes significant immunohistologic changes. There is an infiltration and recruitment of macrophages and marrow-derived stem cells to the interface. Initially, the interface consists of mainly granulation tissue containing type III collagen and produces growth factors like vascular endothelial growth factor (VEGF) and fibroblast growth factor (FGF), stimulating angiogenesis and enlarged fibroblasts at the healing enthesis. Simultaneously, like fractured bone, the bone tunnel starts a process of endochondral ossification and chondroid cells appear from the tunnel wall, which degrade the granulation tissue and produce type II collagen. Gradually, the granulation tissue is replaced by maturing lamellar bone and the chondroid cells decrease in number. Meanwhile, shear stresses between the tunnel and the graft cause Sharpey-like fibers to develop, and from the margins of the hypocellular graft, FGF is expressed, attracting fibroblasts to incorporate into the graft and produce type III collagen.[33]

Although the inflammatory phase is essential for the tendon-to-bone healing process, the phase should be transient and gradually progress to the proliferation phase. Early return to sports or an aggressive rehabilitation protocol may lead to micromotion of the graft inside the tunnel.[34] This relative movement between graft and tunnel may impair healing because of continuous microtrauma of the healing tissues, which results in a sustained inflammatory response at the healing enthesis site. The graft-tunnel motion may also lead to osteoclast activation, which stimulates tunnel widening by bone resorption.[34,35] Although excessive motion impairs healing, some controlled loading has shown to be beneficial in tendon healing (**Fig. 4**).[36] Controlled mechanical loads after a delay to allow resolution of acute postoperative inflammation result in improved mechanical and biological parameters.[37,38]

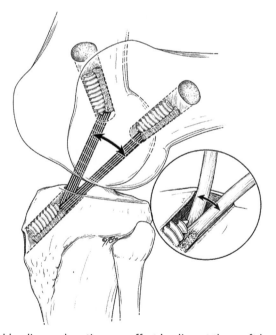

Fig. 4. Mechanical loading and motion can affect healing at the graft-bone interface after ACL reconstruction. The effects can be directly mediated via mechanotransduction by cells at the healing interface or indirectly via local inflammation association with graft motion. (*Courtesy of* Scott Rodeo, MD, New York, NY.)

During the proliferation phase, the stem cells proliferate and differentiate, and matrix metalloproteinases (MMPs) and serine proteases degrade the provisional matrix. The healing cells synthesize and deposit new extracellular matrix with progressive bone ingrowth, which results in an improved load-to-graft failure.[13,39] Gradually, remodeling of the newly formed matrices takes place; the newly formed woven bone, interface tissue, and graft remodel, with establishment of collagen fiber continuity between tendon graft and bone, and cellularity and vascularity at the interface decrease (**Fig. 5**).

TENDON-BONE HEALING: ALLOGRAFT

The use of allograft for soft tissue reconstructive surgery has increased significantly in recent years. The main advantages of using an allograft for ACL reconstruction include the ease of customizing the graft to the desired size and shape, availability, lack of donor-site morbidity, reduced operation times, reduced postoperative pain, and a theoretically lower risk of arthrofibrosis.[40,41] Moreover, some studies have reported no significant difference in clinical outcomes for bone-patellar tendon-bone autografts and allografts, although others have reported significantly greater failure rates in younger patients less than the age of 40 years.[42–44]

Allografts heal through the same biologic pathway of creeping substitutionlike autografts, but at a slower rate. The intra-articular portion of the allograft heals by acting as a type I collagen scaffold, which is populated from the tunnels with host cells derived from the bone and synovial fluid.[45] Angiogenesis is predominately facilitated from the infrapatellar fat pad distally and from the posterior synovial tissues proximally.[46] This angiogenesis is followed by invasion of fibroblasts and synovial cells to repopulate the tendon with host cells and gradually incorporate and remodel the matrix of the graft. As remodeling of the matrix takes place, the tensile strength of the graft is substantially reduced initially and then increases as remodeling is finalized. Allografts lose more of their initial strength during remodeling than autografts, rendering the grafts particularly vulnerable to failure in the subacute phase of postoperative rehabilitation and with a premature return to sport.[47]

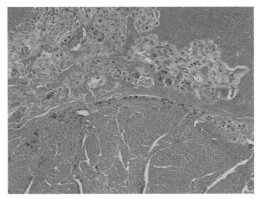

Fig. 5. Axial cross-section of a tendon in a bone tunnel. Note that healing is dependent on osseous ingrowth into the graft at the interface. B, bone; IF, interface tissue; T, tendon. (*From* Gulotta LV, Rodeo SA. Biology of autograft and allograft healing in anterior cruciate ligament reconstruction. Clin Sports Med 2007;26:512; with permission.)

Even although ligaments and tendons are relatively hypocellular, the use of fresh grafts might stimulate the host immune response by lymphocyte invasion, perivascular cuffing, and eventually graft rejection.[48] This immune response is elicited mostly by the expression of major histocompatibility antigens, present on the surface of viable allograft cells. Therefore, fresh tendon allografts are generally not used. Although sterilization can decrease the presence of viable allograft cells, this treatment comes at the expense of decreased biomechanical strength of the graft, which is associated with irradiation or chemical processing.

Tendon allografts can be sterilized by several methods, including chemical sterilization, deep freezing, or γ-irradiation, resulting in decreased graft immunogenicity and reduced risk of disease transmission. However, each method has its own drawbacks, which should be taken into consideration when performing ACL reconstruction with allograft. Chemical sterilization may result in inflammatory reaction, delayed remodeling, and inferior mechanical strength and may not be ideal for soft tissue allograft.[49] Deep freezing is an effective method to kill the donor cell, but may still result in a detectable immune response directed to the matrix antigens, which can also influence graft incorporation and remodeling.[50] Over recent years, γ-irradiation has become the most widely applied allograft sterilization method. Relatively low doses (1.5–2.0 Mrad) can effectively kill bacteria, fungi, and spores, but not viral agents. However, studies have shown that doses more than 2.0 Mrad cause a reduction in the biomechanical properties of the graft and inferior clinical outcomes have been reported.[51,52] Sterilization methods are being further developed and refined to safely sterilizing the tissue, minimizing the risk of disease transmission, and limiting the detrimental effect on the biomechanical properties of the graft. Newer proprietary methods that are currently being studied are typically washes that use a combination of detergents, antibiotics, alcohol, peroxide, and irradiation.

GROWTH FACTOR/CYTOKINE-BASED AUGMENTATION OF TENDON-BONE HEALING

Each phase of the tendon-bone healing process is tightly regulated by a complex cascade of cytokines, promoting cellular proliferation, differentiation, chemotaxis, matrix remodeling, and matrix synthesis, which results in healing. The key chemical regulators are currently believed to include the TGF family, bone morphogenic protein (BMP) family, insulinlike growth factor (IGF) family, MMPs, FGFs, VEGFs, and platelet-derived growth factors (PDGFs). The paracrine and autocrine action of each factor is dependent on multiple variables, including concentration, timing, and synergy with other cytokines and can have both favorable and inhibitory effects depending on the local environment.[53]

TGF-β is a key regulator during embryologic tendon development and also plays a significant role in the modulation of scar tissue formation during connective tissue healing. Three molecular isoforms (TGF-β1, TGF-β2, TGF-β3) have been identified in mammalian tissues. TGF-β1 and TGF-β2 are expressed during the early inflammatory phase of adult tendon healing; stimulating cell migration, proliferation, and collagen synthesis.[54–58] This situation results in scar tissue formation that strengthens the tendon-bone interface, but does not recreate the architecture and mechanical properties of the native tendon enthesis.[59] Recent studies have identified the role of the TGF-β3 isoform in promoting direct tendon healing without scar formation (scarless healing) in the fetal and neonatal environment. Animal models have also shown the ability to improve the collagen ratio, collagen histologic organization, and biomechanical strength in the early healing stages of rotator cuff tendon injuries when treated with TGF-β3 in a calcium phosphate matrix.[57,60] If these results apply to the ACL tendon-bone interface, modulation of the TGF-β family of cytokines may potentially allow for improved healing and recreation of a more anatomic interface.

The BMP molecules are osteoinductive cytokines related to the TGF-β family, and are important for fetal skeletal development.[60] Multiple isoforms of BMP have been identified, with BMP-2 and BMP-7 commercially available for enhancing fracture healing and bone regeneration.[61] BMPs also facilitate the healing of tendon to a bone tunnel by promoting formation of a fibrocartilaginous zone at the bone-tendon interface and stimulating bone ingrowth during the later phases of remodeling.[13,62] The use of BMP-2 delivered via adenovirus has been shown to improve tendon-bone healing during ACL reconstruction in a rabbit model. These studies showed improved collagen organization and osteointegration of the tendon graft with formation of a transitional osteocartilaginous and fibrous tissue matrix compared with a poorly vascularized dense connective tissue in controls. Biomechanical testing of the ACL graft constructs showed significantly higher load to failure and stiffness in the BMP-2–treated group at 8 to 12 weeks after reconstruction.[63,64] Similar results of improved ACL soft tissue graft healing within a bone tunnel with BMP-2 treatment have been reported in canine and porcine models.[65] BMP-12, BMP-13, and BMP-14 have also been found to improve the healing after ligament reconstruction by increasing fibrocartilage formation at the healing enthesis and improving load to failure in animal models, and may have a role in augmenting tendon-to-bone healing after surgery in patients.[66,67]

IGF-1 is a critical cytokine that plays a key role in the inflammatory process at all stages of repair and regeneration of musculoskeletal soft tissue, and the absence of IGF-1 dramatically impairs tissue healing.[68,69] It serves as a chemotactic agent to recruit and stimulate fibroblasts and inflammatory cells to the site of injury. In vitro studies have shown significant increases in DNA synthesis, type 1 and 3 collagen gene expression and synthesis, and proteoglycan synthesis in canine ACL fibroblasts after treatment with IGF-1.[53,70] These stimulatory effects of IGF-1 on in vitro fibroblasts seem to be dose-dependent and have been consistently shown in multiple tendon locations.[53,71] In vivo studies have shown accelerated functional recovery and reduced functional deficit without a change in the tendon biomechanical properties after Achilles transection in rats treated with a single dose of IGF-1 injected into the surgical wound.[72] The investigators concluded that the effects of IGF-1 may occur through modulation of the initial inflammatory response without apparent detriment to the biomechanical strength of the healed tissue. Similar beneficial effects on collagen expression, enthesis architecture, and maximal tendon repair load to failure have been shown in a rotator cuff tear model.[73] The clinical implications of these studies are promising and certainly warrant additional evaluation.

MMPs are zinc-dependent enzymes that are present in connective tissue and are activated from their latent form via a cleavage mechanism, regulating and maintaining the dynamic homeostasis of the extracellular matrix of connective tissues. Their enzymatic activity is balanced by tissue inhibitors of MMP proteins, which assist in coordinating a balance of matrix regeneration and remodeling. MMP production and activation are increased in the presence of inflammatory signals such as interleukin 1b (IL-1b) and TGF-β1, serving as a key component of the early inflammatory and repair phases of healing.[58,74,75] Local and systemic inhibition of MMP activity in a rotator cuff repair model has shown reduced collagen degradation, increased fibrocartilage production, improved collagen fiber organization, and increased mechanical load to failure.[76,77] Regulating the degradative balance of MMPs may play a significant role in improving the quality and rate of healing at the tendon-bone interface during ACL graft incorporation.

The FGF family of cytokines are abundant in normal adult tissue and play an integral role in angiogenesis, mesenchymal cell mitogenesis, and the initiation of granulation tissue formation in the early phases of healing.[78] FGF-2 contributes to fibrous integration at the tendon-bone interface and stimulates vascularization after rabbit ACL transection and reconstruction. Fibroblast expression of FGF during ACL graft healing is highest during the first 6 weeks of healing and coincides with active collagen deposition, progressively declining as the healing changes from fibroblast scar tissue formation to osteoblast deposition of immature, woven bone regulated by BMPs.[62]

VEGF is expressed in the early phase of tendon injury and healing, promoting angiogenesis by stimulating vascular endothelial cells and facilitating recruitment of inflammatory cells. VEGF production is stimulated by local biologic factors, including autocrine and paracrine signaling from inflammatory factors (IL-1b, FGF, prostaglandins) and local tissue hypoxia.[79] Expression of VEGF is highest during the first few weeks after rabbit ACL reconstruction at the bone-tendon interface and continues to be expressed focally by osteoblasts at the bone surface for up to 12 weeks postoperatively.[62] Similarly, VEGF expression is present in multiple sites of tendon injury, and local administration has been shown to improve the biomechanical properties of rat Achilles tendons after repair.[80,81] These beneficial effects of VEGF are most likely caused by angiogenesis and improved transportation of other critical inflammatory mediators to the site of injury or surgical repair.

PDGF is a dimeric molecule consisting of 2 chains (A and B), and is predominantly found in the α granules of platelets. Release of PDGF during the acute inflammatory phase occurs after platelet adherence to the exposed collagen within the vascular endothelial membrane in the setting of injury. It is one of the most potent serum mitogens and promotes early wound healing by stimulating fibroblast, glial, and smooth muscle cell proliferation, initiating the clotting cascade, arachidonic acid synthesis, prostaglandin production, and glycolysis in local tissue. PDGF release is tightly regulated by circulating α-macroglobulin to prevent the biologically active cytokine from entering the systemic circulation.[82] PDGF is not present in normal ACL tissues and has been shown to be present at low levels after ACL transection in a rabbit model. This finding is in contrast to a high level of PDGF present in MCL wounds after surgical transection and may partially account for the lack of clinical healing seen in ACL injuries.[83] After ACL reconstruction with autogenous patellar tendon graft in a canine model, early PDGF deposition is observed in the granulation tissues at the graft-bone tunnel interface and in developing capillary beds within 7 days of surgery. During the early repair and graft incorporation phases of healing (3–6 weeks), PDGF is present in the graft substance and at the bone tunnel interface, gradually decreasing by 12 weeks postoperatively.[84] Li and colleagues[85] investigated the effects of mesenchymal stem cells tranfected for sustained PDGF expression, on allograft incorporation in a rabbit model. This model showed improved granulation tissue formation and neovascularization at 3 weeks and the appearance of more chondrocytelike cells at the healing interface by 6 weeks. Collagen maturation, direct tendon-bone tunnel healing, and allograft incorporation were improved in the PDGF-treated group compared with controls.

Tendon-bone healing is a complex process that is dependent on numerous biological factors, and research on the chemical interactions involved in the healing process have led to promising results in the improvement and acceleration of ACL graft incorporation. Further investigation is required before the routine clinical implementation of cell-based and biological factors is advocated to augment healing after ACL reconstruction, and likely represents a critical frontier to improve outcomes after all soft tissue reconstructive procedures.

SCAFFOLDS AND ACL REPAIR/RECONSTRUCTION

ACL healing after primary repair has not been successful secondary to the unfavorable intra-articular environment and relatively avascular tissue. This situation has led to continued research into novel approaches to manage ACL injuries, including the use of biologic and synthetic scaffolds to augment healing after primary ACL repair or ACL graft incorporation after reconstruction. Multiple materials have been evaluated, including collagen matrices, silk, poly-L-lactic acid polymers, polyglycolic acid constructs, alginate polymers, and chitosan-based polymers. The ideal scaffold supports growth and differentiation of relevant cell populations, directs cellular interactions, promotes formation and maintenance of the extracellular matrix, and possesses adequate mechanical strength to withstand rehabilitation and avoid degradation before incorporation or healing.

To facilitate primary healing of the ACL after repair, an appropriate environment must be present to allow healing and restoration of the native ligament properties. Initial investigation into the use of collagen platelet composites (CPC) has shown successful healing of a central ligament defect in a canine model. Treatment with CPC at the time of ACL injury resulted in robust healing similar to patellar tendon and MCL models, with improved growth factor expression, histologic ligament healing, improved magnetic resonance imaging findings, and significantly increased biomechanical properties compared with untreated ACLs.[86–88] This technique was subsequently validated in vivo with a juvenile pig model treated with complete ACL transection followed by primary ligament repair with absorbable sutures followed by suspension of the collagen scaffold soaked in platelet rich plasma on the suture repair. This technique resulted in a significantly higher repair strength and improved cellularity at 4 weeks and 3 months compared with primary ACL repair without treatment.[89] Further investigations have shown that primary ACL healing with CPC is also dependent on age and time from injury to repair, with younger animals and shorter time from injury to repair showing an improved healing capacity.[90–92] Clinical implications of these findings include the possibility of successful primary ACL healing after repair with an off-the-shelf device, and may represent a future strategy in the management of pediatric ACL injuries without the risk of physeal injury.

Current soft tissue options for ACL reconstruction include hamstring, fascia lata, and quadriceps tendon autografts and various allografts, relying on scar-based healing to the adjacent bone tunnel wall to provide adequate fixation strength. Preliminary results of tissue engineering targeted at enhancing the regeneration of the bone-soft tissue interface by recreating the multitissue transition from tendon/ligament, fibrocartilage, to bone are encouraging. Rabbit studies have shown the ability to improve the tendon-bone interface by incorporating an allogeneic costal cartilage chondrocyte pellet into a surgically created patellar tendon wound and subsequent repair. This technique improved the histologic appearance of the repair site and re-established an anatomic tendon/fibrocartilage/bone enthesis at 8, 12, and 16 weeks compared with control specimen.[93] Spalazzi and colleagues have published their results on a triphasic scaffold consisting of fibroblast, chondrocyte, and osteoblast populations in an attempt to more closely recreate a native tendon insertion. This triphasic scaffold has been evaluated in vitro and in vivo, with phase A consisting of human fibroblasts cultured in a poly(lactic-co-glycolic acid) (PLGA) polymer for soft tissue formation, phase B consisting of a fibrochondrocyte culture in PLGA for transitional tissue, and phase C consisting of human osteoblasts cultured in PLGA combined with sintered glass microspheres to recreate the calcified entheseal layer.[94,95] After subcutaneous incubation in rats, the cellular distribution within the scaffold remained in a phase-specific distribution. The investigators conclude that a triphasic scaffold has the potential to recreate the organization inherent to the ligament-bone interface, and could be used to guide the establishment of an anatomic fibrocartilage interface between a soft tissue graft and a bone tunnel or aperture after ACL surgery.

Clinical interest in avoiding the morbidity of autograft harvest and the risks of allogeneic tissue have stimulated the development of engineered grafts for ACL reconstruction. Ma and colleagues[96] used a sheep model to engineer a bone-ligament-bone construct in cell culture with adequate size to allow for ACL reconstruction. Bone marrow stromal cells were harvested from sheep femurs and treated with specific growth factors to create independent ligament and bone lineages. The ligament cells were allowed to develop into a monolayer and were inserted between 2 20-mm bone monolayers separated by a distance of 30 to 40 mm. Eight individual constructs were combined to form a bone-ligament-bone graft of 60 to 80 mm in length and 3 mm in diameter. ACL reconstruction was then performed with the engineered grafts, followed by harvesting of the native and engineered ACLs at 2, 3, 4, and 6 months postoperatively. At 4 months postoperatively, the graft size was equal to the native ACL, and histologically showed robust vascularity, remodeling, and bone tunnel healing. Biomechanical testing showed a 90-fold increase in graft strength at 6 months, achieving 92% stiffness of the native ACL and similar load to failure. These results represent the successful development of a multiphasic ACL graft with mechanical properties similar to the native adult ACL in sheep and have implications for the future potential of a completely engineered ACL graft for human use.

Synthetic scaffolds or ligament substitutes are another attractive option to avoid graft site morbidity in ACL reconstruction. Previous artificial ligament grafts including polyaramid, carbon fiber, and polyester devices have been largely unsuccessful because of high failure rates and reactive synovitis from wear particles.[97–99] Richmond and Weitzel[98,100] have recently investigated the use of a silk scaffold for ACL reconstruction, with the advantage that manipulation of the fiber properties can control the rate of scaffold degradation and fibrous ingrowth. An in vivo study was performed in a goat model with placement of an artificial ACL ligament constructed of a woven silk fiber composite through 6-mm bone tunnels. Each fiber had a diameter less than 350 μm to facilitate synovial absorption of the degradative products. Histologic results at 12 months showed organized collagen healing with a native crimp pattern and spindle-shaped fibroblasts similar to the native ligament, with Sharpey fibers identified within the bone tunnel at the graft-bone interface. There was no evidence of regional lymph node reactivity of presence of silk particles. Laxity testing revealed up to 4 mm anterior tibial translation at 12 months postoperatively, comparable with the results of autograft and allograft reconstructions reported in a goat model. Human studies have been initiated and preliminary results are pending publication, although the initial goat studies highlight the potential of bioengineered ligament devices to address the requirements of an appropriate synthetic ACL substitute.

SUMMARY

Recent improvements in surgical management options of ACL injuries have called further attention to the importance of new biological strategies to enhance the intra-articular and intraosseous healing process.

Current research trends have focused on both refining existing techniques and developing novel solutions such as augmentation of graft-tunnel healing, primary ACL repair, and use of scaffolds to improve or obviate autogenous or allogeneic grafts for reconstruction. Further research is necessary before widespread clinical adoption; the preliminary results of these modern advances are promising and likely represent the future of ACL injury prevention and management.

REFERENCES

1. Fithian DC, Paxton EW, Stone ML, et al. Prospective trial of a treatment algorithm for the management of the anterior cruciate ligament-injured knee. Am J Sports Med 2005;33:335–46.
2. Bach BR, Levy ME, Bojchuk J, et al. Single-incision endoscopic anterior cruciate ligament reconstruction using patellar tendon autograft. Minimum two-year follow-up evaluation. Am J Sports Med 1998;26:30–40.
3. Beynnon BD, Johnson RJ, Fleming BC, et al. Anterior cruciate ligament replacement: comparison of bone-patellar tendon-bone grafts with two-strand hamstring grafts. A prospective, randomized study. J Bone Joint Surg Am 2002;84-A:1503–13.
4. Yasuda K, Tanabe Y, Kondo E, et al. Anatomic double-bundle anterior cruciate ligament reconstruction. Arthroscopy 2010;26:S21–34.
5. Zelle BA, Beasley LS, Fu FH. The envelope of function in anterior cruciate ligament injuries. Operat Tech Orthop 2005;15:86–8.
6. Ardern CL, Taylor NF, Feller JA, et al. Return-to-sport outcomes at 2 to 7 years after anterior cruciate ligament reconstruction surgery. Am J Sports Med 2012; 40:41–8.
7. Kato Y, Ingham SJ, Kramer S, et al. Effect of tunnel position for anatomic single-bundle ACL reconstruction on knee biomechanics in a porcine model. Knee Surg Sports Traumatol Arthrosc 2010;18:2–10.
8. Xu Y, Liu J, Kramer S, et al. Comparison of in situ forces and knee kinematics in anteromedial and high anteromedial bundle augmentation for partially ruptured anterior cruciate ligament. Am J Sports Med 2011;39:272–8.
9. Wright RW, Gill CS, Chen L, et al. Outcome of revision anterior cruciate ligament reconstruction: a systematic review. J Bone Joint Surg Am 2012;94:531–6.
10. George MS, Dunn WR, Spindler KP. Current concepts review: revision anterior cruciate ligament reconstruction. Am J Sports Med 2006;34:2026–37.
11. Hamner DL, Brown CH, Steiner ME, et al. Hamstring tendon grafts for reconstruction of the anterior cruciate ligament: biomechanical evaluation of the use of multiple strands and tensioning techniques. J Bone Joint Surg Am 1999;81: 549–57.
12. Cooper DE, Deng XH, Burstein AL, et al. The strength of the central third patellar tendon graft. A biomechanical study. Am J Sports Med 1993;21:818–23 [discussion: 823–4].
13. Rodeo SA, Arnoczky SP, Torzilli PA, et al. Tendon-healing in a bone tunnel. A biomechanical and histological study in the dog. J Bone Joint Surg Am 1993; 75:1795–803.
14. Whiston TB, Walmsley R. Some observations on the reactions of bone and tendon after tunnelling of bone and insertion of tendon. J Bone Joint Surg Am 1960;42-B:377–86.
15. Grana WA, Egle DM, Mahnken R, et al. An analysis of autograft fixation after anterior cruciate ligament reconstruction in a rabbit model. Am J Sports Med 1994;22:344–51.
16. Panni AS, Milano G, Lucania L, et al. Graft healing after anterior cruciate ligament reconstruction in rabbits. Clin Orthop Relat Res 1997;343:203–12.

17. Scheffler SU, Unterhauser FN, Weiler A. Graft remodeling and ligamentization after cruciate ligament reconstruction. Knee Surg Sports Traumatol Arthrosc 2008;16:834–42.
18. Ekdahl M, Wang JH, Ronga M, et al. Graft healing in anterior cruciate ligament reconstruction. Knee Surg Sports Traumatol Arthrosc 2008;16:935–47.
19. Bedi A, Kawamura S, Ying L, et al. Differences in tendon graft healing between the intra-articular and extra-articular ends of a bone tunnel. HSS J 2009;5:51–7.
20. Papageorgiou CD, Ma CB, Abramowitch SD, et al. A multidisciplinary study of the healing of an intraarticular anterior cruciate ligament graft in a goat model. Am J Sports Med 2001;29:620–6.
21. Tomita F, Yasuda K, Mikami S, et al. Comparisons of intraosseous graft healing between the doubled flexor tendon graft and the bone-patellar tendon-bone graft in anterior cruciate ligament reconstruction. Arthroscopy 2001;17:461–76.
22. Gulotta LV, Rodeo SA. Biology of autograft and allograft healing in anterior cruciate ligament reconstruction. Clin Sports Med 2007;26:509–24.
23. Gulotta LV, Wiznia D, Cunningham M, et al. What's new in orthopaedic research. J Bone Joint Surg Am 2011;93:2136–41.
24. Sagarriga Visconti C, Kavalkovich K, Wu J, et al. Biochemical analysis of collagens at the ligament-bone interface reveals presence of cartilage-specific collagens. Arch Biochem Biophys 1996;328:135–42.
25. Genin GM, Kent A, Birman V, et al. Functional grading of mineral and collagen in the attachment of tendon to bone. Biophys J 2009;97:976–85.
26. van Eck CF, Lesniak BP, Schreiber VM, et al. Anatomic single- and double-bundle anterior cruciate ligament reconstruction flowchart. Arthroscopy 2010; 6:258–68.
27. van Eck CF, Schreiber VM, Liu TT, et al. The anatomic approach to primary, revision and augmentation anterior cruciate ligament reconstruction. Knee Surg Sports Traumatol Arthrosc 2010;18:1154–63.
28. Goradia VK, Rochat MC, Grana WA, et al. Tendon-to-bone healing of a semitendinosus tendon autograft used for ACL reconstruction in a sheep model. Am J Knee Surg 2000;13:143–51.
29. Kawamura S, Ying L, Kim HJ, et al. Macrophages accumulate in the early phase of tendon-bone healing. J Orthop Res 2005;23:1425–32.
30. Hays PL, Kawamura S, Deng XH, et al. The role of macrophages in early healing of a tendon graft in a bone tunnel. J Bone Joint Surg Am 2008;90:565–79.
31. Shen W, Li Y, Zhu J, et al. Interaction between macrophages, TGF-beta1, and the COX-2 pathway during the inflammatory phase of skeletal muscle healing after injury. J Cell Physiol 2008;214:405–12.
32. Cohen DB, Kawamura S, Ehteshami JR, et al. Indomethacin and celecoxib impair rotator cuff tendon-to-bone healing. Am J Sports Med 2006;34:362–9.
33. Kanazawa T, Soejima T, Murakami H, et al. An immunohistological study of the integration at the bone-tendon interface after reconstruction of the anterior cruciate ligament in rabbits. J Bone Joint Surg Am 2006;88:682–7.
34. Hantes ME, Mastrokalos DS, Yu J, et al. The effect of early motion on tibial tunnel widening after anterior cruciate ligament replacement using hamstring tendon grafts. Arthroscopy 2004;20:572–80.
35. Rodeo SA, Kawamura S, Kim HJ, et al. Tendon healing in a bone tunnel differs at the tunnel entrance versus the tunnel exit: an effect of graft-tunnel motion? Am J Sports Med 2006;34:1790–800.
36. Killian ML, Cavinatto L, Galatz LM, et al. The role of mechanobiology in tendon healing. J Shoulder Elbow Surg 2012;21:228–37.

37. Bedi A, Kovacevic D, Fox AJS, et al. Effect of early and delayed mechanical loading on tendon-to-bone healing after anterior cruciate ligament reconstruction. J Bone Joint Surg Am 2010;92:2387–401.
38. Gardner K, Arnoczky SP, Caballero O, et al. The effect of stress-deprivation and cyclic loading on the TIMP/MMP ratio in tendon cells: an in vitro experimental study. Disabil Rehabil 2008;30:1523–9.
39. Wen CY, Qin L, Lee KM, et al. Peri-graft bone mass and connectivity as predictors for the strength of tendon-to-bone attachment after anterior cruciate ligament reconstruction. Bone 2009;45:545–52.
40. Harner CD, Olson E, Irrgang JJ, et al. Allograft versus autograft anterior cruciate ligament reconstruction: 3- to 5-year outcome. Clin Orthop Relat Res 1996;324:134–44.
41. Cohen SB, Sekiya JK. Allograft safety in anterior cruciate ligament reconstruction. Clin Sports Med 2007;26:597–605.
42. Ghodadra NS, Mall NA, Grumet R, et al. Interval arthrometric comparison of anterior cruciate ligament reconstruction using bone-patellar tendon-bone autograft versus allograft: do grafts attenuate within the first year postoperatively? Am J Sports Med 2012;40:1347–54.
43. Barrett G, Stokes D, White M. Anterior cruciate ligament reconstruction in patients older than 40 years: allograft versus autograft patellar tendon. Am J Sports Med 2005;33:1505–12.
44. Kaeding CC, Aros B, Pedroza A, et al. Allograft versus autograft anterior cruciate ligament reconstruction: predictors of failure from a MOON prospective longitudinal cohort. Sport Health 2010;3:73–81.
45. Min BH, Han MS, Woo JI, et al. The origin of cells that repopulate patellar tendons used for reconstructing anterior cruciate ligaments in man. J Bone Joint Surg Am 2003;85:753–7.
46. Nikolaou PK, Seaber AV, Glisson RR, et al. Anterior cruciate ligament allograft transplantation. Long-term function, histology, revascularization, and operative technique. Am J Sports Med 1986;14:348–60.
47. Jackson DW, Corsetti J, Simon TM. Biologic incorporation of allograft anterior cruciate ligament replacements. Clin Orthop Relat Res 1996;324:126–33.
48. Arnoczky SP, Warren RF, Ashlock MA. Replacement of the anterior cruciate ligament using a patellar tendon allograft. An experimental study. J Bone Joint Surg Am 1986;68:376–85.
49. Scheffler SU, Gonnermann J, Kamp J, et al. Remodeling of ACL allografts is inhibited by peracetic acid sterilization. Clin Orthop Relat Res 2008;466:1810–8.
50. Xiao Y, Parry DA, Li H, et al. Expression of extracellular matrix macromolecules around demineralized freeze-dried bone allografts. J Periodontol 1996;67:1233–44.
51. Guo L, Yang L, Duan XJ, et al. Anterior cruciate ligament reconstruction with bone-patellar tendon-bone graft: comparison of autograft, fresh-frozen allograft, and γ-irradiated allograft. Arthroscopy 2012;28:211–7.
52. Curran AR, Adams DJ, Gill JL, et al. The biomechanical effects of low-dose irradiation on bone-patellar tendon-bone allografts. Am J Sports Med 2004;32:1131–5.
53. DesRosiers EA, Yahia L, Rivard CH. Proliferative and matrix synthesis response of canine anterior cruciate ligament fibroblasts submitted to combined growth factors. J Orthop Res 1996;14:200–8.
54. Chang J, Most D, Stelnicki E, et al. Gene expression of transforming growth factor beta-1 in rabbit zone II flexor tendon wound healing: evidence for dual mechanisms of repair. Plast Reconstr Surg 1997;100:937–44.

55. Kashiwagi K, Mochizuki Y, Yasunaga Y, et al. Effects of transforming growth factor-beta 1 on the early stages of healing of the Achilles tendon in a rat model. Scand J Plast Reconstr Surg Hand Surg 2004;38:193–7.
56. Sporn MB, Roberts AB, Wakefield LM, et al. Transforming growth factor-beta: biological function and chemical structure. Science 1986;233:532–4.
57. Kovacevic D, Fox AJ, Bedi A, et al. Calcium-phosphate matrix with or without TGF-β3 improves tendon-bone healing after rotator cuff repair. Am J Sports Med 2011;39:811–9.
58. Wang Y, Tang Z, Xue R, et al. TGF-β1 promoted MMP-2 mediated wound healing of anterior cruciate ligament fibroblasts through NF-κB. Connect Tissue Res 2011;52:218–25.
59. Campbell BH, Agarwal C, Wang JH. TGF-beta1, TGF-beta3, and PGE(2) regulate contraction of human patellar tendon fibroblasts. Biomech Model Mechanobiol 2004;2:239–45.
60. Lories RJ, Luyten FP. Bone morphogenetic protein signaling in joint homeostasis and disease. Cytokine Growth Factor Rev 2005;16:287–98.
61. Axelrad TW, Einhorn TA. Bone morphogenetic proteins in orthopaedic surgery. Cytokine Growth Factor Rev 2009;20:481–8.
62. Kohno T, Ishibashi Y, Tsuda E, et al. Immunohistochemical demonstration of growth factors at the tendon-bone interface in anterior cruciate ligament reconstruction using a rabbit model. J Orthop Sci 2007;12:67–73.
63. Wang CJ, Weng LH, Hsu SL, et al. pCMV-BMP-2-transfected cell-mediated gene therapy in anterior cruciate ligament reconstruction in rabbits. Arthroscopy 2010;26:968–76.
64. Martinek V, Latterman C, Usas A, et al. Enhancement of tendon-bone integration of anterior cruciate ligament grafts with bone morphogenetic protein-2 gene transfer: a histological and biomechanical study. J Bone Joint Surg Am 2002; 84-A:1123–31.
65. Rodeo SA, Suzuki K, Deng XH, et al. Use of recombinant human bone morphogenetic protein-2 to enhance tendon healing in a bone tunnel. Am J Sports Med 1999;27:476–88.
66. Lou J, Tu Y, Burns M, et al. BMP-12 gene transfer augmentation of lacerated tendon repair. J Orthop Res 2001;19:1199–202.
67. Aspenberg P, Forslund C. Bone morphogenetic proteins and tendon repair. Scand J Med Sci Sports 2000;10:372–5.
68. Steenfos HH, Jansson JO. Gene expression of insulin-like growth factor-I and IGF-I receptor during wound healing in rats. Eur J Surg 1992;158:327–31.
69. Gartner MH, Benson JD, Caldwell MD. Insulin-like growth factors I and II expression in the healing wound. J Surg Res 1992;52:389–94.
70. Gillery P, Leperre A, Maquart FX, et al. Insulin-like growth factor-I (IGF-I) stimulates protein synthesis and collagen gene expression in monolayer and lattice cultures of fibroblasts. J Cell Physiol 1992;152:389–96.
71. Abrahamsson SO, Lohmander S. Differential effects of insulin-like growth factor-I on matrix and DNA synthesis in various regions and types of rabbit tendons. J Orthop Res 1996;14:370–6.
72. Kurtz CA, Loebig TG, Anderson DD, et al. Insulin-like growth factor I accelerates functional recovery from Achilles tendon injury in a rat model. Am J Sports Med 1999;27:363–9.
73. Dines JS, Weber L, Razzano P, et al. The effect of growth differentiation factor-5-coated sutures on tendon repair in a rat model. J Shoulder Elbow Surg 2007;16: S215–21.

74. Tsuzaki M, Guyton G, Garrett W, et al. IL-1 beta induces COX2, MMP-1, -3 and -13, ADAMTS-4, IL-1 beta and IL-6 in human tendon cells. J Orthop Res 2003; 21:256–64.

75. Archambault J, Tsuzaki M, Herzog W, et al. Stretch and interleukin-1beta induce matrix metalloproteinases in rabbit tendon cells in vitro. J Orthop Res 2002;20: 36–9.

76. Bedi A, Fox AJ, Kovacevic D, et al. Doxycycline-mediated inhibition of matrix metalloproteinases improves healing after rotator cuff repair. Am J Sports Med 2010;38:308–17.

77. Bedi A, Kovacevic D, Hettrich C, et al. The effect of matrix metalloproteinase inhibition on tendon-to-bone healing in a rotator cuff repair model. J Shoulder Elbow Surg 2010;19:384–91.

78. Kuang GM, Yau WP, Lu WW, et al. Osteointegration of soft tissue grafts within the bone tunnels in anterior cruciate ligament reconstruction can be enhanced. Knee Surg Sports Traumatol Arthrosc 2010;18:1038–51.

79. Jackson JR, Minton JA, Ho ML, et al. Expression of vascular endothelial growth factor in synovial fibroblasts is induced by hypoxia and interleukin 1beta. J Rheumatol 1997;24:1253–9.

80. Zhang F, Liu H, Stile F, et al. Effect of vascular endothelial growth factor on rat Achilles tendon healing. Plast Reconstr Surg 2003;112:1613–9.

81. Bidder M, Towler DA, Gelberman RH, et al. Expression of mRNA for vascular endothelial growth factor at the repair site of healing canine flexor tendon. J Orthop Res 2000;18:247–52.

82. Deuel TF, Huang JS. Platelet-derived growth factor. Structure, function, and roles in normal and transformed cells. J Clin Invest 1984;74:669–76.

83. Lee J, Harwood FL, Akeson WH, et al. Growth factor expression in healing rabbit medial collateral and anterior cruciate ligaments. Iowa Orthop J 1998;18:19–25.

84. Kuroda R, Kurosaka M, Yoshiya S, et al. Localization of growth factors in the reconstructed anterior cruciate ligament: immunohistological study in dogs. Knee Surg Sports Traumatol Arthrosc 2000;8:120–6.

85. Li F, Jia H, Yu C. ACL reconstruction in a rabbit model using irradiated Achilles allograft seeded with mesenchymal stem cells or PDGF-B gene-transfected mesenchymal stem cells. Knee Surg Sports Traumatol Arthrosc 2007;15: 1219–27.

86. Murray MM, Spindler KP, Devin C, et al. Use of a collagen-platelet rich plasma scaffold to stimulate healing of a central defect in the canine ACL. J Orthop Res 2006;24:820–30.

87. Spindler KP, Murray MM, Devin C, et al. The central ACL defect as a model for failure of intra-articular healing. J Orthop Res 2006;24:401–6.

88. Murray MM, Spindler KP, Ballard P, et al. Enhanced histologic repair in a central wound in the anterior cruciate ligament with a collagen-platelet-rich plasma scaffold. J Orthop Res 2007;25:1007–17.

89. Joshi SM, Mastrangelo AN, Magarian EM, et al. Collagen-platelet composite enhances biomechanical and histologic healing of the porcine anterior cruciate ligament. Am J Sports Med 2009;37:2401–10.

90. Murray MM, Magarian EM, Harrison SL, et al. The effect of skeletal maturity on functional healing of the anterior cruciate ligament. J Bone Joint Surg Am 2010; 92:2039–49.

91. Magarian EM, Fleming BC, Harrison SL, et al. Delay of 2 or 6 weeks adversely affects the functional outcome of augmented primary repair of the porcine anterior cruciate ligament. Am J Sports Med 2010;38:2528–34.

92. Mastrangelo AN, Haus BM, Vavken P, et al. Immature animals have higher cellular density in the healing anterior cruciate ligament than adolescent or adult animals. J Orthop Res 2010;28:1100–6.
93. Wong MW, Qin L, Tai JK, et al. Engineered allogeneic chondrocyte pellet for reconstruction of fibrocartilage zone at bone-tendon junction–a preliminary histological observation. J Biomed Mater Res B Appl Biomater 2004;70:362–7.
94. Spalazzi JP, Doty SB, Moffat KL, et al. Development of controlled matrix heterogeneity on a triphasic scaffold for orthopedic interface tissue engineering. Tissue Eng 2006;12:3497–508.
95. Spalazzi JP, Dagher E, Doty SB, et al. In vivo evaluation of a multiphased scaffold designed for orthopaedic interface tissue engineering and soft tissue-to-bone integration. J Biomed Mater Res A 2008;86:1–12.
96. Ma J, Smietana MJ, Kostrominova TY, et al. Three-dimensional engineered bone-ligament-bone constructs for anterior cruciate ligament replacement. Tissue Eng Part A 2012;18:103–16.
97. Richmond JC, Manseau CJ, Patz R, et al. Anterior cruciate reconstruction using a Dacron ligament prosthesis. A long-term study. Am J Sports Med 1992;20: 24–8.
98. Richmond JC, Weitzel PP. Bioresorbable scaffolds for anterior cruciate ligament reconstruction: do we need an off-the-shelf ACL substitute? Sports Med Arthrosc 2010;18:40–2.
99. Frank CB, Jackson DW. The science of reconstruction of the anterior cruciate ligament. J Bone Joint Surg Am 1997;79:1556–76.
100. Altman GH, Horan RL, Weitzel P, et al. The use of long-term bioresorbable scaffolds for anterior cruciate ligament repair. J Am Acad Orthop Surg 2008;16: 177–87.

Trends in Surgeon Preferences on Anterior Cruciate Ligament Reconstructive Techniques

Kristian Samuelsson, MD, PhD[a], Daniel Andersson, MD[a],
Mattias Ahldén, MD[a], Freddie H. Fu, MD, DSc[b],
Volker Musahl, MD[b], Jón Karlsson, MD, PhD[a],*

KEYWORDS

- Anatomic - Anterior cruciate ligament - Reconstruction - Single-bundle
- Double-bundle - Trends - Preferences - Perspectives

KEY POINTS

- Along with increasing knowledge of anterior cruciate ligament (ACL) anatomy and kine-matics as well as clinical experience, orthopedic surgeons have engaged in and witnessed an amazing evolution regarding surgical reconstructive techniques.
- Today, many surgeons intend to replicate the native ACL as much as possible, aiming at anatomic ACL reconstruction.
- An outline of the new surgical preferences is starting to form; orthopedic surgeons have shifted their preferences in arthroscopic technique, graft type, and fixation during the past decade.

INTRODUCTION

The long and often winding road to today's anatomic anterior cruciate ligament (ACL) reconstruction has been eventful and fascinating. The progress is demonstrated when looking back in the surgical history of the ACL, from the first reported repair of the torn ACL with silk sutures in 1895 by Sir Arthur Mayo-Robson of Leeds to today's

The authors did not receive any outside funding or grants directly related to the research pre-sented in this article. The Department of Orthopaedic Surgery from the University of Pittsburgh receives funding from Smith and Nephew to support research related to reconstruction of the ACL. The authors state that this article is an original work only submitted to this journal. All authors contributed to the preparation of this work.

[a] Department of Orthopaedics, Sahlgrenska University Hospital, Mölndal 431 80, Sweden;
[b] Department of Orthopaedic Surgery, University of Pittsburgh, 3471 Fifth Avenue, Pittsburgh, PA 15213, USA
* Corresponding author. Department of Orthopaedics, Sahlgrenska University Hospital, SE-431 80, Mölndal, Sweden.
E-mail address: jon.karlsson@telia.com

arthroscopic anatomic double-bundle ACL reconstruction.[1] With increasing knowledge of ACL anatomy, the last decade has led to an evolution and a shift in paradigm in the surgical technique for ACL reconstruction. One of the new techniques, double-bundle ACL reconstruction, which aims to reconstruct both functional bundles of the native ACL, has been labeled as anatomic by several investigators.[2,3] However, a reconstruction of both bundles can still be performed nonanatomically. This linguistic confusion has created the need for a definition and guidelines for what constitutes anatomic ACL reconstruction.[4] An outline of the new surgical preferences is starting to form; orthopedic surgeons have shifted their preferences in arthroscopic technique, graft type, and fixation during the past decade.

TECHNICAL AND SURGICAL PERSPECTIVES
Primary Repair and Augmentation

Several clinical attempts of primary repair of the ACL have been tried; but almost all of them report discouraging results, although short-term outcomes are positive.[5,6] These results led orthopedic surgeons onto the path of different augmentation techniques that would theoretically not only promote healing but also prevent elongation and rupture. However, studies on augmentation together with repair revealed high rerupture rates and unfavorable outcomes.[7] The incapacity of the ruptured ACL to heal and discouraging results of primary repair and different augmentation devices made orthopedic surgeons shift from performing ACL repair to reconstructions.

Open and Arthroscopic ACL Reconstruction

The arthroscopic evolution started in 1980 when David Dandy of Cambridge, United Kingdom, performed the first arthroscopic ACL reconstruction with an artificial ligament made out of carbon fibers.[8] Thereafter, several researchers and orthopedic surgeons led the development and employment of the arthroscopic technique. The new technique was appealing because it was less traumatic than reconstruction with arthrotomy. Although it was a difficult procedure because there were no camera or monitors initially, studies revealed improvements in early symptoms.[1,9–12] During the 1980s, the arthroscopic technique was primarily performed with a 2-incision technique whereby one incision was used for drilling the tibial bone tunnel and passing the graft and the other incision was used for drilling the femoral bone tunnel. This technique was also called the rear-entry technique because the second incision was localized posterior to the lateral femur condyle and drilling was performed using a guide, creating the bone tunnel from the outside of the femur condyle into the knee joint. The following decade, a new inside-out technique for femoral drilling was introduced. It was also called an endoscopic, one-incision, and transtibial technique. In this technique, an arthroscopic drill was introduced through the tibial bone tunnel and the femoral tunnel was created via this access. Several potential benefits were identified with this new technique. However, there was a concern that the new drilling technique would result in a nonoptimal femoral tunnel placement. Studies did not reveal any major significant differences between the 1- and 2-incision technique except for the study by Panni and colleagues.[13–18] This study found a more vertical graft placement in the one-incision technique.[18] Thus, the major advantage, transtibial drilling, is also the major limitation of the technique because it creates a restrictive link that prevents free movement of the arthroscopic drill and, therefore, limits the position of the femoral bone tunnel. By the end of the 1990s, most orthopedic surgeons used the transtibial technique, although criticisms of the new technique persisted.[1] During this time period, 3 additional tools were commonly used: isometry, notch plasty, and the o'clock reference.

Isometry

The concept of isometric graft placement was introduced during the 1960s.[1] The term stems from the Greek word for equal measure. The procedure encompasses constant distance between the tunnels in the tibia and femur, or at least as little change as possible, during the knee's range of motion.[19] The reason for aiming at isometric graft placement was that research showed that a graft could be irreversibly stretched if elongated more than 4% and clinical studies revealed positive effects of isometric placement.[20,21] With time and increasing understanding of the native ACL anatomy, researchers and orthopedic surgeons started to criticize the isometric concept. It was clear that the fanlike shape of the native ACL had an anisometric and nonuniform fiber anatomy. Furthermore, none of the bundles in the native ACL are isometric in their own entity.[19,22,23] Also, the revealed isometric points were high and anterior in the femoral notch, far from the native footprint of the ACL (**Fig. 1**).[20,24] It became obvious that the isometric concept was an elusive one, resulting in inferior knee joint kinematics compared with anatomic bone tunnel placement.[24–26] The suboptimal knee joint kinematics were thought to be responsible for inferior clinical results and the development of osteoarthritis.[27] This idea caused a marked decrease in the popularity and use of the isometric concept during the beginning of the twenty-first century.[1] Today, focus is on respecting native anatomy and native tension patterns and not on isometry.[4,26]

Notch Plasty

With the start of the arthroscopic ACL reconstruction, a surgical technique called notch plasty was used. This technique aimed to remove part of the inner wall of the lateral femoral notch to provide a better view of the posterior part of the notch and also to avoid graft impingement. However, notch plasty removes important osseous landmarks aiding in the femoral bone tunnel placement as well as a lateral graft displacement, which can change the kinematics of the graft.[28,29] Furthermore, notch plasty can cause bone overgrowth with graft impingement (**Fig. 2**). With time, orthopedic surgeons started to use new arthroscopic techniques, such as the 3-portal

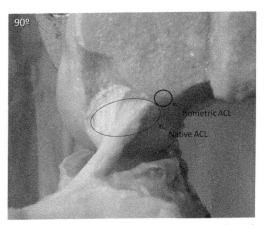

Fig. 1. The localization of the isometric ACL placement and the relation to the native femoral ACL footprint.

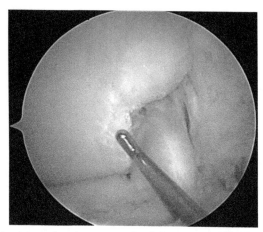

Fig. 2. Arthroscopic picture showing regrowth of the notch after notch plasty.

technique or the 70° arthroscope, which aided in the visualization of the lateral wall of the femoral condyle, thus making notch plasty unnecessary for visualization purposes.[30,31] Because the native ACL does not impinge, anatomically placed ACL grafts will not either. Hence, with increasingly anatomically placed grafts, a decrease should be seen in terms of the use of notch plasty for impingement purposes. Today, new surgical techniques have made the old indications for notch plasty obsolete; notch plasty is, therefore, limited to few and special cases.

O'clock Reference

The development and distribution of arthroscopic ACL reconstruction warranted a new technique for evaluating tunnel position. A reference system using the o'clock face had previously been developed for the assessment of femoral tunnel position on radiographs with the knee in extension, which was found to be reliable in this setting.[32] Most likely because of its simplicity, it also became used for arthroscopic measurements. However, because it is a 2-dimensional reference, it does not take into account the depth and the o'clock position changes depending on the flexion angle of the knee joint.[33] It became clear during the twenty-first century that the o'clock reference is not an adequate method of reporting tunnel position; hence, newer studies have started to use other methods of documenting femoral bone tunnels, such as intraoperative arthroscopic pictures.

Three-Portal Technique and Transportal Drilling

In the late 1990s and the beginning of the twenty-first century, several femoral drilling techniques were developed as the limitations of the transtibial technique were brought to light. During this period of time, it became clear that the nonanatomic transtibial ACL reconstruction did not result in satisfactory knee joint kinematics and seemingly did not prevent long-term osteoarthritis.[1,25,34] Following the increased knowledge of native ACL anatomy and knee joint kinematics, new recommendations and surgical techniques were developed. The restrictive link created when drilling through the tibial tunnel, which could cause inaccurate and nonanatomic femoral tunnel position, was remedied by the development of the so-called transportal drilling.[25,35–43] Initially, arthroscopic drilling was performed through the anteromedial portal; this was developed further to today's 3-portal technique. The 3 portals consist of the lateral portal, central medial portal, and accessory medial portal (**Fig. 3**). These portals aid in both

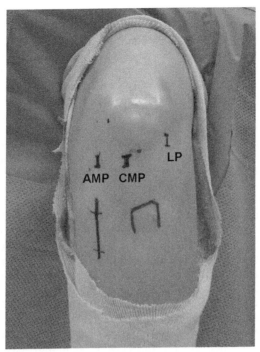

Fig. 3. Before ACL reconstruction with markings for arthroscopic portals. AMP, accessory medial portal; CMP, central medial portal; LP, lateral portal.

improved visualization of the lateral femoral condyle and in drilling of the femoral bone tunnel. In transportal drilling, the femoral tunnel is drilled independently of the tibial tunnel through the medial portal or the accessory medial portal. This technique facilitates anatomic placement of the graft, preservation of the ACL remnants, and isolated reconstruction of either ACL bundle.[44] Several studies have provided data in support of the fact that native femoral footprints are reached more often through transportal drilling than transtibial.[39–42] Interestingly, researchers have also started to promote the previous 2-incision technique once again. Similar to transportal drilling, there are no restrictions in femoral tunnel placement. However, there are 2 more advantages. There is no need for knee hyperflexion during femoral bone tunnel drilling, and it seems that longer femoral bone tunnels can be achieved.[45] Whether these advantages are enough for orthopedic surgeons to start using this technique once again is yet to be seen. Today, transportal drilling has increased in popularity, whereas the transtibial technique has decreased.

Anatomic Single- and Double-Bundle ACL Reconstruction

The 2 functional bundles of the ACL named after their respective tibial insertion, the anteromedial (AM) and the posterolateral (PL) bundle, have been known since the Weber brothers' thorough description of the ACL in 1836.[1] The first reported double-bundle ACL reconstruction was performed in 1983 by William Mott in Wyoming. However, this reconstructive technique and the others that followed most likely did not replicate the native bundle tension patterns or footprints. In 1994, a review was published by Andersen and Amis[46] that analyzed studies concerning tension on the natural and the reconstructed ACL. The investigators reported that different grafts required different tension and that graft placement and tensioning angle was important to restore normal stability.[46] In 1997, Sakane and colleagues[47] published on the in situ forces of the respective bundles. This article was the first of its kind and revealed that the in situ forces of the PL bundle were affected by knee flexion angle, in contrast to the AM bundle. It became clear later on that the AM bundle is taut throughout knee flexion and tightened to its maximum at 45° to 60° and that the PL bundle is tightened to its maximum when the knee is near full extension.[26] Consequently, the PL bundle plays an important role when the knee is near extension and the same applies to the AM bundle when the knee is in flexion. Thus, one part of the ACL will always be taut during movement. These data created a shift in focus toward reconstructing 2 bundles instead of 1 bundle. At this time, double-bundle ACL reconstruction was called anatomic because it aimed to recreate functional bundle anatomy. However, at the beginning of the twenty-first century, it became obvious that double-bundle ACL reconstruction was actually not necessarily anatomic.[3] Most studies may have tried to replicate the tension patterns of the native ACL; however, the placement of the femoral tunnel was probably not always in the native femoral footprint. This idea became evident as the footprints were more thoroughly studied both in the clinical setting and in research in general. This newfound research also changed the bone tunnel placement for single-bundle ACL reconstruction to the native footprints of the ACL. Both biomechanical studies and a systematic review on randomized controlled trials found that double-bundle ACL reconstruction was more successful in restoring rotatory laxity.[25,48] However, additional research was undertaken when it became evident that investigations performing double-bundle ACL reconstruction did not necessarily do it with respect to the native footprint.[2,3] To increase homogeneity of the studies, the concepts of anatomic ACL reconstruction has been presented.[4] New studies found that anatomic double-bundle ACL reconstruction is superior to anatomic single-bundle ACL reconstruction, which in turn is superior to the conventional single-bundle ACL reconstruction.[49] Today, there are guidelines and principles for both anatomic single- and double-bundle ACL reconstruction.[4]

GRAFT TYPE
Synthetic Grafts

The use of synthetics when reconstructing the ACL is theoretically very appealing, allowing surgeons to use custom made off-the-shelf grafts while also shortening operating time by avoiding time-consuming graft harvest. Accordingly, patients undergoing reconstructive surgery would be free of donor site morbidity, such as muscle weakness and pain. However, more than a century later, through several clinical attempts with silk, silver wire, Teflon (DuPont, Wilmington, Delaware), polyester, carbon fibers, the polypropylene ligament augmentation device, and GORE-TEX (W.L. Gore & Associates, Inc, Newark, Delaware) synthetic graft materials have not proven to be the revolution once thought to be. This finding is mainly attributable to graft failures because the biologic and mechanical properties of synthetic grafts never measure up to biologic grafts.[1,5,50,51] Therefore, the use of synthetic grafts over the past 3 decades has rightfully decreased and is probably only applied in experimental settings.

Allografts

Like synthetic graft materials, allografts are associated with the absence of harvest site symptoms, leaving the flexor and extensor muscles intact. Although operating time is shortened, the use of allografts demand thorough processing methods to reduce the risk of transmitted viral disease. The most commonly chosen allografts are patellar tendon, Achilles tendon, and tibialis anterior tendon, which offer off-the-shelf availability but are unfortunately associated with a higher risk of graft failure in young and active patients.[52,53] Today, the main indications for allograft reconstruction is ACL revision surgery, multiple ligament reconstruction, older patients, and athletes with high demands on knee function and low tolerance for leg muscle deficits.[4] With time, the processing techniques have improved and the demand for allografts has increased; however, they will naturally always be inferior to autografts in terms of healing (**Fig. 4**).

Patellar Tendon

Jones pioneered the ACL reconstruction development with his paper in 1963, describing a new surgical technique for ligament reconstruction.[54] Jones used the central third of the patellar tendon but still left the graft attached to the tibial tubercle. A decade later, Artmann[55] concluded that distally attached patellar grafts were not long enough to reach an anatomic insertion, which prompted studies on free patellar tendon grafts that would eventually lead to its status as the gold standard in ACL reconstruction following the work of Franke.[1,55,56] The advantage of the free patellar tendon graft is the bone plugs in each end, making it ideal for fixation and osseointegration (**Fig. 5**). It is a more rigid reconstruction than the hamstring grafts, which might promote earlier return to strenuous sport activities.[48] Furthermore, it allows for preoperative graft dimension assessment through magnetic resonance imaging (MRI). The patellar tendon autografts are, however, not suitable for double-bundle ACL reconstruction. As a result of the harvesting technique, reconstruction with the patellar tendon is associated with particular donor site morbidity, such as anterior knee pain, kneeling pain, and quadriceps weakness, and maybe even osteoarthritis in the long term when compared with hamstring grafts.[48,57–59]

Quadriceps Tendon

Considering the potential complications following the patellar tendon graft reconstruction, knee surgeons turned their attention proximally to the quadriceps tendon, following the studies of Blauth and Fulkerson and Langeland.[60,61] The quadriceps tendon graft design is somewhat similar to that of the patellar tendon graft with its bone-attachment possibilities and the chance to assess graft dimensions preoperatively. The quadriceps tendon is substantially thicker, which facilitates more coverage of the femoral footprint than the patellar tendon. Furthermore, the structure of the quadriceps tendon with rectus and vastus intermedius portions makes it suitable for both single- and double-bundle ACL reconstruction. The large cross-sectional area

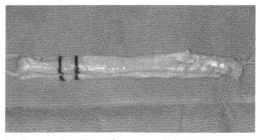

Fig. 4. A doubled tibialis anterior allograft prepared for ACL reconstruction.

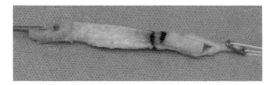

Fig. 5. A patellar tendon allograft prepared for ACL reconstruction. An Endobutton is attached to the bone block for the femoral tunnel.

is also considered when performing revision surgery on patients with potentially widened bone tunnels.

Hamstring Tendon

Since the early works by Edwards on cadavers in 1927, the hamstring tendon has continuously increased in popularity.[1,62] In the 1980s, the hamstring autograft reconstruction was modernized by Friedman (after the introduction of arthroscopic instrumentation) by going one step further and using a quadrupled hamstring graft, eventually making it the most frequently used graft type today (**Fig. 6**).[4] In Sweden, the quadrupled hamstring graft accounts for 98% of the graft choice in all ACL reconstructions.[63] In Norway, the graft accounts for 60%; in the Multicenter Orthopedic Outcomes Network cohort from the United States, it accounts for 44% of all ACL reconstructions.[64] The comparison of the patellar tendon and hamstring tendon graft has been a topic of great interest and source of numerous publications throughout the past few decades aiming to appoint the optimal graft of choice.[48,65] However, as it turned out, the reality is more complicated and the different graft choices simply represent different characteristics. A systematic review concluded that in terms of clinical outcome, there are no major differences between the patellar tendon and the hamstring tendon graft.[48] A recently published long-term cohort study by Leys and colleagues[57] could, however, point out that the patellar tendon graft reconstruction was associated with more radiological osteoarthritis and contralateral ACL rupture, although patient satisfaction and activity level were excellent. Today, the hamstrings tendon graft is used in both single- and double-bundle ACL reconstruction. However, the hamstrings tendon puts the surgical skill of the orthopedic surgeon to test because it is not possible to preoperatively asses the graft dimensions of the tendon, which can be done both with the patellar tendon and the quadriceps tendon. Also, complete footprint coverage of the femoral ACL insertion site is not always possible.

FIXATION TECHNIQUES

For the purpose of understanding the rapid development in graft fixation techniques, one must appreciate that the reconstructed ACL is no stronger than its weakest link,

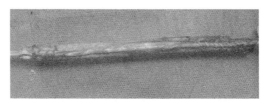

Fig. 6. A quadrupled semitendinosus and gracilis tendon graft prepared for ACL reconstruction.

which is the graft fixation, as noted by Kurosaka and colleagues.[66] The patellar tendon autograft with an interference screw fixation technique has enjoyed a status of gold standard since the latter part of the twentieth century.[4] However, with the emerging world-wide popularity of the hamstring graft and lesser used graft types, such as the quadriceps tendon autograft and Achilles tendon allograft, graft fixation techniques have developed accordingly, producing an amazing range of methods of how to anchor the newly reconstructed ACL to the housing of its new environment.[65]

Metal Interference Screws

Kurosaka et al performed a cadaveric study in 1987 helped bring forth the metal interference screws to wider attention, becoming the standard fixation technique when reconstructing the ACL with a patellar tendon graft (**Fig. 7**).[66] A decade later, Pinczewski and colleagues[67] published the results of a hamstring graft reconstruction with a round-headed cannulated interference (RCI) screw. The RCI screw reconstruction entailed histologic signs of osseointegration with collagen fiber continuity between bone and graft, proving the RCI screw to be universally suitable for soft tissue graft fixation. It is important to note that interference screws are aperture fixators and, therefore, a possible cause of altered grafts kinematics because they press the graft against the bone tunnel wall. However, aperture fixators produce a more rigid complex, yielding less bone tunnel widening.[65] Finally, metal interference screws prevent 360° tunnel healing and, thus, less bone-to-tendon interface.

Bioabsorbable Screws

Using bioabsorbable interference screws is increasingly popular when fixating a hamstring graft on the femoral side. There are basically 2 different types of bioabsorbable screws: the poly-L-lactic acid (PLLA) screw and the polyglyconate screw.[65] They offer the advantage of disappearing at some point after reconstruction, producing less interference with MRI, although their disappearance might take considerably longer than expected.[68,69] In addition, future knee surgery, such as graft revision, is theoretically simplified by not having to consider removal of previously inserted metal objects.[65] In fact, a systematic review showed that biodegradable screws seem to produce equal clinical results to those of metal screws with no higher

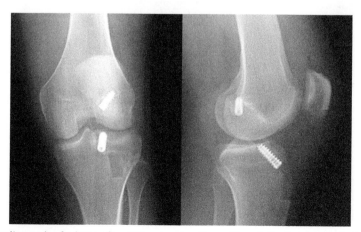

Fig. 7. Radiograph of a knee after ACL reconstruction with patellar tendon graft fixed with metal inference screws on the femur and the tibia.

incidence of osteoarthritis. Adverse effects are, however, tunnel widening and the risk of breakage on insertion.[65]

Endobutton

The Endobutton (Smith & Nephew Endoscopy, Andover, Massachusetts) is an extracortical suspensory fixation technique, which has gained popularity and widespread use along with the hamstring graft. Introduced in 1994, the Endobutton was initially designed to anchor the hamstring graft at the femoral tunnel aperture. Proving to be very useful and easy to handle, the Endobutton has gone through many adaptations over the years and is also now used in conjunction with the patellar tendon graft (**Fig. 8**). Anchoring a graft far away from the knee joint does, however, induce some micromobility of the graft inside the bone tunnel during loading and may be a cause of tunnel widening.[65] At the same time, the extracortical fixation creates a long bone–tendon interface, making it suitable for many types of ACL reconstruction techniques as well as single- and double-bundle reconstruction.

EndoPearl and Staples

When reconstructing the ACL using the hamstring or quadriceps tendon graft, it is possible to enhance the fixation technique both proximally and distally. The EndoPearl (Linvatec, Largo, Florida), which basically is a plastic bead sewn to the graft, is used as an adjunct to a bioabsorbable screw to prevent the graft from slipping inside the femoral tunnel.[70–72] Recently, the EndoPearl device was also shown to work on the tibial side.[73] Yet another technique for fixating the graft on the tibial side is the use of a staple, which is inserted distally to the tibial screw, below the tibial tunnel opening. The use of a staple, however, increases kneeling pain after ACL reconstruction.[74]

Cross-pins

Cross-pins offer the advantage of high failure loads while also producing less femoral and tibial tunnel widening, which may be attributable to fixation closer to the joint. Fixating the graft closer to the joint is thought to counteract graft motion inside the bone tunnel. Clinical results are, however, comparable with interference screws and

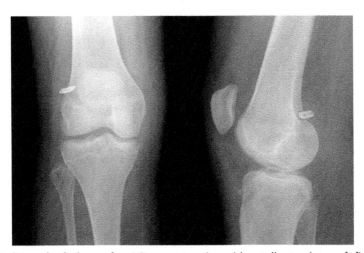

Fig. 8. Radiograph of a knee after ACL reconstruction with patellar tendon graft fixed with an Endobutton on the femur.

the Endobutton when used in hamstring and patellar tendon reconstruction, respectively.[75–82] Cross-pins together with the transtibial technique were once the gold standard. This position has changed with the increased use of transportal drilling because there are only guidelines available for the use of cross-pins in conjunction with the transtibial drilling technique.

SUMMARY

There has been an amazing evolution in the knowledge of ACL anatomy and the surgical techniques for ACL reconstruction from open to arthroscopic reconstruction. An outline of the new surgical preferences is starting to form, yet another shift in paradigm is identified, the anatomic reconstructive concept. Today, orthopedic knee surgeons performing ACL reconstruction have a wide array of graft choices and fixation techniques at hand, which enables them to specifically tailor each reconstruction to patients' anatomy and specific needs.

REFERENCES

1. Schindler OS. Surgery for anterior cruciate ligament deficiency: a historical perspective. Knee Surg Sports Traumatol Arthrosc 2012;20(1):5–47.
2. van Eck CF, Samuelsson K, Vyas SM, et al. Systematic review on cadaveric studies of anatomic anterior cruciate ligament reconstruction. Knee Surg Sports Traumatol Arthrosc 2011;19(Suppl 1):S101–8.
3. van Eck CF, Schreiber VM, Mejia HA, et al. "Anatomic" anterior cruciate ligament reconstruction: a systematic review of surgical techniques and reporting of surgical data. Arthroscopy 2010;26(Suppl 9):S2–12.
4. Karlsson J, Irrgang JJ, van Eck CF, et al. Anatomic single- and double-bundle anterior cruciate ligament reconstruction, part 2: clinical application of surgical technique. Am J Sports Med 2011;39(9):2016–26.
5. Grontvedt T, Engebretsen L, Benum P, et al. A prospective, randomized study of three operations for acute rupture of the anterior cruciate ligament. Five-year follow-up of one hundred and thirty-one patients. J Bone Joint Surg Am 1996; 78(2):159–68.
6. Sandberg R, Balkfors B, Nilsson B, et al. Operative versus non-operative treatment of recent injuries to the ligaments of the knee. A prospective randomized study. J Bone Joint Surg Am 1987;69(8):1120–6.
7. Grøntvedt T, Engebretsen L. Comparison between two techniques for surgical repair of the acutely torn anterior cruciate ligament. A prospective, randomized follow-up study of 48 patients. Scand J Med Sci Sports 1995;5(6):358–63.
8. Dandy DJ. Arthroscopic surgery of the knee. Br J Hosp Med 1982;27(4):360, 362, 365.
9. Buss DD, Warren RF, Wickiewicz TL, et al. Arthroscopically assisted reconstruction of the anterior cruciate ligament with use of autogenous patellar-ligament grafts. Results after twenty-four to forty-two months. J Bone Joint Surg Am 1993;75(9):1346–55.
10. Cameron SE, Wilson W, St Pierre P. A prospective, randomized comparison of open vs arthroscopically assisted ACL reconstruction. Orthopedics 1995;18(3): 249–52.
11. Raab DJ, Fischer DA, Smith JP, et al. Comparison of arthroscopic and open reconstruction of the anterior cruciate ligament. Early results. Am J Sports Med 1993;21(5):680–3 [discussion: 3–4].

12. Shelbourne KD, Wilckens JH. Intraarticular anterior cruciate ligament reconstruction in the symptomatic arthritic knee. Am J Sports Med 1993;21(5):685–8 [discussion: 8–9].
13. Hess T, Duchow J, Roland S, et al. Single-versus two-incision technique in anterior cruciate ligament replacement: influence on postoperative muscle function. Am J Sports Med 2002;30(1):27–31.
14. Gerich TG, Lattermann C, Fremerey RW, et al. One- versus two-incision technique for anterior cruciate ligament reconstruction with patellar tendon graft. Results on early rehabilitation and stability. Knee Surg Sports Traumatol Arthrosc 1997;5(4):213–6.
15. Harner CD, Marks PH, Fu FH, et al. Anterior cruciate ligament reconstruction: endoscopic versus two-incision technique. Arthroscopy 1994;10(5):502–12.
16. Brandsson S, Faxen E, Eriksson BI, et al. Reconstruction of the anterior cruciate ligament: comparison of outside-in and all-inside techniques. Br J Sports Med 1999;33(1):42–5.
17. Reat JF, Lintner DM. One-versus two-incision ACL reconstruction. A prospective, randomized study. Am J Knee Surg 1997;10(4):198–208.
18. Panni AS, Milano G, Tartarone M, et al. Clinical and radiographic results of ACL reconstruction: a 5- to 7-year follow-up study of outside-in versus inside-out reconstruction techniques. Knee Surg Sports Traumatol Arthrosc 2001;9(2):77–85.
19. Amis AA, Zavras TD. Isometricity and graft placement during anterior cruciate ligament reconstruction. Knee 1995;2(1):5–17.
20. Zavras TD, Race A, Bull AM, et al. A comparative study of 'isometric' points for anterior cruciate ligament graft attachment. Knee Surg Sports Traumatol Arthrosc 2001;9(1):28–33.
21. Sommer C, Friederich NF, Muller W. Improperly placed anterior cruciate ligament grafts: correlation between radiological parameters and clinical results. Knee Surg Sports Traumatol Arthrosc 2000;8(4):207–13.
22. Amis AA, Dawkins GP. Functional anatomy of the anterior cruciate ligament. Fibre bundle actions related to ligament replacements and injuries. J Bone Joint Surg Br 1991;73(2):260–7.
23. Kurosawa H, Yamakoshi K, Yasuda K, et al. Simultaneous measurement of changes in length of the cruciate ligaments during knee motion. Clin Orthop Relat Res 1991;265:233–40.
24. Musahl V, Plakseychuk A, VanScyoc A, et al. Varying femoral tunnels between the anatomical footprint and isometric positions: effect on kinematics of the anterior cruciate ligament-reconstructed knee. Am J Sports Med 2005;33(5):712–8.
25. Yagi M, Wong EK, Kanamori A, et al. Biomechanical analysis of an anatomic anterior cruciate ligament reconstruction. Am J Sports Med 2002;30(5):660–6.
26. Yasuda K, van Eck CF, Hoshino Y, et al. Anatomic single- and double-bundle anterior cruciate ligament reconstruction, part 1: basic science. Am J Sports Med 2011;39(8):1789–99.
27. Jonsson H, Riklund-Ahlstrom K, Lind J. Positive pivot shift after ACL reconstruction predicts later osteoarthrosis: 63 patients followed 5-9 years after surgery. Acta Orthop Scand 2004;75(5):594–9.
28. Markolf KL, Hame SL, Hunter DM, et al. Biomechanical effects of femoral notchplasty in anterior cruciate ligament reconstruction. Am J Sports Med 2002;30(1):83–9.
29. May DA, Snearly WN, Bents R, et al. MR imaging findings in anterior cruciate ligament reconstruction: evaluation of notchplasty. AJR Am J Roentgenol 1997;169(1):217–22.

30. Cohen SB, Fu FH. Three-portal technique for anterior cruciate ligament reconstruction: use of a central medial portal. Arthroscopy 2007;23(3):325.e1–5.
31. Bedi A, Dines J, Dines DM, et al. Use of the 70 degrees arthroscope for improved visualization with common arthroscopic procedures. Arthroscopy 2010;26(12): 1684–96.
32. Yamazaki J, Muneta T, Koga H, et al. Radiographic description of femoral tunnel placement expressed as intercondylar clock time in double-bundle anterior cruciate ligament reconstruction. Knee Surg Sports Traumatol Arthrosc 2011; 19(3):418–23.
33. van Eck CF, Lesniak BP, Schreiber VM, et al. Anatomic single- and double-bundle anterior cruciate ligament reconstruction flowchart. Arthroscopy 2010;26(2): 258–68.
34. Woo SL, Kanamori A, Zeminski J, et al. The effectiveness of reconstruction of the anterior cruciate ligament with hamstrings and patellar tendon. A cadaveric study comparing anterior tibial and rotational loads. J Bone Joint Surg Am 2002;84(6): 907–14.
35. Yasuda K, Kondo E, Ichiyama H, et al. Anatomic reconstruction of the anteromedial and posterolateral bundles of the anterior cruciate ligament using hamstring tendon grafts. Arthroscopy 2004;20(10):1015–25.
36. Loh JC, Fukuda Y, Tsuda E, et al. Knee stability and graft function following anterior cruciate ligament reconstruction: comparison between 11 o'clock and 10 o'clock femoral tunnel placement. 2002 Richard O'Connor Award paper. Arthroscopy 2003;19(3):297–304.
37. Scopp JM, Jasper LE, Belkoff SM, et al. The effect of oblique femoral tunnel placement on rotational constraint of the knee reconstructed using patellar tendon autografts. Arthroscopy 2004;20(3):294–9.
38. Yamamoto Y, Hsu WH, Woo SL, et al. Knee stability and graft function after anterior cruciate ligament reconstruction: a comparison of a lateral and an anatomical femoral tunnel placement. Am J Sports Med 2004;32(8):1825–32.
39. Arnold MP, Kooloos J, van Kampen A. Single-incision technique misses the anatomical femoral anterior cruciate ligament insertion: a cadaver study. Knee Surg Sports Traumatol Arthrosc 2001;9(4):194–9.
40. Hantes ME, Zachos VC, Liantsis A, et al. Differences in graft orientation using the transtibial and anteromedial portal technique in anterior cruciate ligament reconstruction: a magnetic resonance imaging study. Knee Surg Sports Traumatol Arthrosc 2009;17(8):880–6.
41. Dargel J, Schmidt-Wiethoff R, Fischer S, et al. Femoral bone tunnel placement using the transtibial tunnel or the anteromedial portal in ACL reconstruction: a radiographic evaluation. Knee surgery, sports traumatology. Arthroscopy 2009;17(3):220–7.
42. Gavriilidis I, Motsis EK, Pakos EE, et al. Transtibial versus anteromedial portal of the femoral tunnel in ACL reconstruction: a cadaveric study. Knee 2008;15(5): 364–7.
43. Heming JF, Rand J, Steiner ME. Anatomical limitations of transtibial drilling in anterior cruciate ligament reconstruction. Am J Sports Med 2007;35(10):1708–15.
44. Cha PS, Chhabra A, Harner CD. Single-bundle anterior cruciate ligament reconstruction using the medial portal technique. Operat Tech Orthop 2005;15(2): 89–95.
45. Lubowitz JH, Konicek J. Anterior cruciate ligament femoral tunnel length: cadaveric analysis comparing anteromedial portal versus outside-in technique. Arthroscopy 2010;26(10):1357–62.

46. Andersen HN, Amis AA. Review on tension in the natural and reconstructed anterior cruciate ligament. Knee Surg Sports Traumatol Arthrosc 1994;2(4): 192–202.
47. Sakane M, Fox RJ, Woo SL, et al. In situ forces in the anterior cruciate ligament and its bundles in response to anterior tibial loads. J Orthop Res 1997;15(2): 285–93.
48. Samuelsson K, Andersson D, Karlsson J. Treatment of anterior cruciate ligament injuries with special reference to graft type and surgical technique: an assessment of randomized controlled trials. Arthroscopy 2009;25(10):1139–74.
49. Hussein M, van Eck CF, Cretnik A, et al. Prospective randomized clinical evaluation of conventional single-bundle, anatomic single-bundle, and anatomic double-bundle anterior cruciate ligament reconstruction: 281 cases with 3- to 5-year follow-up. Am J Sports Med 2012;40(3):512–20.
50. Murray AW, Macnicol MF. 10-16 year results of Leeds-Keio anterior cruciate ligament reconstruction. Knee 2004;11(1):9–14.
51. Moyen B, Lerat JL. Artificial ligaments for anterior cruciate replacement. A new generation of problems. J Bone Joint Surg Br 1994;76(2):173–5.
52. Carey JL, Dunn WR, Dahm DL, et al. A systematic review of anterior cruciate ligament reconstruction with autograft compared with allograft. J Bone Joint Surg Am 2009;91(9):2242–50.
53. van Eck CF, Schkrohowsky JG, Working ZM, et al. Prospective analysis of failure rate and predictors of failure after anatomic anterior cruciate ligament reconstruction with allograft. Am J Sports Med 2012;40(4):800–7.
54. Jones KG. Reconstruction of the anterior cruciate ligament. A technique using the central one-third of the patellar ligament. J Bone Joint Surg Am 1963;45:925–32.
55. Artmann M, Wirth CJ. Is the length of the patellar ligament sufficient for the repair of the anterior cruciate ligament? A roentgenologic analysis (author's transl). Arch Orthop Unfallchir 1974;79(2):149–52 [in German].
56. Franke K. Clinical experience in 130 cruciate ligament reconstructions. Orthop Clin North Am 1976;7(1):191–3.
57. Leys T, Salmon L, Waller A, et al. Clinical results and risk factors for reinjury 15 years after anterior cruciate ligament reconstruction: a prospective study of hamstring and patellar tendon grafts. Am J Sports Med 2012;40(3):595–605.
58. Keays SL, Newcombe PA, Bullock-Saxton JE, et al. Factors involved in the development of osteoarthritis after anterior cruciate ligament surgery. Am J Sports Med 2010;38(3):455–63.
59. Sajovic M, Strahovnik A, Dernovsek MZ, et al. Quality of life and clinical outcome comparison of semitendinosus and gracilis tendon versus patellar tendon autografts for anterior cruciate ligament reconstruction: an 11-year follow-up of a randomized controlled trial. Am J Sports Med 2011;39(10):2161–9.
60. Blauth W. 2-strip substitution-plasty of the anterior cruciate ligament with the quadriceps tendon. Unfallheilkunde 1984;87(2):45–51 [in German].
61. Fulkerson JP, Langeland R. An alternative cruciate reconstruction graft: the central quadriceps tendon. Arthroscopy 1995;11(2):252–4.
62. Edwards AH. Operative repair of cruciate ligaments in severe trauma of knee. Br J Surg 1926;13(51):432–8.
63. XBase, the Swedish national knee ligament register: annual report 2010. 2011. Available online at: www.aclregister.nu.
64. Magnussen RA, Granan LP, Dunn WR, et al. Cross-cultural comparison of patients undergoing ACL reconstruction in the United States and Norway. Knee Surg Sports Traumatol Arthrosc 2010;18(1):98–105.

65. Andersson D, Samuelsson K, Karlsson J. Treatment of anterior cruciate ligament injuries with special reference to surgical technique and rehabilitation: an assessment of randomized controlled trials. Arthroscopy 2009;25(6):653–85.

66. Kurosaka M, Yoshiya S, Andrish JT. A biomechanical comparison of different surgical techniques of graft fixation in anterior cruciate ligament reconstruction. Am J Sports Med 1987;15(3):225–9.

67. Pinczewski LA, Clingeleffer AJ, Otto DD, et al. Integration of hamstring tendon graft with bone in reconstruction of the anterior cruciate ligament. Arthroscopy 1997;13(5):641–3.

68. Drogset JO, Grontvedt T, Myhr G. Magnetic resonance imaging analysis of bioabsorbable interference screws used for fixation of bone-patellar tendon-bone autografts in endoscopic reconstruction of the anterior cruciate ligament. Am J Sports Med 2006;34(7):1164–9.

69. Stener S, Ejerhed L, Sernert N, et al. A long-term, prospective, randomized study comparing biodegradable and metal interference screws in anterior cruciate ligament reconstruction surgery: radiographic results and clinical outcome. Am J Sports Med 2010;38(8):1598–605.

70. Arneja S, Froese W, MacDonald P. Augmentation of femoral fixation in hamstring anterior cruciate ligament reconstruction with a bioabsorbable bead: a prospective single-blind randomized clinical trial. Am J Sports Med 2004;32(1):159–63.

71. Cheung P, Chan WL, Yen CH, et al. Femoral tunnel widening after quadrupled hamstring anterior cruciate ligament reconstruction. J Orthop Surg (Hong Kong) 2010;18(2):198–202.

72. Kim SJ, Kumar P, Oh KS. Anterior cruciate ligament reconstruction: autogenous quadriceps tendon-bone compared with bone-patellar tendon-bone grafts at 2-year follow-up. Arthroscopy 2009;25(2):137–44.

73. Kocabey Y, Nawab A, Caborn DN, et al. Endopearl augmentation of bioabsorbable interference screw fixation of a soft tissue tendon graft in a tibial tunnel. Arthroscopy 2004;20(6):658–61.

74. Hill PF, Russell VJ, Salmon LJ, et al. The influence of supplementary tibial fixation on laxity measurements after anterior cruciate ligament reconstruction with hamstring tendons in female patients. Am J Sports Med 2005;33(1):94–101.

75. Fauno P, Kaalund S. Tunnel widening after hamstring anterior cruciate ligament reconstruction is influenced by the type of graft fixation used: a prospective randomized study. Arthroscopy 2005;21(11):1337–41.

76. Harilainen A, Sandelin J. A prospective comparison of 3 hamstring ACL fixation devices–Rigidfix, BioScrew, and Intrafix–randomized into 4 groups with 2 years of follow-up. Am J Sports Med 2009;37(4):699–706.

77. Harilainen A, Sandelin J, Jansson KA. Cross-pin femoral fixation versus metal interference screw fixation in anterior cruciate ligament reconstruction with hamstring tendons: results of a controlled prospective randomized study with 2-year follow-up. Arthroscopy 2005;21(1):25–33.

78. Marks P, O'Donnell S, Yee G. A pilot clinical evaluation comparing the Mitek bone-tendon-bone cross pin and bioabsorbable screw in anterior cruciate ligament reconstruction fixation, a randomized double blind controlled trial. Knee 2008;15(3):168–73.

79. Price R, Stoney J, Brown G. Prospective randomized comparison of Endobutton versus cross-pin femoral fixation in hamstring anterior cruciate ligament reconstruction with 2-year follow-up. ANZ J Surg 2010;80(3):162–5.

80. Rose T, Hepp P, Venus J, et al. Prospective randomized clinical comparison of femoral transfixation versus bioscrew fixation in hamstring tendon ACL

reconstruction–a preliminary report. Knee Surg Sports Traumatol Arthrosc 2006; 14(8):730–8.

81. Sabat D, Kundu K, Arora S, et al. Tunnel widening after anterior cruciate ligament reconstruction: a prospective randomized computed tomography–based study comparing 2 different femoral fixation methods for hamstring graft. Arthroscopy 2011;27(6):776–83.

82. Stengel D, Casper D, Bauwens K, et al. Bioresorbable pins and interference screws for fixation of hamstring tendon grafts in anterior cruciate ligament reconstruction surgery: a randomized controlled trial. Am J Sports Med 2009;37(9): 1692–8.

Augmentation Technique for Anterior Cruciate Ligament Injury

Hiromi Kazusa, MD, Atsuo Nakamae, MD, PhD,
Mitsuo Ochi, MD, PhD*

KEYWORDS

- Anterior cruciate ligament (ACL) • Augmentation technique • Partial rupture
- Remnant-preserving technique • Double bundle

KEY POINTS

- The anterior cruciate ligament (ACL) augmentation technique has potential advantages in terms of proprioceptive function of the knee, revascularization of the graft, and contribution to knee stability.
- The decision of whether the remaining bundle represents partial rupture or complete rupture of the ACL was made on the basis of physical, magnetic resonance imaging, and arthroscopic findings in a comprehensive manner.
- Single-bundle ACL reconstruction with remnant-preserving technique is performed in cases of partial rupture of the anteromedial (AM) or posterolateral (PL) bundle of the ACL, and double-bundle ACL reconstruction with remnant-preserving technique is done mainly for patients with continuity of the ACL remnant between the tibia and either the femur or posterior cruciate ligament after complete rupture of the ACL.
- The femoral and tibial bone tunnel opening should not be placed at the center of the anatomic attachment of the bundle when using hamstring tendons, because the graft shifts to the anterodistal side in the femoral tunnel opening and to the PL side in the tibial tunnel opening.
- In cases of partial rupture of the AM or PL bundle of the ACL, surgeons should keep in mind that the remaining bundle is not completely intact and it is likely that the biomechanical function of the remaining bundle declines to some extent.

Anterior cruciate ligament (ACL) reconstruction has become a common treatment in orthopedic sports medicine. The normal ACL consists of 2 major functional bundles: the anteromedial (AM) bundle and the posterolateral (PL) bundle. Traditional single-bundle ACL reconstruction has concentrated mainly on the functional restoration of the AM bundle.

Recently, several studies have shown that the central anatomic single-bundle ACL reconstruction can restore normal knee function.[1–3] With this method, the tibial and

Conflict of interest: The authors report no conflict of interest.
Department of Orthopaedic Surgery, Integrated Health Sciences, Institute of Biomedical & Health Sciences, Hiroshima University, 1-2-3 Kasumi, Minami-ku, Hiroshima 734-8551, Japan
* Corresponding author.
E-mail address: ochim@hiroshima-u.ac.jp

femoral tunnels are well placed in the center of their respective ACL footprints. More-over, interest in double-bundle ACL reconstruction has been growing because of its greater potential to restore knee kinematics.[4–8] Double-bundle ACL reconstruction can mimic more closely the normal structure of the ACL. Restoration of the biome-chanical function is essential in ACL reconstruction. However, biological healing of the graft is vital to the achievement of satisfying clinical results. Accelerated biological healing is necessary not only for early return to sports but also for reliable remodeling of the grafted tendon.

ACL AUGMENTATION
Potential Advantages

Arthroscopic examination for ACL reconstruction occasionally demonstrates a rela-tively thick and abundant ACL remnant. In standard single-bundle or double-bundle ACL reconstruction, the ACL remnant is totally debrided to enable clear visualization of the femoral and tibial bone tunnels. However, recent studies have shown that human ACL remnants contain several types of mechanoreceptors. These mechanore-ceptors may provide positive effects on the proprioceptive function of the knee.[9–12] In addition, some studies have shown that the ACL remnants provide some biomechan-ical stability to the knee.[13,14] Therefore, ACL reconstruction that preserves the remnant by using the ACL augmentation technique might have several advantages:

1. The ACL remnant may contribute to knee stability and guarantee mechanical strength in the early postoperative period.
2. With respect to the proprioceptive function of the knee, nerve fibers may originate from the preserved ACL remnant and regenerate mechanoreceptors around the augmented graft.
3. The ACL remnant may accelerate cellular proliferation and revascularization of the grafted tendon.

Indications

The ACL remnant often maintains a bridge between the tibia and either the intercon-dylar notch or posterior cruciate ligament (PCL). Even when the substantial remnant maintains a bridge between the tibia and the intercondylar notch, the femoral attach-ment of the ACL remnant is often positioned abnormally. These cases represent a complete rupture of the ACL. However, sometimes a partial rupture of the AM or PL bundle of the ACL can be observed. In the authors' previous studies, the frequency of partial rupture was 10% during 2002 and 2005,[15] and 20% during 2006 and 2008.[13] In these cases, although rupture of the AM bundle or PL bundle could be seen, the other bundle was well preserved, with an attachment of anatomic femoral origin.

Partial rupture of the AM or PL bundle of the ACL
Previously, the authors performed the ACL augmentation procedure only for cases of partial rupture of the ACL. In these cases, single-bundle reconstruction of the ruptured bundle is desirable to minimize damage to the femoral attachment of the remaining bundle. Therefore, isolated AM bundle or PL bundle rupture is an indication for the single-bundle augmentation technique.

Continuity of the ACL remnant between the tibia and either the femur or PCL after complete rupture of the ACL
In 2008, the authors began performing the ACL augmentation procedure even for patients with continuity of the ACL remnant between the tibia and either the femur or PCL after complete rupture of the ACL. In this complete rupture group, the

indication for the procedure comprises cases whose ACL remnant maintains a ligamentous bridge between the tibia and either the intercondylar notch or PCL. Initially, central single-bundle ACL reconstruction with the remnant-preserving technique was performed for patients with a complete rupture. Recently, double-bundle reconstruction with the remnant-preserving technique has been performed to mimic more closely the normal structure of the ACL.

Preoperative and Intraoperative Evaluation

It is sometimes difficult to decide whether the remaining bundle represents a partial or complete rupture of the ACL. The decision was made after thorough consideration of physical, magnetic resonance imaging (MRI), and arthroscopic findings.[13] Quantitative evaluation of anteroposterior knee laxity can be one indicator for this decision. Partial rupture of the ACL was suspected when the side-to-side difference in the anterior displacement of the tibia was less than about 5 mm and a delayed firm end point was noted. The anterior displacement of the tibia was measured by the KT-2000 knee arthrometer or Kneelax-3 at 30 lb (13.6 kg). MRI also provides important information for evaluation of the femoral attachment of the bundles. However, the final decision was made after arthroscopic confirmation of the status of the injured ACL.

Evaluation by Arthroscopy

Arthroscopic intra-articular inspection was performed through the standard AM portal, anterolateral portal, and the far AM portal. A thorough arthroscopic probing is needed to precisely assess the ACL remnant patterns. Careful probing on the femoral side is important because most ACL ruptures occur in the proximal half. Partial rupture of the ACL was suspected when ligamentous continuous fibers were observed between the tibia and the anatomic femoral insertion of the ACL. Furthermore, arthroscopic examination should be performed in a figure-of-4 position and at various knee-flexion angles to consider the different tension patterns of the 2 bundles.[16–19]

Classification of the ACL Remnant

The ACL remnant pattern was thoroughly examined to determine the treatment strategy, and was classified (**Box 1**). Groups 1a and 1b indicate single-bundle reconstruction with the remnant-preserving technique. Groups 1c, 2a, 2b, and 2c indicate double-bundle reconstruction with the remnant-preserving technique. It is important for surgeons to keep in mind that, even in the partial rupture cases, the remaining bundle is invariably not completely intact. It is likely that the biomechanical function of the remaining bundle declines to some extent.

SURGICAL TECHNIQUE

Since 1992, the senior author has performed the ACL augmentation technique when indicated.[20] However, the early procedures required 2 incisions at the medial aspect of the proximal tibia and at the lateral femoral condyle, because the grafted tendon was fixed to the femur through the over-the-top route. This early technique had a serious flaw, because it was not a true reconstruction that restored normal ACL anatomy. Therefore, Ochi started to perform the 1-incision technique for ACL augmentation in 1996. Compared with the 2-incision technique, the 1-incision technique is less invasive and enabled reconstruction of the ACL in the anatomic portion. Here the authors introduce the ACL augmentation technique for partial and complete rupture of the ACL.[15,21–23]

Box 1
Classification of the ACL remnant

Group 1: Partial rupture of the ACL

   Group 1a: Partial rupture of the PL bundle

      The ligamentous AM bundle of the ACL had an attachment of femoral origin and was well preserved.

   Group 1b: Partial rupture of the AM bundle

      The ligamentous PL bundle of the ACL had an attachment of femoral origin and was well preserved.

   Group 1c: Partial rupture of the ACL but the remaining bundle could not be ascribed to either the AM or PL bundles

Group 2: Complete rupture of the ACL

   Group 2a: ACL remnant bridging the PCL and tibia

      The normal attachment of the ACL to the intercondylar notch was entirely lost.

   Group 2b: ACL remnant bridging the roof of the intercondylar notch and tibia

      There were no ligamentous continuous fibers in the normal attachment of the ACL to the femur. Diameter of the remnant was somewhat attenuated.

   Group 2c: ACL remnant bridging lateral wall of the intercondylar notch and tibia

      Attenuated ACL remnant healed to the lateral wall more arthroscopically anterior than its anatomic origin. There were no ligamentous continuous fibers in the normal attachment of the ACL to the femur.

   Group 2d: No substantial ACL remnants bridging the tibia and either the femur or the PCL

Patient Positioning and Graft Harvest

The patient was placed supine on the operating table, and a tourniquet was applied around the upper thigh. The knee was placed at 90° of flexion with a foot support and lateral thigh support, and full range of motion was possible. A longitudinal skin incision of approximately 4 cm was made on the anteromedial aspect of the proximal tibia. Semitendinosus and gracilis tendons were identified, and only the semitendinosus tendon was harvested using an open tendon stripper. For the preparation of a tibial bone tunnel, the periosteum was divided longitudinally and reflected medially, just medial to the tibial tubercle.

Graft Preparation

In the cases of single-bundle reconstruction with the remnant-preserving technique, a quadrupled semitendinosus tendon was used as the graft for the augmentation. An appropriate size of the EndoButton CL (Acufex; Smith & Nephew, Mansfield, MA) was determined according to the length of the femoral bone tunnel. The quadrupled semitendinosus tendon was connected to the EndoButton CL at the femoral side and to the polyester tapes (EndoButton tape; Acufex; Smith & Nephew) at the tibial side.

In the cases of double-bundle augmentation, 2 pieces of doubled semitendinosus tendon were used as a graft. The semitendinosus tendon was divided in half. Each tendon was then doubled, and EndoButton tapes were mechanically connected in series to each free end of the graft. The EndoButton CLs were then connected to each loop end.

Portal Placement

A 3-portal technique was used. The anterolateral portal was placed as medial (close to the lateral edge of the patellar tendon) as possible to allow visualization of the entire lateral wall of the notch. The AM portal was placed above the joint line, adjacent to the medial edge of the patellar tendon. Finally, the far AM portal was placed as inferior (close to the anterior portion of the medial meniscus) as possible, and 2.5 to 3 cm medial to the medial border of the patellar tendon. The use of this far AM portal for instrumentation allows the AM portal to be used to view the lateral wall of the intercondylar notch.

Femoral Bone Tunnel Preparation

There are 2 major techniques for creating a femoral tunnel. One is drilling through the tibial tunnel (transtibial technique) and the other is drilling through the far AM portal (far AM portal technique). The authors regularly use the far AM portal technique, because this technique allows more flexibility in accurate anatomic positioning for femoral tunnel drilling than the transtibial technique. It has been confirmed that the far AM portal technique is as effective as the transtibial technique and results in good restoration of joint stability and knee scores, despite a shorter femoral tunnel length and an inferoposterior position of the EndoButton.[24]

Excision of the femoral stump using a motorized shaver system was kept to a minimum. No notchplasty was performed. The targeted point for the femoral tunnel was marked with a microfracture awl with the knee at 90°. When performing single-bundle or double-bundle ACL reconstruction using hamstring tendons, the authors hold that the femoral and tibial bone tunnel opening should not be placed at the center of the anatomic attachment of the bundle. The graft is pulled and shifts to the anterodistal side of the femoral tunnel opening and to the PL side of the tibial tunnel opening. When the femoral tunnel is created at the center of the bundle's femoral footprint, the point of application of force at the tunnel opening shifts from the center of the femoral footprint to an anterodistal direction. The same can be said for the tibial tunnel. Thus, one must recognize that the center of the ACL's footprint is different from the optimal center of the bone tunnel. The center of the tunnel opening is not the central point of the application of force. It may be true that the biomechanical main part of the femoral attachment of the ACL is on the resident's ridge, and the remaining part is attached to the posterior portion of the ridge. However, although the femoral tunnel opening can partially include the resident's ridge, the authors maintain that the center of the femoral tunnel opening should be placed behind the resident's ridge, for reasons discussed previously (**Figs. 1** and **2**).

Single-bundle reconstruction with the remnant-preserving technique (Groups 1a and 1b)

In cases of PL bundle rupture (group 1a), the aim was to position the central portion of the femoral tunnel between 2 o'clock and 2:30 (left knee) or between 9:30 and 10 o'clock (right knee).[23] The marked position indicated that approximately one-quarter of the femoral tunnel opening should include the femoral attachment of the AM bundle (see **Fig. 1A**). Once again, surgeons should keep in mind that the remaining bundle is not intact and that the biomechanical function of the remaining bundle probably declines to some extent. It is unsuitable to create a bone tunnel at the center of the PL bundle attachment. A passing pin was inserted using the far AM portal technique to create a femoral tunnel with 110° to 120° of knee flexion. The length of the tunnel was calculated after increasing the diameter to 4.5 mm with the EndoButton drill. Then a femoral bone socket was created using a headed cannulated reamer of the same diameter as that of the proximal portion of the graft.

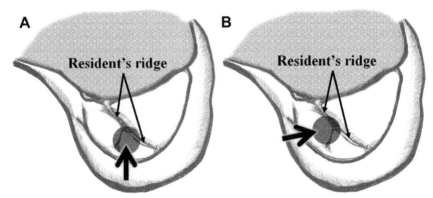

Fig. 1. Femoral bone tunnel placement (*short arrow*) in single-bundle ACL reconstruction with remnant-preserving technique. (*A*) In cases of posterolateral (PL) bundle rupture (group 1a), the center of the femoral tunnel was aimed at clock positions between 2:00 and 2:30 (*left knee*) or between 9:30 and 10:00 (*right knee*). The marked position (*short arrow*) indicated that approximately one-quarter of the femoral tunnel opening should include the femoral attachment of the anteromedial (AM) bundle. (*B*) In cases of AM bundle rupture (group 1b), the aim is to position the center of the femoral tunnel between 1:30 and 2:00 (*left knee*) or between 10:00 and 10:30 (*right knee*). The marked position (*short arrow*) indicated that approximately one-quarter of the femoral tunnel opening should include the femoral attachment of the PL bundle.

In cases of AM bundle rupture (group 1b), the aim was to position the center of the femoral tunnel between 1:30 and 2 o'clock (left knee) or between 10 o'clock and 10:30 (right knee).[23] The marked position indicated that approximately one-quarter of the femoral tunnel opening should include the femoral attachment of the PL bundle (see **Fig. 1**B).

Double-bundle reconstruction with remnant-preserving technique (Groups 1c, 2a, 2b, and 2c)

Through the far AM portal, a passing pin was directed at the targeted point, and the femoral tunnel was subsequently drilled through this portal. Furthermore, the centers of the femoral tunnel openings should be placed posterior to resident's ridge (see **Fig. 2**).[22] In group 2b, both the targeted points for the AM and PL femoral tunnels are posterior to the femoral attachment of the ACL remnant. In groups 1c and 2c, although the targeted point for the PL femoral tunnel is distal and posterior to the femoral attachment of the ACL remnant, the targeted point for the AM femoral tunnel is proximal and anterior to the ACL remnant, because the positions of the ACL remnants in groups 1c and 2c are more posterior than those in groups 2a and 2b. Therefore, in groups 1c and 2c, the ACL remnant is sandwiched between the 2 grafted tendons.

The passing pin was drilled through the femur to emerge on the lateral aspect of the thigh. After the passing pin was drilled, the procedure was the same as for single-bundle augmentation (see **Fig. 2**C).

Tibial Bone Tunnel Preparation

Tibial attachment of the ACL remnant is a useful landmark for orientation because in most cases the tibial side of the ACL remnant is almost normal. A longitudinal slit was made at the center of the ACL remnant through the AM portal (**Fig. 3**A). The tip of the tibial drill guide (Director Drill Guide System; Acufex; Smith & Nephew) was inserted

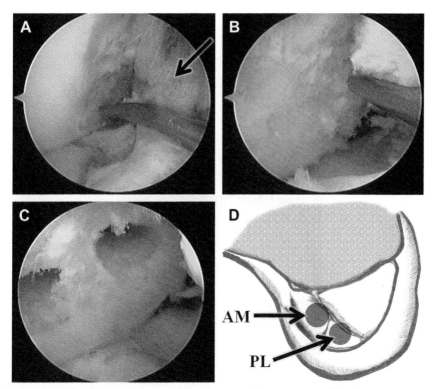

Fig. 2. Femoral bone tunnel preparation in group 2b (ACL remnant [*black arrow*] bridging the roof of the intercondylar notch and tibia; right knee). (*A*) The targeted point for the PL femoral tunnel was marked with a microfracture awl with the knee at 90°. (*B*) The point for the AM femoral tunnel. (*C*) Femoral bone tunnels for double-bundle augmentation. (*D*) Schematic (left knee) of femoral tunnel placement for AM and PL bundle.

through the AM portal. The tip was then put through the slit of the ACL remnant at an angle of up to 65° to the tibial plateau to allow visualization of the tip of the Kirschner wire (**Fig. 3**B).[22]

Single-bundle reconstruction with remnant-preserving technique (Groups 1a and 1b)
In cases of PL bundle rupture (group 1a), the tip of the drill guide was positioned in the center of the tibial insertion of the whole ACL. Then a 2.0-mm Kirschner wire was inserted using the drill guide. When the position of the Kirschner wire was satisfactory, the wire was carefully advanced by a conventional cannulated reamer to create a tibial bone tunnel. The size of the reamer was 0.5 mm smaller than the diameter of the distal portion of the graft. The tibial tunnel was then enlarged to the graft diameter with the appropriate tunnel dilator. In cases of AM bundle rupture (group 1b), the tibial tunnel opening should be positioned as anterior as possible within the tibial footprint of the ACL.[23] The position of the guide wire was then checked with the knee extended, to see if the guide wire impinged on the roof of the intercondylar notch.

Double-bundle reconstruction with remnant-preserving technique (Groups 1c, 2a, 2b, and 2c)
The tip of the tibial drill guide was put through the slit of the ACL remnant. Two 2.0-mm Kirschner wires were inserted into the tibial attachment of the ACL remnant using the

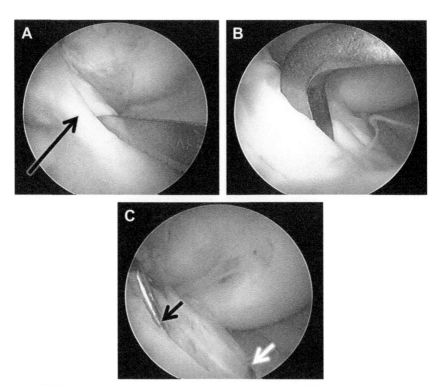

Fig. 3. Tibial bone tunnel preparation in group 2c (ACL remnant [*long black arrow*] bridging lateral wall of the intercondylar notch and tibia; right knee). (*A*) A longitudinal slit was made at the center of the ACL remnant. (*B*) The tip of the tibial drill guide was put through the slit of the ACL remnant. (*C*) The Kirschner wire for the PL bundle (*short black arrow*) was inserted at 8 mm posterior to the wire for the AM bundle (*short white arrow*).

drill guide. The drill guide was set at an angle of up to 65° to the tibial plateau, to allow visualization of the tip of the wires. The Kirschner wire for the AM bundle should be inserted to enable the tibial tunnel opening of the AM bundle to be positioned as anterior as possible within the tibial footprint of the ACL.[22] The Kirschner wire for the PL bundle was inserted at 8 mm posterior to the wire for the AM bundle to keep 2 to 3 mm thick of bony wall between the tibial bone tunnels (**Fig. 3**C).

Therefore, it is necessary to make a longitudinal slit in the ACL remnant to visualize the tips of the guide wires. In addition, when using the transtibial technique, it is difficult to find the tip of the Kirschner wire for the PL bundle in the slit, because this technique requires the wire to be inserted at a shallower angle to the tibial plateau. As a result, the wire for the PL bundle will be parallel to the preserved ACL remnant. Therefore, the use of an image intensifier is required for intraoperative localization of the wire when using the transtibial technique. However, the use of an image intensifier has several risks including radiation exposure, extended time in surgery, infection, and lower accuracy of measuring the distance between the wires than arthroscopy. The authors recommend the far AM portal technique, because it does not impose any restrictions on the angle of the tibial tunnel. Increasing the inclination of the tibial tunnels to 65° allows for better visualization of the tips of the guide wires. After the passing pin was drilled, the procedure was the same as for single-bundle augmentation.

Graft Passage and Fixation

Graft passage depends on the patterns of the ACL remnant and can be either through or above the slit of the ACL remnant.[22]

Graft passing through the slit of the ACL remnant

For cases such as partial rupture of the PL bundle, if the graft passes above the ACL remnant, the positional relationship is anatomically incorrect and there is a danger of impingement, whereby the graft should pass through the slit of the ACL remnant. To prepare for this method, a curved hemostat was passed through the slit to create a passage to the intra-articular aperture of the femoral tunnel. All of the grafts for the PL bundle as well as grafts for the AM bundle in groups 2a and 2b are indications of this method. **Fig. 4** shows an example of a graft passage for the PL bundle in group 2c. The creation of a passage through the ACL remnant allows minimal impingement of the ACL remnant against the reconstruction graft and the roof of the intercondylar notch.

Graft passing above the ACL remnant

As for the grafts for the AM bundle in groups 1b, 1c, and 2c, a looped Ethibond suture passed above the ACL remnant (**Fig. 5**). The graft composites were introduced from the tibial tunnel to the femoral tunnel using the looped Ethibond suture (**Fig. 6**). The

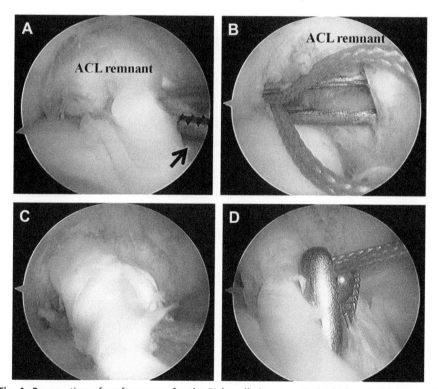

Fig. 4. Preparation of graft passage for the PL bundle in group 2c (right knee). (*A*) A curved hemostat was passed through the slit (*arrow*) to create a passage to the intra-articular aperture of the femoral tunnel. (*B, C*) A looped Ethibond suture for later introduction of the graft for the PL bundle was retrieved by the curved hemostat through the longitudinal slit in the ACL remnant. (*D*) An arthroscopic grasper was subsequently used to pass the retrieved Ethibond suture for the PL bundle into the created tibial tunnel for the PL bundle.

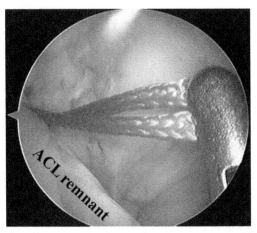

Fig. 5. Preparation of graft passage for the AM bundle in group 2c (right knee). A looped Ethibond suture for later introduction of the graft for the AM bundle was passed above the ACL remnant and was retrieved into the created tibial tunnel for the AM bundle by an arthroscopic grasper.

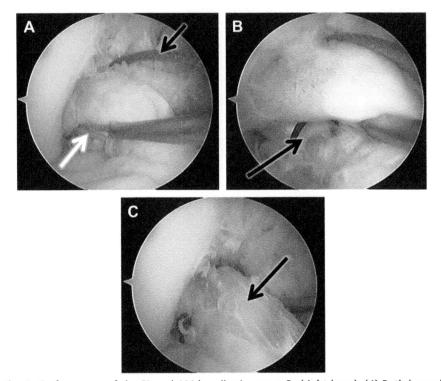

Fig. 6. Graft passage of the PL and AM bundles in group 2c (right knee). (A) Both looped Ethibond sutures for introduction of the PL bundle graft (*white arrow*) and AM bundle grafts (*black arrow*) passed under and above the ACL remnant, respectively. (B) First, the graft for the PL bundle (*arrow*) was introduced from the tibial tunnel to the femoral tunnel. (C) Second, the graft for the AM bundle (*arrow*) was introduced into the joint. In groups 2c and 1c, the ACL remnant was sandwiched between the 2 grafted tendons.

proximal side of the graft was fixed to the lateral femoral cortex by flipping the Endo-button and pulling the graft distally. Change in the length of the graft was examined during knee flexion-extension motion. In single-bundle augmentation, a tension force of 50 N was applied to the distal Endobutton tape connected to the graft and this was secured with 2 staples (Meira, Nagoya, Japan) at 30° of knee flexion. In double-bundle augmentation, a tension force of 30 N was applied to the EndoButton tape of each graft. The EndoButton tapes were fixed with 2 staples each at a knee flexion angle of 15° for the PL bundle and 40° for the AM bundle. Finally, the separated ACL remnant at the slit was sutured onto the graft to create a closed tube (**Fig. 7**). The authors first performed the ACL augmentation technique in 2011, using a quadriceps tendon–patellar bone autograft. Bone–patellar tendon–bone and quadriceps tendon can be good options for the augmentation technique (**Fig. 8**).

CLINICAL RESULTS IN THE LITERATURE

In 2000, Adachi and colleagues[20] reported that the joint stability and proprioceptive function in 40 patients who underwent the ACL augmentation procedure were superior to those of 40 patients who underwent standard ACL reconstruction during the same period. However, as mentioned, the early procedures needed 2 incisions and were not true reconstructions that restored normal ACL anatomy. Therefore, Ochi and colleagues[15] started to perform the ACL augmentation 1-incision technique for the partial rupture of the AM or PL bundle of the ACL, publishing their first report in 2006. Later, Ochi and colleagues[21] also showed that ACL augmentation using the 1-incision technique substantially improved joint stability, the joint position sense, and the Lysholm score postoperatively in cases of partial ACL rupture.

Recently, other orthopedic surgeons also demonstrated favorable clinical results using the ACL augmentation technique.[16,25–29] The preliminary results from Siebold and Fu[16] using autologous doubled or tripled semitendinosus tendon showed good clinical outcomes for AM and PL bundle augmentation at an average of 1 year postoperatively. Ahn and colleagues[28] reported good clinical and MRI results for

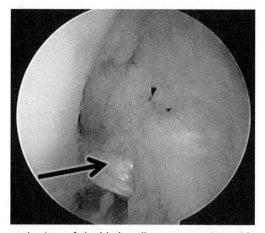

Fig. 7. Final arthroscopic view of double-bundle reconstruction with remnant-preserving technique in group 2b (right knee). In this group, both grafts for the AM bundle (*hidden*) and PL bundle (*arrow*) passed under the ACL remnant. The separated ACL remnant at the slit was sutured onto the graft.

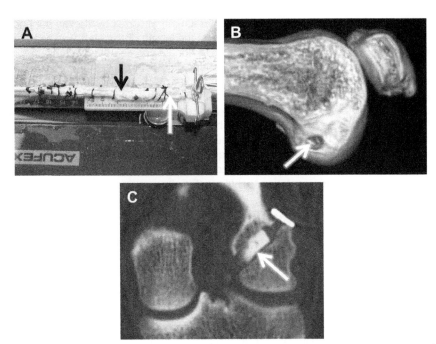

Fig. 8. ACL augmentation technique using quadriceps tendon–patellar bone autograft. (*A*) Quadriceps tendon–patellar bone autograft (*black arrow*, quadriceps tendon; *white arrow*, patellar bone). (*B*) Three-dimensional computed tomography image of the femoral side (*arrow*, bone block in the femoral tunnel). (*C*) Coronal computed tomography image of the femoral side (*arrow*, bone block in the femoral tunnel).

single-bundle ACL reconstruction using the remnant preservation and femoral tensioning technique.

Longer follow-up is necessary before a definitive conclusion can be reached, especially regarding the double-bundle augmentation technique. Nevertheless, the authors believe that this technique of preserving the remnant tissue of the ACL is a valuable procedure, especially in terms of biological healing of the grafted tendon. In the near future, a navigation system may play an important role in the ACL augmentation procedure.

SUMMARY

In ACL reconstruction, biological healing of the graft is vital to the achievement of satisfactory clinical results. The ACL augmentation technique has potential advantages in terms of proprioceptive function of the knee, revascularization of the graft, and contribution to knee stability. The decision of whether the remaining bundle represents partial or complete rupture of the ACL has to be made on the basis of thorough and comprehensive physical examination, MRI, and arthroscopic findings. Single-bundle reconstruction with the remnant-preserving technique is performed in cases of partial rupture of either AM or PL bundle, and double-bundle reconstruction with the remnant-preserving technique is performed mainly for patients with continuity of the ACL remnant between the tibia and either the femur or PCL after complete rupture of the ACL. However, in cases of partial rupture of the AM or PL bundle, surgeons should keep in mind that the remaining bundle is not completely intact and that the biomechanical function of the remaining bundle probably declines to some extent. Although longer follow-up is necessary before a definitive conclusion can be reached, the authors believe that this technique is a valuable procedure.

REFERENCES

1. Ho JY, Gardiner A, Shah V, et al. Equal kinematics between central anatomic single-bundle and double-bundle anterior cruciate ligament reconstructions. Arthroscopy 2009;25:464–72.
2. Asagumo H, Kimura M, Kobayashi Y, et al. Anatomic reconstruction of the anterior cruciate ligament using double-bundle hamstring tendons: surgical techniques, clinical outcomes, and complications. Arthroscopy 2007;23:602–9.
3. Kanaya A, Ochi M, Deie M, et al. Intraoperative evaluation of anteroposterior and rotational stabilities in anterior cruciate ligament reconstruction: lower femoral tunnel placed single-bundle versus double-bundle reconstruction. Knee Surg Sports Traumatol Arthrosc 2009;17:907–13.
4. Kondo E, Merican AM, Yasuda K, et al. Biomechanical comparisons of knee stability after anterior cruciate ligament reconstruction between 2 clinically available transtibial procedures: anatomic double bundle versus single bundle. Am J Sports Med 2010;38:1349–58.
5. Petersen W, Tretow H, Weimann A, et al. Biomechanical evaluation of 2 techniques for double-bundle anterior cruciate ligament reconstruction. Am J Sports Med 2007;35:228–34.
6. Hussein M, van Eck CF, Cretnik A, et al. Prospective randomized clinical evaluation of conventional single-bundle, anatomic single-bundle, and anatomic double-bundle anterior cruciate ligament reconstruction: 281 cases with 3- to 5-year follow-up. Am J Sports Med 2011;40:512–20.
7. Buoncristiani AM, Tjoumakaris FP, Starman JS, et al. Anatomic double-bundle anterior cruciate ligament reconstruction. Arthroscopy 2006;22:1000–6.
8. Fu FH, Shen W, Starman JS, et al. Primary anatomic double-bundle anterior cruciate ligament reconstruction: a preliminary 2-year prospective study. Am J Sports Med 2008;36:1263–74.
9. Adachi N, Ochi M, Uchino Y, et al. Contribution of mechanoreceptors in the anterior cruciate ligament to the joint position sense knee. Acta Orthop Scand 2002;73:330–4.
10. Denti M, Monteleone M, Berardi A, et al. Anterior cruciate ligament mechanoreceptors. Histologic studies on lesions and reconstruction. Clin Orthop Relat Res 1994;308:29–32.
11. Ochi M, Iwasa J, Uchino Y, et al. The regeneration of sensory neurones in the reconstruction of the anterior cruciate ligament. J Bone Joint Surg Br 1999;81:902–6.
12. Ochi M, Iwasa J, Uchino Y, et al. Induction of somatosensory evoked potentials by mechanical stimulation in reconstructed human anterior cruciate ligaments. J Bone Joint Surg Br 2002;84:761–6.
13. Nakamae A, Ochi M, Deie M, et al. Biomechanical function of anterior cruciate ligament remnants: how long do they contribute to knee stability after injury in patients with complete tears? Arthroscopy 2010;26:1577–85.
14. Crain EH, Fithian DC, Paxton EW, et al. Variation in anterior cruciate ligament scar pattern: does the scar pattern affect anterior laxity in anterior cruciate ligament-deficient knees? Arthroscopy 2005;21:19–24.
15. Ochi M, Adachi N, Deie M, et al. Anterior cruciate ligament augmentation procedure with a 1-incision technique: anteromedial bundle or posterolateral bundle reconstruction. Arthroscopy 2006;22:463.e1–5.

16. Siebold R, Fu FH. Assessment and augmentation of symptomatic anteromedial or posterolateral bundle tears of the anterior cruciate ligament. Arthroscopy 2008; 24:1289–98.
17. Petersen W, Zantop T. Partial rupture of the anterior cruciate ligament. Arthroscopy 2006;22:1143–5.
18. Sonnery-Cottet B, Chambat P. Arthroscopic identification of the anterior cruciate ligament posterolateral bundle: the figure-of-four position. Arthroscopy 2007;23: 1128.e1–3.
19. Sonnery-Cottet B, Barth J, Graveleau N, et al. Arthroscopic identification of isolated tear of the posterolateral bundle of the anterior cruciate ligament. Arthroscopy 2009;25:728–32.
20. Adachi N, Ochi M, Uchio Y, et al. Anterior cruciate ligament augmentation under arthroscopy. A minimum 2-year follow-up in 40 patients. Arch Orthop Trauma Surg 2000;120:128–33.
21. Ochi M, Adachi N, Uchio Y, et al. A minimum 2-year follow-up after selective anteromedial or posterolateral bundle anterior cruciate ligament reconstruction. Arthroscopy 2009;25:117–22.
22. Ochi M, Abouheif MM, Kongcharoensombat W, et al. Double bundle arthroscopic anterior cruciate ligament reconstruction with remnant preserving technique using a hamstring autograft. Sports Med Arthrosc Rehabil Ther Technol 2011;3:30.
23. Nakamae A, Deie M, Adachi N, et al. Augmentation procedure for partial rupture of the anterior cruciate ligament. Tech Knee Surg 2010;9:194–200.
24. Nakamae A, Ochi M, Adachi N, et al. Clinical comparisons between the transtibial technique and the far anteromedial portal technique for posterolateral femoral tunnel drilling in anatomic double-bundle anterior cruciate ligament reconstruction. Arthroscopy 2012;28:658–66.
25. Kim SJ, Jo SB, Kim TW, et al. A modified arthroscopic anterior cruciate ligament double-bundle reconstruction technique with autogenous quadriceps tendon graft: remnant-preserving technique. Arch Orthop Trauma Surg 2009;129:403–7.
26. Yoon KH, Bae DK, Cho SM, et al. Standard anterior cruciate ligament reconstruction versus isolated single-bundle augmentation with hamstring autograft. Arthroscopy 2009;25:1265–74.
27. Sonnery-Cottet B, Lavoie F, Ogassawara R, et al. Selective anteromedial bundle reconstruction in partial ACL tears: a series of 36 patients with mean 24 months follow-up. Knee Surg Sports Traumatol Arthrosc 2010;18:47–51.
28. Ahn JH, Wang JH, Lee YS, et al. Anterior cruciate ligament reconstruction using remnant preservation and a femoral tensioning technique: clinical and magnetic resonance imaging results. Arthroscopy 2011;27:1079–89.
29. Lee BI, Kwon SW, Kim JB, et al. Comparison of clinical results according to amount of preserved remnant in arthroscopic anterior cruciate ligament reconstruction using quadrupled hamstring graft. Arthroscopy 2008;24:560–8.

ACL Reconstruction and Extra-articular Tenodesis

Victoria B. Duthon, MD[a],*, Robert A. Magnussen, MD[b],
Elvire Servien, MD, PhD[c], Philippe Neyret, MD[c]

KEYWORDS

- ACL reconstruction • Extra-articular tenodesis • ACL revision

KEY POINTS

- Historically, anterior laxity in anterior cruciate ligament (ACL)-deficient knees was treated surgically by isolated extra-articular tenodesis, as described by Lemaire or MacIntosh.
- This procedure effectively limited rotation of the tibial plateau relative to the femur; however, isolated extra-articular reconstructions provided only moderate control of anterior laxity.
- The procedure was largely abandoned when single-bundle intra-articular ACL reconstruction emerged as the gold standard surgical treatment of ACL tear.

INTRODUCTION

Historically, anterior laxity in ACL-deficient knees was treated surgically by isolated extra-articular tenodesis, as described by Lemaire or MacIntosh.[1,2] This procedure effectively limited rotation of the tibial plateau relative to the femur; however, isolated extra-articular reconstructions provided only moderate control of anterior laxity. The procedure was largely abandoned when single-bundle intra-articular ACL reconstruction emerged as the gold standard surgical treatment of ACL tear. Some patients, however, experience persistent rotatory laxity after such reconstructions. Double-bundle ACL reconstruction was developed in part to allow improved control of rotational laxity through independent reconstruction and tensioning of the posterolateral (PL) bundle of the ACL. Although this procedure has been shown to produce excellent results in the hands of experienced surgeons, it is technically challenging, particularly in patients with smaller ACL footprints. Excessive rotatory laxity can also be controlled

Funding sources: Nil.
Conflict of interest: Nil.
[a] Department of Orthopaedic Surgery, Orthopaedic Surgery and Traumatology, University Hospital of Geneva, Rue Gabrielle-Perret-Gentil 14, Genève 1205, Switzerland; [b] Department of Orthopaedic Surgery, The Ohio State University College of Medicine, 2050 Kenny Road, Suite 3100, Columbus, OH 43221, USA; [c] Department of Orthopaedic Surgery, Hôpital de la Croix-Rousse, Centre Albert Trillat, 103 Grande rue de la Croix-Rousse, Lyon 69004, France
* Corresponding author.
E-mail address: victoria.duthon@hcuge.ch

sportsmed.theclinics.com

by the addition of an extra-articular lateral tenodesis to a single-bundle intra-articular ACL reconstruction. Recent studies report comparable results of double-bundle ACL reconstruction and single-bundle reconstruction augmented with lateral extra-articular tenodesis. The aims of this article are to review the clinical indications, surgical techniques, and reported results of augmentation of intra-articular ACL reconstruction with lateral extra-articular tenodesis.

BACKGROUND
Single-Bundle ACL Reconstruction

Single-bundle ACL reconstruction is performed to restore control of anterior and rotational knee laxity that is lost with rupture of the native ACL. Stabilizing the knee aims to prevent further injury to articular cartilage and the menisci and to maximize patient function. This technique provides good to excellent results in most cases and reliably restores function in activities of daily living and athletic activities in most cases. A meta-analysis of 48 studies (5770 participants) on return to sport after ACL reconstruction showed that 90% of participants achieved normal or nearly normal knee function; 82% of participants had returned to some kind of sports participation, 63% had returned to their preinjury level of participation; and 44% had returned to competitive sport at final follow-up.[3] Recurrent or persistent instability after ACL reconstruction, however, several studies report 11% to 30% of recurrent and persistent instability after ACL reconstruction.[4–6]

Failure of ACL Reconstruction

Reasons for instability after ACL reconstruction are varied[7] and include technical error (frequently tunnel malposition or failure to address associated injuries), inadequate graft material or fixation, traumatic reinjuries, and biologic failure.[8] Recurrent or persistent laxity, in particular rotational laxity associated with a positive pivot shift test, has been associated with poorer patient-reported outcomes after ACL reconstruction.[4] This rotatory laxity has been reported even without failure of the ACL graft, suggesting that in some patients a single-bundle intra-articular reconstruction is not sufficient to completely restore rotational knee stability.[9]

Double-Bundle ACL Reconstruction

Several approaches have been developed in recent years to improve rotational control after ACL reconstruction. First, the concept of anatomic ACL reconstruction has been advanced as a possible solution to persistent rotational laxity. The native ACL is composed of 2 bundles: the anteromedial (AM) bundle and the PL bundle. Traditional single-bundle ACL reconstructions often resulted in nonanatomic vertical graft placement or at best only recreated the AM bundle.[10] Vertical graft placement fails to recreate the PL bundle (which functions to resist tibial internal rotation near full-knee extension), possibly contributing to persistent rotatory laxity in some patients undergoing this procedure. More anatomically placed single-bundle reconstructions as well as anatomic double-bundle ACL reconstructions have been developed to better restore the function of the PL bundle. Biomechanical studies have demonstrated better rotational control with anatomic double-bundle reconstructions, leading to the increased popularity of these techniques.[10,11] Clinical superiority of this technique, however, has not been definitively demonstrated.[12]

Lateral Extra-Articular Tenodesis

Another approach to improve rotational control after ACL reconstruction is based on the concept that anterolateral capsular injury is frequently associated with ACL tears.

The capsular avulsion is termed a Segond fracture[13,14] when associated with bony avulsion of the lateral tibial plateau but does not always include an osseous fragment. This lesion has been shown to be present in the vast majority of acute ACL injuries and its presence is associated with significantly increased rotational knee laxity. Furthermore, when chronic anterior laxity is left untreated, rotatory laxity can develop due to a progressive stretching of secondary restrains in the lateral aspect of the knee.[15] This stretching can further increase anterior laxity. To address the contributions of anterolateral capsule injury to rotational knee laxity, some investigators have proposed the addition of a lateral extra-articular tenodesis to the standard intra-articular ACL reconstruction.[16] Several techniques classically used for isolated lateral tenodesis have been modified and used as an adjunct to intra-articular ACL reconstruction in this manner. These combined procedures are advantageous for several reasons. First, the longer lever arm of the lateral reconstruction allowed for efficient control of tibial rotation. Second, the lateral tenodesis may effectively control rotational laxity even in the face of failure of the intra-articular graft, provided a backup for the intra-articular graft in such cases.[17] Finally, the addition of a lateral tenodesis has been shown to decrease the stress seen by the associated intra-articular reconstruction by more than 40%.[18] These advantages are especially useful in cases of revision ACL reconstruction. One contraindication to lateral extra-articular tenodesis is the presence of a PL corner injury. In such cases, the tenodesis may tether the tibia in a PL subluxated position.

SURGICAL TECHNIQUES

Many lateral extra-articular tenodesis techniques have been described in the literature. The most common are summarized according to the type of graft used. The common goal of these different procedures is to diminish tibial internal rotation and anterior translation of the lateral tibia.

Iliotibial Band

Lemaire procedure

The Lemaire procedure was first described in 1967.[1] This extra-articular tenodesis uses a strip of iliotibial band measuring 18 cm long and 1 cm wide that is left attached to the Gerdy tubercle. Two osseous tunnels are prepared to anchor this graft: the first is in the femur, just above the lateral epicondyle and proximal to the lateral collateral ligament (LCL) insertion; the other is through the Gerdy tubercle on the proximal lateral tibia. Once the strip of iliotibial band is harvested and the bony tunnels are prepared, the graft is passed under the LCL, through the femoral bone tunnel, and back under the LCL and finally inserted into Gerdy tubercle via the second bone tunnel. Graft fixation is done at 30° of knee flexion, with neutral rotation (**Fig. 1**). When this technique is performed in association with a standard ACL reconstruction, a technical problem can be encountered in the lateral distal femur when the femoral tunnel made for the ACL graft interferes with the femoral tunnel made to anchor the iliotibial band graft. To avoid this problem, the bone-tendon-bone ACL graft can be prepared with a hole in the tibial bone block that is fixed in the femoral tunnel. The iliotibial band graft (**Fig. 2**A) can be passed through this bone block and is thus automatically anchored in the femur when the ACL graft is fixed in the femur (see **Fig. 2**B).

Modified Lemaire procedure

Christel and Djian[19] described a modified Lemaire procedure in order to simplify the classic Lemaire technique. First, the length of the iliotibial band graft is diminished in order to decrease the required skin incision and subcutaneous dissection on the

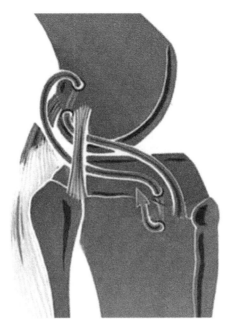

Fig. 1. Isolated lateral extra-articular tenodesis procedure as described by Lemaire.

lateral thigh. Christel and Djian described a graft measuring 75 mm long and 12 mm wide, again left attached distally on the Gerdy tubercle. The proximal portion of the graft is then passed to an isometric point on the lateral femoral condyle determined by a compass and secured in a femoral tunnel with an interference screw. To avoid possible devascularization of the LCL, the graft is not passed under the ligament. The graft is twisted 180° because this method has been shown by Draganish and colleagues[17] to yield more homogenous graft forces and better isometry.

MacIntosh procedure
The first described MacIntosh procedure[2] (MacIntosh 1) was similar to the Lemaire procedure; however, femoral fixation was achieved not via a bone tunnel but through suture fixation to the lateral intermuscular septum. This procedure was modified

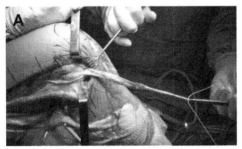
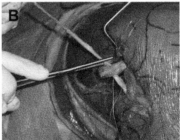

Fig. 2. Bone-tendon-bone ACL reconstruction and lateral extra-articular tenodesis with iliotibial band. (A) A strip of iliotibial band measuring 18 cm long and 1 cm wide is harvested and left attached to the Gerdy tubercle. (B) The strip of iliotibial band is passed through the bone block of the ACL graft before the bone block is press-fit into the femoral tunnel, securing it to the femur.

(MacIntosh 2) to include passage of the graft into the joint via the over-the-top position, through the notch, and into a tibial tunnel. In 1979, the Marshall-MacIntosh procedure[20] (MacIntosh 3) was described. The central third of the entire extensor mechanism is harvested with a wider portion taken from the prepatellar aponeurotic tissue. This graft was used to reconstruct the intra-articular ACL via a tibial tunnel and passage over the top of the lateral femoral condyle, and to complete the extra-articular tenodesis by fixing it in Gerdy tubercule. This same concept of using one graft to reconstruct both the ACL and perform the extra-articular tenodesis is used now with hamstring tendons (discussed later), although current techniques use a femoral tunnel rather than passing the tendons over the top.

Hamstrings

Hamstrings can be used to perform the extra-articular tenodesis alone or associated with an intra-articular reconstruction performed with other tissue or can be used for both the ACL reconstruction and the extra-articular tenodesis. Both techniques are described.

Hamstrings for both ACL reconstruction and extra-articular tenodesis

Colombet,[21] in 2011, described a mini-invasive technique using the same hamstring graft for intra-articular reconstruction and extra-articular tenodesis. The gracilis and semitendinosus tendons are harvested and stripped of muscle fibers. Then, the graft is prepared in 1 of 2 possible configurations according to the length or the tendons: 4 + 2 or 2 + 2. The overall length graft should measure at least 21 cm. When the gracilis and semitendinosus tendons are long enough to form a 9-cm segment containing 4 strands (which are used to reconstruct the ACL) and a 12-cm segment containing 2 strands (which are used to do the extra-articular tenodesis), the 4 + 2 configuration is used. If not, the 2 + 2 configuration is used. The tibial and femoral tunnel tunnels are drilled via an outside-in approach and absorbable interference screws are used in both tunnels to secure the graft. The remaining extra-articular graft is then passed under the iliotibial band and anchored with an interference screw in a tibial tunnel made in the Gerdy tubercle. Navigation can be used to optimize tunnel placement.

Bone-tendon-bone graft for ACL reconstruction and hamstrings for extra-articular tenodesis (authors' preferred technique)

Neyret[22] has reported a technique based on 3 articles,[1,23,24] described in detail by Magnussen and colleagues[25] in *Techniques in Knee Surgery*. A patellar tendon autograft is used for an intra-articular reconstruction of the ACL and a gracilis autograft is used for the extra-articular tenodesis. The semitendinosus tendon is preserved. The gracilis is passed through the tibial bone block of the ACL graft, making a single graft for both ACL reconstruction and extra-articular tenodesis (**Fig. 3**). The ACL graft is introduced into the knee through the femoral tunnel and the tibial bone block is impacted into the tunnel and press-fit. This procedure also fixes the gracilis in the femoral tunnel as it was previously passed through the bone block (**Fig. 4**A). The distal insertion of the gracilis is secured by a drill hole in the Gerdy tubercle on the tibia. The 2 free ends of the gracilis graft are passed distally. The most posterior is passed under the LCL, superficial to the popliteus tendon and through the bony tunnel in the Gerdy tubercle from posterior to anterior. The most anterior is passed under the LCL, superficial to the popliteus tendon and under the posterior portion of the iliotibial band and then through the same tunnel in the Gerdy tubercle from anterior to posterior. Tensioning of the graft is done at 30° of knee flexion and in neutral rotation. The 2 limbs of the graft are sutured to one another, side to side (see **Fig. 4**B).

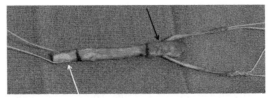

Fig. 3. Combined bone-tendon-bone: gracilis graft for reconstruction of the intra-articular ACL and lateral extra-articular tenodesis. The white arrow indicates the patellar bone block that will be fixed in tibial tunnel whereas the black arrow indicates the tibial bone block with gracilis tendon that will be press-fit into the femoral tunnel.

RESULTS

The results of the different techniques used to control both anterior tibial translation and rotatory laxity are discussed. A recent literature review article by Dodds and colleagues[26] summarized the results of 10 studies on isolated extra-articular tenodesis and of 13 studies on combined intra-articular ACL reconstruction with associated extra-articular tenodesis.

Isolated Extra-Articular Tenodesis

The overall long-term results of isolated extra-articular tenodesis are poor and only half of patients reported good to excellent results. The main problem with this technique is that it is a nonanatomic procedure that does not restore the function of the ACL in preventing anterior tibial translation. Amis and Scammell[27] showed an inability of isolated extra-articular tenodesis to restore normal anterior tibial translation while maintaining normal rotational laxity. In addition, increased degenerative changes of the lateral tibiofemoral compartment have been described after this procedure.[28] This degeneration may be due to overtensioning of the graft leading to overconstraint of this compartment or to the standard 4 to 6 weeks' postoperative cast immobilization that was standard at that time. Isolated extra-articular tenodesis in an ACL-deficient knee is no longer recommended.[29]

ACL Reconstruction and Extra-articular Tenodesis

Lateral extra-articular tenodesis does have a role when performed in association with a standard intra-articular reconstruction of the ACL, particularly in revision cases.

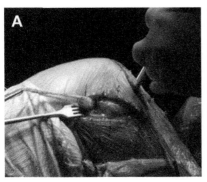
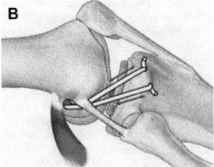

Fig. 4. Intra-operative picture (A) and schematic drawing (B) demonstrating the bone-tendon-bone: gracilis graft in place, reconstructing both the intra-articular ACL and completing the lateral extra-articular tenodesis.

Twelve of the 13 studies reviewed by Dodds and colleagues[26] reported good to excellent results in 80% to 90% of patients. The remaining study[30] performed an advancement of the biceps femoris tendon as an extra-articular restraint, which is different from the extra-articular tenodesis techniques described previously. Marcacci and colleagues[31] prospectively studied 54 high-level athletes who underwent ACL reconstruction with an associated extra-articular tenodesis. The hamstring tendons with intact tibial insertions were used for intra-articular ACL reconstruction and extra-articular reconstruction was performed with the remnant part of the tendons. They reported highly satisfactory results, with 90.7% of patients classified as International Knee Documentation Committee (IKDC) A or B 11 years after surgery. They did not find more knee osteoarthritis in this group compared with patients who did not have extra-articular tenodesis.

ACL Single-Bundle Reconstruction and Extra-articular Tenodesis Versus ACL Double-Bundle Reconstruction

Two studies have been published comparing double-bundle ACL reconstruction and single-bundle reconstruction with extra-articular augmentation.

Zaffagnini and colleagues[32] compared the static and dynamic behavior of the knee after either single-bundle ACL reconstruction with extra-articular tenodesis or anatomic double-bundle technique in 35 patients with an isolated ACL tear. A surgical navigation system was used to quantify knee laxity and the pivot shift phenomenon before and after surgery. They found that single-bundle reconstruction with extra-articular tenodesis better controlled valgus/varus laxity at full extension and internal/external rotation at 90° of flexion, whereas double-bundle reconstruction better controlled pivot shift phenomenon and restored the dynamic behavior of the knee. They conclude that extra-articular tenodesis is an easy surgical procedure that can be added to ACL reconstructions in patients not involved in highly demanding sport activities.

Monaco and colleagues[33] studied a group of 20 patients with ACL tear. Half of them underwent a double-bundle ACL reconstruction and half underwent a single-bundle reconstruction with extra-articular tenodesis. The goal was to evaluate the effect of both techniques on the internal rotation of the tibia. They found that both techniques significantly reduced anteroposterior displacement as well as internal and external rotation of the tibia compared with the preoperative condition. But the single-bundle with extra-articular tenodesis technique was more effective in reducing the internal rotation of the tibia at 30° of knee flexion compared with an anatomic double-bundle reconstruction.

Extra-articular Tenodesis in Revision ACL Reconstruction

Extra-articular reconstruction can also function as a backup to the ACL graft in cases of revision surgery. Trojani and colleagues,[34] in a multicenter French study on revision ACL reconstruction, assessed the influence of an associated lateral extra-articular tenodesis on knee stability and IKDC score; 163 patients with 2-year minimum follow-up were included. They found that when a lateral tenodesis was performed, 80% of patients had a negative pivot shift test, versus 63% in those without a tenodesis ($P = .03$). There was no significant difference, however, in the IKDC score. They conclude that the addition of a lateral extra-articular tenodesis in cases of revision ACL reconstruction increases knee stability but does not significantly improve the IKDC score.

DISCUSSION

Recent studies have shown that lateral extra-articular tenodesis increases knee stability when combined with intra-articular ACL reconstruction and shows a benefit in patients with combined anterior laxity and increased internal rotation of the lateral compartment. This control of rotation can be explained by the lever arm of lateral extra-articular tenodesis relative to the center of rotation of the knee. It efficiently controls tibial internal rotation while the ACL graft controls anterior translation of the tibia. The addition of a lateral tenodesis also has a benefit in revision ACL reconstruction.

Unfortunately, there are no well-validated clinical or radiologic criteria indicating which patients will experience persistent instability after isolated single-bundle intra-articular ACL reconstruction. Similarly, there is little evidence to guide the choice between a double-bundle ACL reconstruction and a single-bundle ACL reconstruction with extra-articular augmentation in such patients. It is possible that patients with associated lateral capsular injuries or increased preoperative pivot shift are more likely to benefit from additional stabilization. Current imaging studies, however, have not demonstrated the ability to identify lateral capsular injuries nor has it been proved that patients with an increased pivot shift preoperatively benefit more from these procedures. If a precise ligament of the anterolateral capsule was described as torn in certain ACL-deficient knees, the extra-articular tenodesis could be thought of as an anatomic procedure and it would be easier to determine which patients could benefit from this technique.

Surgical Indications for ACL Reconstruction and Extra-articular Tenodesis

In primary ACL reconstruction

To help surgeons deciding whether an extra-articular tenodesis should be added to the ACL reconstruction, some investigators have suggested potential clinical and radiologic clues.

Giraud and colleagues[35] compared patients who had isolated ACL reconstruction with patients who had ACL reconstruction and extra-articular tenodesis. At 7 years' follow-up, they found that extra-articular tenodesis improved the results in patients with increased anterior laxity of the lateral compartment preoperatively. Pivoting was better controlled in the lateral plasty group ($P = .23$) but there was no significant difference in direct anterior translation with the addition of the lateral plasty. They concluded that extra-articular tenodesis should be considered in patients with increased anterior laxity of the lateral compartment. Precise measurement of anterior knee laxity and tibial rotation, however, are still difficult to obtain. Several devices have been described for evaluation of static and dynamic knee laxity.[36–39] Further refinement of these techniques will greatly improve their ability to guide future treatment protocols.[40]

Imaging techniques have also been proposed to help guide treatment decisions. Lerat and colleagues[41] described a dynamic radiologic protocol for quantifying anterior and posterior displacement of the medial and lateral compartments of the knee. They classified anterior knee laxity based on the differential anterior translation of the medial compartment. They identified 4 grades for anterior laxity (1–4) in each of which 4 subgrades for laxity of the lateral compartment (A–D) have been distinguished. Based on this classification, they proposed an algorithm of treatment to help surgeons decide whether an extra-articular tenodesis should be added to the intra-articular ACL reconstruction. Among patients classified as grade 1 or 2 (up to 8 mm of anterior translation of the medial compartment), patients subclassified as subgrade A or B (up to 8 mm of anterior translation of the lateral compartment) can be treated with isolated intra-articular ACL reconstruction. Those subclassififed as subgrade C or D (more than 8 mm of anterior translation of the lateral compartment) may benefit from the addition of a lateral extra-articular procedure.

To objectively quantify this rotatory laxity of the knee, Espregueira-Mendes and colleagues[42] developed a porto-knee testing device. It allows evaluation of both anteroposterior and rotatory laxity of the knee during MRI examinations. The porto-knee testing device proved a reliable tool in assessment of anteroposterior translation (compared with KT-1000 arthrometer) and rotatory laxity (compared with lateral pivot shift under anesthesia) of the ACL-deficient knee during MRI examination.

Computer-assisted measurement techniques are also being developed to identify patients who may benefit from additional procedures to control rotational knee laxity. Branch and colleagues[43] showed that tibial internal rotation varies greatly among patients. In their study, patients with a contralateral ACL injury demonstrated significantly increased tibial internal rotation (20.6° vs 11.4°, $P<.001$) and reduced external rotation (16.7° vs 26.6°, $P<.001$) compared with healthy volunteers. Female patients demonstrated significantly increased internal and external rotation as well as significantly increased rotational compliance compared with male patients ($P<.05$). The investigators concluded that highly accurate and reliable computer-assisted rotational measurements allow surgeons to preoperatively target patients who may require surgical techniques that provide the greatest rotational stability, as adding an extra-articular tenodesis to the ACL reconstruction.

In revision ACL reconstruction

Because results of revision ACL reconstruction are generally considered inferior to those of primary ACL reconstruction,[7] some investigators have considered the addition of a lateral extra-articular tenodesis in these patients to improve knee stability. Although the evidence for such an approach is currently sparse, the few published studies on the topic suggest a role for this procedure in a revision population. Ferretti and colleagues[44] reported 90% good and very good results with revision ACL with doubled semitendinosus and gracilis tendons and lateral extra-articular reconstruction. Trojani and colleagues[34] reported the results of a retrospective multicenter study of 189 patients under revision ACL reconstruction, 14% of whom had a concomitant lateral extra-articular tenodesis. They found that the addition of a lateral tenodesis to revision ACL reconstruction did not improve the global IKDC score but did decrease the incidence of a positive pivot shift postoperatively and decrease the failure rate. It has been further suggested that the addition of lateral extra-articular augmentation may be a useful adjunct procedure in cases of re-revision ACL reconstruction, particularly in cases in which no clear reason for failure of the previous grafts (tunnel malposition, missed associated injuries, and so forth) was evident.[45,46]

Is Lateral Extra-articular Tenodesis an Anatomic Procedure?

An ACL-deficient knee presents with anterior laxity and a variable degree of associated rotational laxity. Variable degrees of injury to the lateral capsuloligamentous structures have been hypothesized as contributing to the degree of rotational laxity that is present.[47] Lateral extra-articular procedures to control knee laxity have classically been considered biomechanical rather than anatomic procedures because they do not reconstruct a clearly defined ligament in the manner of an intra-articular reconstruction.[48–50]

Anatomic studies have identified structures in the lateral capsule that could play a role in rotational knee stability. Segond[13] described a reinforcement of the lateral joint capsule by fibers of the iliotibial band. Terry and LaPrade[51] referred to this reinforcement as the "capsulo-osseous layers" of the iliotibial band and associated its injury with increasingly abnormal Lachman, pivot shift, and anterior drawer tests. LaPrade and colleagues[52] described the same structure as the "midthird lateral capsular ligament." Campos and colleagues[14] called it the "lateral capsular ligament" and Vieira and colleagues[53] referred to it as the "anterolateral ligament."

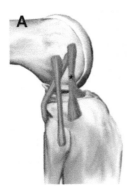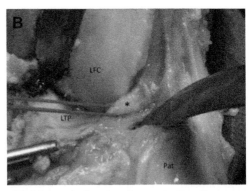

Fig. 5. The anterolateral ligament. (*A*) Schematic drawing demonstrating the course of the anterolateral ligament (*asterisk*). (*B*) Intraoperative photo demonstrating the anterolateral ligament (*asterisk*) in a patient undergoing total knee arthroplasty. LFC, lateral femoral condyle; LTP, lateral tibial plateau; Pat, patella.

The authors' team recently evaluated the anatomy of this structure anatomically and called it the "anterolateral ligament."[54] It was present in all 40 knees studied. It originated from the lateral femoral condyle, just anterior to the popliteus tendon, and inserted on the anterolateral tibial plateau. Its tibial insertion was posterior to the posterior border of the Gerdy tubercle. It can be supposed that it can be torn or avulsed during traumatic ACL injuries (**Fig. 5**). No biomechanical study has been done yet on this ligament. The anterolateral ligamentous structures of the knee are under significant load when the lateral tibia is translated anteriorly and could act as a secondary restraint, supplementing the primary role of the ACL in preventing tibial rotation and anterior translation. Therefore, an extra-articular tenodesis may be an anatomic procedure, reconstructing the injured anterolateral ligament.

SUMMARY

Extra-articular tenodesis may improve rotational stability when added to a standard single intra-articular ACL reconstruction in patients with explosive pivot shift test, patients involved in high-impact pivoting-sports, and in cases of revision ACL reconstruction. The surgical indications for this technique need to be improved to help surgeons select patients who would most benefit of this technique.

REFERENCES

1. Lemaire M, Combelles F. Plastic repair with fascia lata for old tears of the anterior cruciate ligament (author's transl). Rev Chir Orthop Reparatrice Appar Mot 1980; 66:523–5 [in French].
2. Ireland J, Trickey EL. Macintosh tenodesis for anterolateral instability of the knee. J Bone Joint Surg Br 1980;62:340–5.
3. Ardern CL, Webster KE, Taylor NF, et al. Return to sport following anterior cruciate ligament reconstruction surgery: a systematic review and meta-analysis of the state of play. Br J Sports Med 2011;45:596–606.
4. Kocher MS, Steadman JR, Briggs K, et al. Determinants of patient satisfaction with outcome after anterior cruciate ligament reconstruction. J Bone Joint Surg Am 2002;84:1560–72.

5. Anderson AF, Snyder RB, Lipscomb AB Jr. Anterior cruciate ligament reconstruction. A prospective randomized study of three surgical methods. Am J Sports Med 2001;29:272–9.
6. Eriksson E. How good are the results of ACL reconstruction? Knee Surg Sports Traumatol Arthrosc 1997;5:137.
7. Kamath GV, Redfern JC, Greis PE, et al. Revision anterior cruciate ligament reconstruction. Am J Sports Med 2011;39:199–217.
8. Menetrey J, Duthon VB, Laumonier T, et al. "Biological failure" of the anterior cruciate ligament graft. Knee Surg Sports Traumatol Arthrosc 2008;16:224–31.
9. Tashman S, Collon D, Anderson K, et al. Abnormal rotational knee motion during running after anterior cruciate ligament reconstruction. Am J Sports Med 2004; 32:975–83.
10. Yagi M, Wong EK, Kanamori A, et al. Biomechanical analysis of an anatomic anterior cruciate ligament reconstruction. Am J Sports Med 2002;30:660–6.
11. Schreiber VM, van Eck CF, Fu FH. Anatomic double-bundle ACL reconstruction. Sports Med Arthrosc 2010;18:27–32.
12. Yasuda K, Tanabe Y, Kondo E, et al. Anatomic double-bundle anterior cruciate ligament reconstruction. Arthroscopy 2010;26:S21–34.
13. Segond P. Recherches cliniques et experimentales sur les épanchements sanguins du genou par entorse. Progr Med 1879;7:297–341.
14. Campos JC, Chung CB, Lektrakul N, et al. Pathogenesis of the Segond fracture: anatomic and MR imaging evidence of an iliotibial tract or anterior oblique band avulsion. Radiology 2001;219:381–6.
15. Logan M, Dunstan E, Robinson J, et al. Tibiofemoral kinematics of the anterior cruciate ligament (ACL)-deficient weightbearing, living knee employing vertical access open "interventional" multiple resonance imaging. Am J Sports Med 2004;32:720–6.
16. Pearl AJ, Bergfeld JA, editors. Extraarticular reconstruction in the anterior cruciate ligament deficient knee. American Orthopaedic Society for Sports Medicine. Champaign (IL): Human Kinetics; 1992.
17. Draganich LF, Reider B, Ling M, et al. An in vitro study of an intraarticular and extraarticular reconstruction in the anterior cruciate ligament deficient knee. Am J Sports Med 1990;18:262–6.
18. Engebretsen L, Lew WD, Lewis JL, et al. The effect of an iliotibial tenodesis on intraarticular graft forces and knee joint motion. Am J Sports Med 1990;18:169–76.
19. Christel P, Djian P. Anterio-lateral extra-articular tenodesis of the knee using a short strip of fascia lata. Rev Chir Orthop Reparatrice Appar Mot 2002;88:508–13 [in French].
20. Marshall JL, Warren RF, Wickiewicz TL, et al. The anterior cruciate ligament: a technique of repair and reconstruction. Clin Orthop Relat Res 1979;143:97–106.
21. Colombet PD. Navigated intra-articular ACL reconstruction with additional extra-articular tenodesis using the same hamstring graft. Knee Surg Sports Traumatol Arthrosc 2011;19:384–9.
22. Neyret P, Verdonk P, Aït Selmi T. Chirurgie du genou, my knee practice. Paris: Masson; 2007.
23. Dejour H, Walch G, Neyret P, et al. Results of surgically treated chronic anterior laxities. Apropos of 251 cases reviewed with a minimum follow-up of 3 years. Rev Chir Orthop Reparatrice Appar Mot 1988;74:622–36 [in French].
24. Chambat PWG, Deschamps G, Dejour H. Acute lesions of the anterior cruciate ligament of the knee. A propos of 71 follow-up cases. Rev Chir Orthop Reparatrice Appar Mot 1984;70:152–5.

25. Magnussen RA, Jacobi M, Demey G, et al. Lateral Extra-articular Augmentation of ACL Reconstruction Techniques in Knee Surgery 2011;10:224–30.
26. Dodds AL, Gupte CM, Neyret P, et al. Extra-articular techniques in anterior cruciate ligament reconstruction: a literature review. J Bone Joint Surg Br 2011; 93:1440–8.
27. Amis AA, Scammell BE. Biomechanics of intra-articular and extra-articular reconstruction of the anterior cruciate ligament. J Bone Joint Surg Br 1993;75:812–7.
28. Strum GM, Fox JM, Ferkel RD, et al. Intraarticular versus intraarticular and extra-articular reconstruction for chronic anterior cruciate ligament instability. Clin Orthop Relat Res 1989;245:188–98.
29. Neyret P, Palomo JR, Donell ST, et al. Extra-articular tenodesis for anterior cruciate ligament rupture in amateur skiers. Br J Sports Med 1994;28:31–4.
30. Roth JH, Kennedy JC, Lockstadt H, et al. Intra-articular reconstruction of the anterior cruciate ligament with and without extra-articular supplementation by transfer of the biceps femoris tendon. J Bone Joint Surg Am 1987;69:275–8.
31. Marcacci M, Zaffagnini S, Giordano G, et al. Anterior cruciate ligament reconstruction associated with extra-articular tenodesis: A prospective clinical and radiographic evaluation with 10- to 13-year follow-up. Am J Sports Med 2009;37:707–14.
32. Zaffagnini S, Signorelli C, Lopomo N, et al. Anatomic double-bundle and over-the-top single-bundle with additional extra-articular tenodesis: an in vivo quantitative assessment of knee laxity in two different ACL reconstructions. Knee Surg Sports Traumatol Arthrosc 2012;20:153–9.
33. Monaco E, Labianca L, Conteduca F, et al. Double bundle or single bundle plus extraarticular tenodesis in ACL reconstruction? A CAOS study. Knee Surg Sports Traumatol Arthrosc 2007;15:1168–74.
34. Trojani C, Beaufils P, Burdin G, et al. Revision ACL reconstruction: influence of a lateral tenodesis. Knee Surg Sports Traumatol Arthrosc 2012;20:1565–70.
35. Giraud B, Besse JL, Cladiere F, et al. Intra-articular reconstruction of the anterior cruciate ligament with and without extra-articular supplementation by quadricipital tendon plasty: seven-year follow-up. Rev Chir Orthop Reparatrice Appar Mot 2006;92:788–97 [in French].
36. Mouton C, Seil R, Agostinis H, et al. Influence of individual characteristics on static rotational knee laxity using the Rotameter. Knee Surg Sports Traumatol Arthrosc 2012;20:645–51.
37. Lorbach O, Brockmeyer M, Kieb M, et al. Objective measurement devices to assess static rotational knee laxity: focus on the Rotameter. Knee Surg Sports Traumatol Arthrosc 2012;20:639–44.
38. Okazaki K, Tashiro Y, Izawa T, et al. Rotatory laxity evaluation of the knee using modified Slocum's test in open magnetic resonance imaging. Knee Surg Sports Traumatol Arthrosc 2012;20:679–85.
39. Haughom BD, Souza R, Schairer WW, et al. Evaluating rotational kinematics of the knee in ACL-ruptured and healthy patients using 3.0 Tesla magnetic resonance imaging. Knee Surg Sports Traumatol Arthrosc 2012;20:663–70.
40. Ahlden M, Hoshino Y, Samuelsson K, et al. Dynamic knee laxity measurement devices. Knee Surg Sports Traumatol Arthrosc 2012;20:621–32.
41. Lerat JL, Moyen BL, Cladiere F, et al. Knee instability after injury to the anterior cruciate ligament. Quantification of the Lachman test. J Bone Joint Surg Br 2000;82:42–7.
42. Espregueira-Mendes J, Pereira H, Sevivas N, et al. Assessment of rotatory laxity in anterior cruciate ligament-deficient knees using magnetic resonance imaging with Porto-knee testing device. Knee Surg Sports Traumatol Arthrosc 2012;20:671–8.

43. Branch TP, Browne JE, Campbell JD, et al. Rotational laxity greater in patients with contralateral anterior cruciate ligament injury than healthy volunteers. Knee Surg Sports Traumatol Arthrosc 2010;18:1379–84.
44. Ferretti A, Conteduca F, Monaco E, et al. Revision anterior cruciate ligament reconstruction with doubled semitendinosus and gracilis tendons and lateral extra-articular reconstruction. J Bone Joint Surg Am 2006;88:2373–9.
45. Wegrzyn J, Chouteau J, Philippot R, et al. Repeat revision of anterior cruciate ligament reconstruction: a retrospective review of management and outcome of 10 patients with an average 3-year follow-up. Am J Sports Med 2009;37:776–85.
46. Magnussen RA. Third time's a charm? Improving re-revision ACL reconstruction by addressing reasons for prior failures. Eur Orthop Traumatol 2012;3:55–60.
47. Terry GC, Norwood LA, Hughston JC, et al. How iliotibial tract injuries of the knee combine with acute anterior cruciate ligament tears to influence abnormal anterior tibial displacement. Am J Sports Med 1993;21:55–60.
48. Noyes FR, Barber SD. The effect of an extra-articular procedure on allograft reconstructions for chronic ruptures of the anterior cruciate ligament. J Bone Joint Surg Am 1991;73:882–92.
49. Goertzen M, Schulitz KP. Isolated intraarticular plasty of the semitendinosus or combined intra- and extra-articular plasty in chronic anterior laxity of the knee. Rev Chir Orthop Reparatrice Appar Mot 1994;80:113–7 [in French].
50. Lerat JL, Mandrino A, Besse JL, et al. Effect of external extra-articular ligament plasty on the results of anterior cruciate ligament reconstruction with patellar tendon, a 4 years follow-up. Rev Chir Orthop Reparatrice Appar Mot 1997;83: 591–601 [in French].
51. Terry GC, LaPrade RF. The posterolateral aspect of the knee. Anatomy and surgical approach. Am J Sports Med 1996;24:732–9.
52. LaPrade RF, Gilbert TJ, Bollom TS, et al. The magnetic resonance imaging appearance of individual structures of the posterolateral knee. A prospective study of normal knees and knees with surgically verified grade III injuries. Am J Sports Med 2000;28:191–9.
53. Vieira EL, Vieira EA, da Silva RT, et al. An anatomic study of the iliotibial tract. Arthroscopy 2007;23:269–74.
54. Vincent JP, Magnussen RA, Gezmez F, et al. The anterolateral ligament of the human knee: an anatomic and histologic study. Knee Surg Sports Traumatol Arthrosc 2012;20:147–52.

Anatomic Anterior Cruciate Ligament Reconstruction with Quadriceps Tendon Autograft

Stephen J. Rabuck, MD*, Volker Musahl, MD,
Freddie H. Fu, MD, Robin V. West, MD

KEYWORDS

• Anterior cruciate ligament • Quadriceps tendon • Autograft • Harvest

KEY POINTS

- Preoperative measurement of tendon dimensions on magnetic resonance imaging is helpful.
- Measure scalpel depth to approximate depth of incision.
- Begin with medial incision, which has less risk of violating the suprapatellar pouch.
- Avoid cutting bone block more than 10 × 15 mm to minimize risk of fracture.
- Avoiding violation of the suprapatellar pouch can minimize fluid extravasation.
- Incision 1 cm proximal to the superior pole of the patella to 5 cm in length proximally.
- Skin flaps allow visualization through a smaller incision.
- Slight flexion assists with stabilization of the patella during bone cuts.
- A natural plane between the rectus femoris and vastus intermedius allows for harvesting single-bundle or double-bundle grafts).
- May harvest soft tissue graft alone.
- Autologous bone graft (from drill tunnels) into patella harvest defect is recommended.

INTRODUCTION

Reconstruction of the ruptured anterior cruciate ligament (ACL) requires selection of a graft that best accommodates the patient's individual needs. Numerous grafts, including allograft and autograft options, have been described. These options include grafts consisting of soft tissue alone and grafts allowing for osseous healing. Research

Funding sources: There were no funding sources for this study.
Conflict of interest: The authors report no conflict of interest.
Center for Sports Medicine, Department of Orthopaedic Surgery, University of Pittsburgh Medical Center, 3200 South Water Street, Pittsburgh, PA 15203, USA
* Corresponding author. Department of Orthopaedic Surgery, Center for Sports Medicine, University of Pittsburgh Medical Center, 3200 South Water Street, Pittsburgh, PA 15203, USA.
E-mail address: rabucksj@upmc.edu

surrounding ACL reconstruction has led to a further understanding of the native anatomy of the ACL. The function of the anteromedial (AM) and posterolateral (PL) bundles of the ACL have led to a better understanding of not only the translational but also the rotational stability provided by the native ACL. As a result, ACL reconstruction may be better approached with a versatile graft that can reproduce the stability provided by the native ACL and allow for graft incorporation and healing. The quadriceps tendon autograft is a versatile option, which takes advantage of osseous healing and allows for both single-bundle and double-bundle reconstruction.

Blauth[1] first described use of the quadriceps tendon for ACL reconstruction in 1984. The original description of this technique describes a double-bundle reconstruction, by which the central third quadriceps tendon is harvested with a bone block from the superior pole of the patella. The bone block was then fixed within the tibia; 1 bundle was fixed to the medial wall of the lateral femoral condyle and the other bundle of the quadriceps tendon was fixed in the over-the-top position. Staubli and colleagues[2] elaborated on this technique, including fluoroscopic evaluation and the development of a press fit, outside in modification. This technique was further popularized because studies reported biomechanical advantages and good clinical outcomes comparing the patellar tendon and quadriceps tendon grafts.[2–4] Harvesting quadriceps tendon grafts showed promise, with less apparent anterior knee pain when compared with patellar tendon grafts.[5,6] Still, a risk of patellar fracture exists not only during harvest but as a result of the defect within the patella postoperatively.[6] Fulkerson and Langeland[7] later described harvesting of the central third quadriceps tendon as a free-tendon graft, thereby reducing the morbidity of harvest regarding anterior knee pain and patellar fracture.[5] The effect of patellar tendon and quadriceps tendon graft harvest on extensor mechanism strength has not been clearly answered, because some studies show an apparent benefit for quadriceps tendon harvest, whereas others show no difference.[8,9]

ANATOMY AND BIOMECHANICS
Anatomy and Biomechanics of the Native ACL

The ACL acts as a primary restraint to anterior translation and tibial rotation. Recent research has led to a more profound understanding of the native ACL. The AM and PL bundles of the ACL provide differential tensioning as the ACL moves through a normal range of motion, with the AM bundle resisting translation and the PL bundle resisting rotation.

The ACL originates on the medial wall of the lateral femoral condyle. Osseous landmarks have been described to improve anatomic ACL reconstruction.[10] The lateral intercondylar ridge identifies the anterior border of the ACL, whereas the bifurcate ridge marks the junction of the AM and PL bundles. The AM and PL bundles are named for their relative insertion on the tibia. Anatomic landmarks used to locate the tibial insertion of the ACL include the intercondylar eminence, anterior horn of the lateral meniscus, and the posterior cruciate ligament. The insertion of the ACL is variable, especially with regartd to the orientation of the AM and PL bundles. As a result, preserving the ACL remnant can aid in determining tunnel position, and may be even more important when a double-bundle reconstruction is planned.[11]

Anatomy and Biomechanics of the Quadriceps Tendon

The quadriceps tendon is formed by the tendinous insertion of the anterior thigh musculature, with the central third primarily consisting of a confluence of the rectus femoris and vastus intermedius. The resultant insertion maintains this relationship by maintaining a natural plane within the tendon. This division within the tendon can be useful, especially in double-bundle ACL reconstructions. The quadriceps tendon inserts directly onto the anterior half of the patella in an oblique orientation.[3] The quadriceps tendon has an average thickness of 8 mm, which is nearly twice the thickness of the patellar tendon and more closely replicates the dimensions of the native ACL. Furthermore, the quadriceps tendon has shown similar biomechanic properties, capable of exceeding those of the intact ACL (**Table 1**).[4,12]

FIXATION OPTIONS

The method of fixation for quadriceps tendon graft can vary based on surgeon preference. The presence of osseous and soft tissue components allows for a variety of options. Interference screw fixation can be used on both osseous and soft tissue components. Suspensory fixation for a bone plug within the femoral tunnel has been successfully used, including the ENDOBUTTON (Smith and Nephew, Andover, MA). On the tibial side, suspensory fixation may be used alone, or to reinforce interference screw fixation. In cases of a short graft, suspensory fixation such as tying over a post may be advantageous. All inside systems with unique fixation have been described as well.

The versatility of the quadriceps tendon for methods of fixation makes it desirable for revision cases as well. If a bone block is used, it can be secured within the defect. In addition, with the increased cross-sectional area of the quadriceps tendon, apposition can be achieved circumferentially within the tunnel.

The quadriceps tendon can be used for over-the-top ACL reconstructions as well. If a bone block is used in these cases, it is secured within the tibial tunnel. The tendinous portion can be secured proximally over a post. It is critical to be sure that adequate graft is harvested when over-the-top reconstructions are performed.

SURGICAL TECHNIQUE: HARVEST

The patient is positioned supine on the operating room table. The central quadriceps tendon can be harvested using a leg-holder with the end of the bed flexed or with the foot on the table and a post for lateral support. When using a post, 2.26-kg and 4.53-kg (5-pound and 10-pound) sand bags can be used for the foot to rest at variable knee flexion angles during graft harvest. Doing so allows for varied exposure of the quadriceps tendon and patella through the incision.

The incision is made longitudinal at the proximal pole of the patella, following the central axis of the quadriceps tendon 5 cm proximal (**Fig. 1**). During exposure, care is taken to maintain meticulous hemostasis. Skin flaps are developed to allow for adequate visualization of the quadriceps tendon origin proximally, the patella distally,

Table 1			
Biomechanical characteristics of selected grafts. Comparison of quadriceps tendon, patellar tendon, and quadrupled hamstring with the native ACL			
Graft	**Tensile Load (N)**	**Stiffness (N/mm)**	**Cross-Sectional Area (mm²)**
Quadriceps tendon[4,12]	2352	463	62
Patellar tendon[13]	2977	620	35
Quadruple hamstring[14]	4090	776	53
Native ACL[15]	2160	242	44

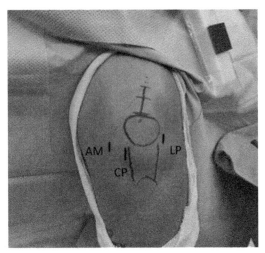

Fig. 1. Incision and portals for quadriceps tendon harvest. A longitudinal incision is planned in line with the fibers of the quadriceps tendon to a point 3 to 5 cm proximal to the patella. A far lateral portal (LP) is placed above the patellar fat pad, whereas a central portal (CP) and an accessory medial portal (AM) are placed medially.

and the medial and lateral aspects of the quadriceps tendon and patella. The central fibers of the quadriceps tendon are followed to a point 6 to 7 cm proximal to the superior edge of the patella. A 10-mm-wide tendon segment is incised using a number 10 blade, taking care to avoid violating the suprapatellar pouch. A Kelly clamp can be passed under the distalmost quadriceps tendon to develop the plane between the quadriceps tendon and suprapatellar pouch.

The patellar cuts are planned next, extending the 10-mm-wide segment distally to a point 15 mm distal from the superior pole of the patella. Needle-tip electrocautery is used to extend the incisions and remove any intervening soft tissue for saw cuts. Using a small oscillating saw, longitudinal bone cuts are made to a depth of 8 to 10 mm, angled 20° to 40° toward midline, creating a trapezoid bone plug. The final transverse bone cut is made after confirming the length of the bone plug. Care must be taken to avoid creation of stress risers. A curved 0.6-cm (0.25-inch) osteotome is used to complete the cuts and free the bone plug.

Another option to avoid creating a patellar stress riser is to perform an undercut on the patellar bone plug. The same angled cuts are created, and the soft tissue graft is released proximally and extended distally. The tendon insertion is well visualized on the proximal patella, then a small sagittal saw is used to make an undercut at the insertion, creating a true trapezoidal bone plug.

The soft tissue component of the graft is then released at least 7 cm from the superior pole of the patella to ensure an adequate soft tissue component to the graft. The graft is then taken to the back table for preparation (**Fig. 2**). Any defect made in the suprapatellar pouch is closed before arthroscopy to avoid extravasation of fluid and potential complications therein. The tendon defect is reapproximated and a standard closure with nonbraided suture is performed. The patellar defect can be bone grafted using bone chips from the graft preparation or from the bone debris from tunnel drilling. Alternatively, a core reamer can be used on the tibial side and that bone can be grafted into the patellar defect.

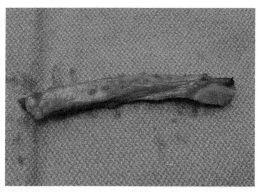

Fig. 2. Quadriceps tendon autograft. Harvested quadriceps tendon harvest with superior pole patella bone block.

Alternatively, a graft consisting of soft tissue alone may be harvested. In this case, careful attention must be paid to the proximal extent of the graft and harvesting a tendon of adequate length. If an adequate length graft can be harvested, the central 10-mm segment is longitudinally incised. Depending on the thickness of the tendon and surgeon preference, the harvest can incorporate the entire rectus femoris and a partial-thickness vastus intermedius tendon (leaving some on the synovial layer), or a full-thickness graft may be obtained by taking the entire vastus intermedius through the synovial layer. After releasing the distal attachment to the superior pole of the patella, the graft is released proximally, as described earlier.

The graft harvest can be modified to a more cosmetic horizontal incision at the superior pole of the patella. Skin flaps are mobilized to expose the superior pole of the patella and quadriceps tendon. A bone plug may be harvested as above. Special tools such as a double-bladed scalpel can aid in proximal tendon harvest with minimal exposure, however care must be taken to avoid violating the nearby musculature. Finally, an accessory incision is made proximally for release of the tendinous portion.

SURGICAL TECHNIQUE OF ACL RECONSTRUCTION
Portals

The basic principles of anatomic ACL reconstruction are followed when quadriceps tendon autograft is used. As discussed earlier, both single-bundle and double-bundle ACL reconstruction can be performed. Standard arthroscopy portals are created, including lateral, central, and accessory medial portals (see **Fig. 1**). By using a central and accessory medial portal, adequate visualization of the native origin from the lateral femoral condyle can be appreciated and a safe tunnel trajectory maintained (**Fig. 3**).

Arthroscopic Evaluation

During diagnostic arthroscopy, evaluation of the ACL remnant and notch dimensions allows for decision making of the optimal method of reconstruction. Measurements of ACL insertion length as well as bundle width for both the femoral and tibial insertions are obtained (**Fig. 4**). Measurements of both notch width and height are obtained as well. Generally, for patients with a tibial insertion of less than 14 mm, a single-bundle reconstruction is recommended, whereas with lengths of more than 18 mm, a double-bundle reconstruction is recommended. In addition, for those patients with a notch width less than 12 mm, a single-bundle reconstruction is recommended.

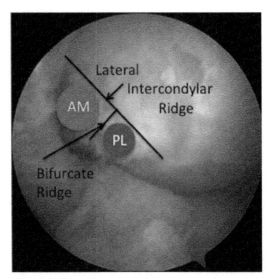

Fig. 3. The native ACL origin from the lateral femoral condyle as viewed from the central portal. Adequate visualization allows for identification of osseous landmarks, including the lateral intercondylar ridge and the bifurcate ridge. These landmarks assist in identification of the native AM and PL bundles.

Femoral Tunnel Preparation

When performing ACL reconstructions with the quadriceps tendon, a single femoral tunnel is used regardless of whether a single-bundle or double-bundle reconstruction is planned. First, the native AM and PL bundles are identified (see **Fig. 3**). Next, the single femoral tunnel is placed at a midpoint between the centers of the femoral AM

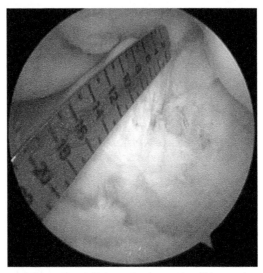

Fig. 4. Measurement of the native ACL insertion onto the tibia, as viewed from the lateral portal. Careful evaluation of the native ACL anatomy assists in surgical planning for the optimal technique to reproduce the native ACL anatomy.

and PL insertion. An awl is used to mark the desired entry point for a guide pin, with the knee hyperflexed. The distance to the lateral femoral cortex is determined, and the tunnel is expanded to accommodate the graft.

Tibial Tunnel Preparation

Preparation of the tibial tunnels is performed after defining the anatomic centers of the tibial AM and PL attachments. The native anatomy of the tibial insertion is identified before planning guide pin and tunnel placement. The centers of the AM and PL bundles are identified. Before guide pin passage, a longitudinal incision is performed at the desired location over the proximal tibia.

For cases in which a double-bundle reconstruction is planned, 2 tibial tunnels are created, taking care to avoid tunnel convergence and maintain the native anatomic orientation. Assessment of pin spread is performed before tunnel preparation with traditional guide pin placement. Another option for surgeons is to use a RetroDrill (Arthrex, Naples, FL) system to prevent tunnel convergence, because the 2 tunnels can be drilled simultaneously. For preparation of the PL tunnel, the tibial guide is set at 45°, centered within the PL remnant, and positioned over the AM tibia at the juncture of the posterior one-third and anterior two-thirds. Next, the guide is adjusted to 55°, centered within the AM insertion, and positioned at the juncture of the anterior one-third and posterior two-thirds over the medial aspect of the tibia. It is important to be mindful of tunnel positioning as the obliquity of these tunnels may result in convergence on the articular side.

For some patients, a single-bundle reconstruction best reproduces the native anatomy. If a single-bundle reconstruction is planned, a central point midway between the tibial AM and PL anatomic centers is cleared of soft tissue. A guide set at 55°, centered between the AM and PL bundles is used to pass a guide pin drilled in a retrograde fashion from the proximal tibia. A traditional tibial guide or a RetroDrill can be used to create the tibial tunnel.

Graft Passage and Fixation

Graft passage is performed maintaining the orientation of the graft to reproduce the orientation of AM and PL bundles whether 1 or 2 tibial tunnels are created. First, the bone block is passed from the accessory medial portal into the femoral tunnel, maintaining the AM and PL bundles in their anatomic orientation. If a single-bundle reconstruction is performed, the sutures of the graft are pulled into the tibial tunnel, and the graft is passed in an antegrade fashion. The graft is then fixed in 15° to 20° of flexion. When a double-bundle reconstruction is performed, the PL bundle is passed before the AM bundle. The PL bundle is secured in full extension while the AM bundle is secured in 45 degrees of flexion.

OUTCOMES/COMPLICATIONS

The outcomes of ACL reconstruction have focused primarily on hamstring, patellar tendon, and allograft options. Increasing evidence is showing the benefits of the quadriceps tendon graft as well as recognizing inherent risks in the graft harvest.

ACL reconstruction with the central third quadriceps tendon has shown excellent stability in follow-up.[6] Good outcomes have been shown in follow-up of not only primary but also revision surgery when quadriceps autograft has been used.[16–18] Hamstring and allograft tissue has raised concern of long-term graft stability and maintenance of graft integrity, which has not been shown in cases undergoing quadriceps tendon autograft.

Quadriceps tendon harvest does not seem to be as detrimental to the extensor mechanism as patellar tendon harvest. Several studies have found quadriceps harvest

Table 2
Complications of selected grafts for ACL reconstruction. Incidence of anterior knee pain and patellar fracture as well as the resultant weakness after quadriceps tendon, patellar tendon, and hamstring tendon after graft harvest

Graft	Anterior Knee Pain (%)	Weakness (% Loss)	Patellar Fracture (%)
Quadriceps tendon	5[21]	11[6]	1.2[6]
Patellar tendon	17–26[21,22]	10–18[23]	0.2–1.8[24,25]
Hamstring	11[22]	10[23]	Not applicable

to result in less of a decrease in extensor mechanism strength than patellar tendon harvest.[8,19] Lee and colleagues[6] also found excellent stability with quadriceps tendon grafts and muscle recovery of 80% to 82% at 1 year and 89% at 2 years after surgery.[20]

Anterior knee pain is a well-recognized sequela of patellar tendon harvest. Recent studies comparing quadriceps tendon with patellar tendon have shown less anterior knee pain.[21] In addition, these patients have not shown the patellar tendon shortening and infrapatellar contracture associated with patellar tendon autograft.[21]

Complications related specifically to graft harvest include weakness, patella fracture, donor site-related pain as well as cosmetic consequences of an additional incision proximal to the patella (**Table 2**). The quadriceps tendon is a hypervascular region with an inherent risk of bleeding and careful attention should be paid to hemostasis. As outlined earlier, the insult to the extensor mechanism and incidence of anterior knee pain does seem to be lessened in patients undergoing quadriceps tendon harvest. The risk of fracture seems to be similar for patellar tendon and quadriceps tendon grafts, with an incidence of 0.2% to 2.0% for patellar tendon and 1.2% for quadriceps tendon.[6,24,25]

SUMMARY

The quadriceps tendon is an excellent option for autograft ACL reconstruction, with structural properties approximating those of more traditional grafts. As we understand more about the native anatomy of the ACL and how to best restore that anatomy, the graft options must advance as well as the methods of fixation to allow for reliable incorporation and healing of the graft after surgical reconstruction. The quadriceps tendon shows promise as a graft for ACL reconstruction because its anatomic and biomechanical characteristics closely approximate the native ACL. Also, the quadriceps tendon can be used to perform both single-bundle and double-bundle reconstruction and shows tremendous potential for revision cases. The versatility of this graft may prove to be more beneficial as understanding of the restoration of knee kinematics after ACL reconstruction improves. Long-term clinical outcome studies will help to assess the relative advantages and disadvantages of grafts used for ACL reconstruction. The goal of anatomic ACL reconstruction using quadriceps tendon autograft is an individualized, functional ACL reconstruction that allows for safe return to full activity.

REFERENCES

1. Blauth W. A new drill template for the operative treatment of injuries of the anterior cruciate ligament. Unfallheilkunde 1984;87(11):463–6 [in German].

2. Staubli HU, Jakob RP. Central quadriceps tendon for anterior cruciate ligament reconstruction. Part I: morphometric and biochemical evaluation. Am J Sports Med 1997;25(5):725–7.

3. Staubli HU, Schatzmann L, Brunner P, et al. Quadriceps tendon and patellar ligament: cryosectional anatomy and structural properties in young adults. Knee Surg Sports Traumatol Arthrosc 1996;4(2):100–10.

4. Staubli HU, Schatzmann L, Brunner P, et al. Mechanical tensile properties of the quadriceps tendon and patellar ligament in young adults. Am J Sports Med 1999; 27(1):27–34.

5. DeAngelis JP, Fulkerson JP. Quadriceps tendon–a reliable alternative for reconstruction of the anterior cruciate ligament. Clin Sports Med 2007;26(4):587–96.

6. Lee S, Seong SC, Jo H, et al. Outcome of anterior cruciate ligament reconstruction using quadriceps tendon autograft. Arthroscopy 2004;20(8):795–802.

7. Fulkerson JP, Langeland R. An alternative cruciate reconstruction graft: the central quadriceps tendon. Arthroscopy 1995;11(2):252–4.

8. Adams DJ, Mazzocca AD, Fulkerson JP. Residual strength of the quadriceps versus patellar tendon after harvesting a central free tendon graft. Arthroscopy 2006;22(1):76–9.

9. Pigozzi F, Di Salvo V, Parisi A, et al. Isokinetic evaluation of anterior cruciate ligament reconstruction: quadriceps tendon versus patellar tendon. J Sports Med Phys Fitness 2004;44(3):288–93.

10. Ferretti M, Ekdahl M, Shen W, et al. Osseous landmarks of the femoral attachment of the anterior cruciate ligament: an anatomic study. Arthroscopy 2007;23(11): 1218–25.

11. Kopf S, Musahl V, Tashman S, et al. A systematic review of the femoral origin and tibial insertion morphology of the ACL. Knee Surg Sports Traumatol Arthrosc 2009;17(3):213–9.

12. Harris NL, Smith DA, Lamoreaux L, et al. Central quadriceps tendon for anterior cruciate ligament reconstruction. Part I: morphometric and biomechanical evaluation. Am J Sports Med 1997;25(1):23–8.

13. Noyes FR, Butler DL, Grood ES, et al. Biomechanical analysis of human ligament grafts used in knee-ligament repairs and reconstructions. J Bone Joint Surg Am 1984;66(3):344–52.

14. Hamner DL, Brown CH Jr, Steiner ME, et al. Hamstring tendon grafts for reconstruction of the anterior cruciate ligament: biomechanical evaluation of the use of multiple strands and tensioning techniques. J Bone Joint Surg Am 1999;81(4):549–57.

15. Woo SL, Hollis JM, Adams DJ, et al. Tensile properties of the human femur-anterior cruciate ligament-tibia complex. The effects of specimen age and orientation. Am J Sports Med 1991;19(3):217–25.

16. Chen CH, Chuang TY, Wang KC, et al. Arthroscopic anterior cruciate ligament reconstruction with quadriceps tendon autograft: clinical outcome in 4-7 years. Knee Surg Sports Traumatol Arthrosc 2006;14(11):1077–85.

17. Garofalo R, Djahangiri A, Siegrist O. Revision anterior cruciate ligament reconstruction with quadriceps tendon-patellar bone autograft. Arthroscopy 2006; 22(2):205–14.

18. Joseph M, Fulkerson J, Nissen C, et al. Short-term recovery after anterior cruciate ligament reconstruction: a prospective comparison of three autografts. Orthopedics 2006;29(3):243–8.

19. Shoemaker SC, Adams D, Daniel DM, et al. Quadriceps/anterior cruciate graft interaction. An in vitro study of joint kinematics and anterior cruciate ligament graft tension. Clin Orthop 1993;294:379–90.

20. Chen CH, Chen WJ, Shih CH. Arthroscopic anterior cruciate ligament reconstruction with quadriceps tendon-patellar bone autograft. J Trauma 1999;46(4):678–82.
21. Geib TM, Shelton WR, Phelps RA, et al. Anterior cruciate ligament reconstruction using quadriceps tendon autograft: intermediate-term outcome. Arthroscopy 2009;25(12):1408–14.
22. Freedman KB, D'Amato MJ, Nedeff DD, et al. Arthroscopic anterior cruciate ligament reconstruction: a metaanalysis comparing patellar tendon and hamstring tendon autografts. Am J Sports Med 2003;31(1):2–11.
23. Nakamura N, Horibe S, Sasaki S, et al. Evaluation of active knee flexion and hamstring strength after anterior cruciate ligament reconstruction using hamstring tendons. Arthroscopy 2002;18(6):598–602.
24. Christen B, Jakob RP. Fractures associated with patellar ligament grafts in cruciate ligament surgery. J Bone Joint Surg Br 1992;74(4):617–9.
25. Viola R, Vianello R. Three cases of patella fracture in 1,320 anterior cruciate ligament reconstructions with bone-patellar tendon-bone autograft. Arthroscopy 1999;15(1):93–7.

Rehabilitation and Return to Play After Anatomic Anterior Cruciate Ligament Reconstruction

Mohammad A. Yabroudi, MS, PT[a,b],
James J. Irrgang, PhD, PT, ATC, FAPTA[a,b],*

KEYWORDS

- Anterior cruciate ligament • Surgery • Knee • Rehabilitation

KEY POINTS

- Anterior cruciate ligament (ACL) reconstruction is one of the most common orthopedic surgical procedures.
- Evidence-based rehabilitation after ACL reconstruction is important to permit the individual to return to their previous level of activity and to minimize the risk for reinjury or injury to the contralateral knee.
- Rehabilitation after ACL reconstruction should consider control of postoperative pain and swelling, protection of the healing graft, restoration of full range of motion symmetric to the contralateral knee, strengthening of the muscles that stabilize the knee, hip, and trunk, enhancing neuromuscular control, and a gradual progression to functional activities that are required for return to sports.
- Recent advances towards anatomic ACL reconstruction, which focuses on restoring normal anatomy and function of the ACL, have important implications for rehabilitation.

INTRODUCTION

Rehabilitation after anterior cruciate ligament (ACL) reconstruction has evolved over the past 20 years and continues to advance rapidly. The evolution in rehabilitation after ACL reconstruction is in part a result of the development of different surgical procedures that address ACL injuries. In particular, recent efforts to anatomically reconstruct the ACL, which is defined as the functional restoration of the ACL to its native dimensions, collagen orientation, and insertion sites[1] is an important consideration for postoperative rehabilitation. Anatomic ACL reconstruction may result in a more

Funding Sources: Nil.
Conflict of Interest: Nil.
[a] Department of Physical Therapy, School of Health and Rehabilitation Sciences, University of Pittsburgh, 6035 Forbes Tower, Pittsburgh, PA 15260, USA; [b] Department of Orthopaedic Surgery, School of Medicine, University of Pittsburgh, 3471 Fifth Avenue, Suite 911, Kaufmann Building, Pittsburgh, PA 15213, USA
* Corresponding author.
E-mail address: jirrgang@pitt.edu

Clin Sports Med 32 (2013) 165–175
http://dx.doi.org/10.1016/j.csm.2012.08.016   **sportsmed.theclinics.com**

rapid return of range of motion (ROM); however, the in situ forces in an anatomically placed graft are greater (comparable with the native ACL) than those in a nonanatomically placed graft (less force than the native ACL as a result of nonanatomic position of the graft).[2] As a result, rehabilitation and return to sport after anatomic ACL reconstruction may need to be progressed slower than after traditional, nonanatomic ACL reconstruction.

Other factors that have influenced advances in rehabilitation after ACL reconstruction include our understanding of the importance of early motion, prevention of joint stiffness, development of neuromuscular control, and the influence of the trunk and hips on function of the knee has greatly influenced the evolution of ACL rehabilitation. However, despite the advances in surgery and rehabilitation, the optimal rehabilitation program is still debatable and depends on the surgical procedure to reconstruct the ACL, concomitant surgical procedures that were performed, the individual's previous level of activity and fitness, response to surgery and rehabilitation, and desired activity level after surgery.

The safety and speed of returning patients to activity and sports after ACL reconstruction depends on the rehabilitation protocol. Initial protocols for ACL rehabilitation favored immobilization and only limited protected motion. Based on the observed problems with joint stiffness, more aggressive accelerated protocols that allowed early full ROM and immediate weight bearing became more widely accepted.[3–5] A randomized clinical trial conducted by Beynnon and colleagues[6] reported that no adverse effects were associated with accelerated versus traditional nonaccelerated rehabilitation in patients who underwent bone-patellar tendon-bone ACL reconstruction. In a recent systematic review, Wright and colleagues[7] evaluated studies that investigated accelerated rehabilitation. In addition to the randomized trial conducted by Beynnon and colleagues,[6] the systematic review identified 1 other study that reported no significant differences between a 6-month or 8-month rehabilitation program at 12 months.

The progression of rehabilitation after ACL reconstruction is affected by several factors. These factors include whether the surgical procedure was anatomic or nonanatomic, graft type, the presence of associated injuries (eg, meniscus tear, multiple ligament injury, chondral damage), and individual patient variation. Several goals remain constant for rehabilitation after ACL reconstruction regardless of the surgical procedure. Emphasis is placed on early ROM, preservation of quadriceps function, and progression of functional activities and not exceeding the limits of the involved tissue healing properties.

In this article, the rehabilitation program after (anatomic) ACL reconstruction is divided into 3 phases:

- Early postoperative stage
- Strengthening and neuromuscular control stage
- Return to activity and sports stage.

EARLY POSTOPERATIVE STAGE (FIRST 4–6 WEEKS AFTER SURGERY)

The main goals of this stage (**Table 1**) are to control pain and swelling, protect the healing graft, minimize the effects of immobilization, obtain full passive and active extension of the knee symmetric to the noninvolved knee, achieve 100° to 120° of knee flexion, preserve quadriceps muscle function, restore the ability to perform a straight-leg raise (SLR) without a quadriceps lag, progression to full weight bearing, and achieve normal gait. To progress to the next stage, an individual should be able to walk normally without crutches or gait deviation; have full passive knee extension

Table 1
Summary of the primary goals for each stage of rehabilitation after anatomic ACL reconstruction

Early Postoperative	Strengthening and Neuromuscular Control	Return to Activity and Sports
Controlling pain and edema	Progression of strengthening	Complete the entire
Protecting the healing graft	Neuromuscular control	functional rehabilitation
Minimizing the effects of	Improving balance	spectrum
immobilization	Preparation for the return to	Make a full return to the
Obtaining full passive and	activity and sports stage	patient's previous level of
active extension of the		daily, occupational and
knee symmetric to the		athletic activity, and sport
noninvolved knee		participation
Achieving 100° to 120° of		
knee flexion		
Preserving quadriceps muscle		
function		
Restore the ability to perform		
straight-leg raise without		
a quadriceps lag		
Progression to full weight		
bearing		
Achieving normal gait		

symmetric to the noninvolved knee, and 100° to 120° of knee flexion; have no evidence of an extensor lag, and minimal effusion or other signs of active inflammation (**Table 2**).

Controlling pain and swelling is one of the most important goals in the early postoperative rehabilitation stage after ACL reconstruction. Reducing pain and swelling leads to improved ROM and quadriceps function and reduces the risk of limited ROM and contracture, which could later cause gait abnormalities and delay in the progression to the next stage. Control of pain and swelling can be achieved by following the ICE (ice, compression, and elevation) principle. A combination of these techniques results in better outcomes. Cryotherapy has been found to cause significant decrease in

Table 2
Summary of the critical milestones for progression of rehabilitation after anatomic ACL reconstruction

Early Postoperative	Strengthening and Neuromuscular Control	Return to Activity and Sports
Patients should be able to	Patients should have no	Patients should achieve
walk normally without	difficulty with daily	a quadriceps index of 85%
crutches or gait deviation	activities	or greater
Have full passive knee	Should tolerate all strength	Have satisfied all the previous
extension symmetric to the	and flexibility exercises	criteria (appropriate ROM,
noninvolved knee	without evidence of joint	strength, proprioception,
Have at least 100°–120° of	pain or inflammation	and endurance) for
knee flexion	Should be able to jog 3.2 km	functional progression
Have no evidence of an	(2 miles) (if possible	Able to tolerate full-effort
extensor lag	previous to injury) and	sprinting, cutting,
Have minimal effusion or	tolerate submaximal	pivoting, jumping, and
other signs of active	multidirectional functional	hopping drills
inflammation	activities	

postoperative pain.[8] In some challenging cases, nonsteroidal antiinflammatory drugs may be prescribed to control postoperative swelling and inflammation.

To protect the graft early after surgery, crutches and a postoperative brace are used. Patients typically ambulate with axillary crutches weight bearing as tolerated (WBAT), with knee brace locked in full extension for 1 week. After 1 week, unless the patient has a concomitant meniscus repair, the brace can be unlocked for ambulation. If the patient had a meniscus repair, the brace should remain locked in extension for ambulation for 4 to 6 weeks to reduce shear stresses on healing meniscus during ambulation.[9] The brace is continued until the patient has comfortably achieved at least 100° to 120° of knee flexion.

Restoration of ROM is also crucial in this stage. Achieving full extension symmetric to noninvolved knee and 100° to 120° of flexion is important in the early postoperative stage of rehabilitation. If the patient had a concomitant meniscus repair, they progress more slowly because knee flexion should be limited to less than 90° for 4 weeks after surgery. Failure to achieve these ranges may lead to gait abnormalities, patellofemoral pain, and in the long-term may contribute to degenerative joint disease. Activities to increase ROM after ACL reconstruction include the immediate initiation of heel slides, gastrocnemius and hamstring stretches, and passive, active-assisted, and active knee flexion exercises. Pedaling a stationary bicycle through a partial revolution progressing to a full revolution is also beneficial for restoring the range of knee flexion. A continuous passive motion (CPM) device may be used for select cases; however, 2 systematic reviews have shown no substantial advantage for the use of CPM except for a possible decrease in postoperative pain.[10,11] Patellar mobilization is used to maintain or increase patellar mobility. Inferior mobilization for the patella should be used if the patient has loss of passive flexion and decreased inferior patellar translation during mobility testing. Superior glide of the patella is important to ensure full active knee extension, which requires the quadriceps to pull the patella superiorly.

Preservation of quadriceps function in the early postoperative stage of rehabilitation after ACL reconstruction should be emphasized. Early initiation of isometric quadriceps setting exercises that result in superior translation of the patella are begun during the early rehabilitation period. SLR exercises are also initiated at this time. The ability to perform an SLR with the knee at the end range of full extension should be emphasized. The use of high-intensity electrical stimulation after ACL reconstruction has been shown to improve quadriceps strength,[12,13] gait,[13] and patient-reported outcomes.[12,14]

Activities that prepare the individual for progression to full weight bearing and ambulation, improving balance and postural control, and achieving normal gait should also be emphasized during this stage. Weight-shifting exercises should allow the individual to begin accommodating loads through the surgical knee and should be progressed to basic single-leg balance activities as tolerated. Gait training is performed as necessary to ensure that the individual uses a normal heel-toe gait and does not walk with a flexed knee during the midstance of gait.

Progression to full weight bearing and achieving a normal gait are necessary steps before progression to the strengthening and neuromuscular control stage. The patient initially starts walking WBAT with a postoperative rehabilitation brace and crutches, and later may progress to cane as necessary. Criteria for progression to ambulation without assistive devices includes minimal pain and swelling, full passive knee extension symmetric to the noninvolved side, ability to perform an SLR without a quadriceps lag, and demonstration of the ability to walk with a normal gait pattern without assistive devices.

As the patient continues to progress toward full weight-bearing status, therapeutic activities for all other muscles of the lower extremity should be advanced. Flexibility and strengthening exercises for the hip muscles, hamstring, gastrocnemius, and soleus muscles should be initiated and emphasized. SLR exercises in all planes of motion and use of a stationary bicycle with low resistance are advocated. However, individuals with a medial collateral ligament (MCL) injury or who underwent MCL repair should defer hip adduction exercises for 4 to 6 weeks after surgery, and those undergoing ACL reconstruction with a hamstring tendon or those who have undergone concomitant meniscus repair should defer resisted hamstring exercises until 6 weeks after surgery.

STRENGTHENING AND NEUROMUSCULAR CONTROL STAGE

The main goals during this stage of rehabilitation are continued progression of strengthening, neuromuscular control, balance activities, and preparation for the return to activity and sports stage (see **Table 1**).

Weight-bearing (closed kinetic chain [CKC]) and nonweight-bearing (open kinetic chain [OKC]) strengthening activities are initiated and progressed during this stage of rehabilitation. The effectiveness, safety, and functional implications of OKC versus CKC exercises have been discussed in the literature. Earlier protocols often emphasized early use of CKC exercises based on assumptions such as CKC activities being more functionally relevant and producing less graft strain secondary to joint compression and cocontraction of the quadriceps and hamstrings. It has been suggested that the OKC knee extension should be avoided because of increased ACL strain with extension in the range of 45° to full extension. However, evidence suggests that CKC and OKC activities produce similar levels of strain on the ACL and graft.[15,16] During OKC knee extension, the amount of strain increases as resistance is added, whereas ACL strain does not increase with increased loading of CKC activities. Patellofemoral contact stress increases between 45° and 20° of extension during OKC knee extension, and with increasing knee flexion during CKC activities. The effect of graft strain during OKC or CKC on graft healing is still unknown. A recent systematic review by Trees and colleagues[17] found no differences between groups using CKC and OKC exercises after ACL reconstruction in knee function, patellofemoral pain severe enough to restrict activity at 1 year, or knee laxity at 1 year. Although there is a debate in the literature regarding the advantages and disadvantages of nonweight-bearing and weight-bearing exercises, a review of available data suggests that a combination of both OKC and CKC exercises is helpful when appropriate precautions are taken to protect the healing graft and avoid excessive stress to the patellofemoral joint.[18–21] Also, the combination of these 2 exercises resulted in more frequent return to sport 2.5 years after ACL reconstruction compared with weight-bearing exercise only.[17]

To minimize strain on the healing graft, limited arc of motion between 90° and 60° for nonweight-bearing knee extension exercises for the first 3 months after surgery are recommended. After 3 to 4 months, we encourage OCK knee extension exercises through the full arc of motion as tolerated by the patellofemoral joint. OKC knee flexion can be performed to increase strength of the hamstrings, but is avoided for the first 4 to 6 weeks after surgery when a meniscus repair has been performed.

For the first 3 months after surgery, weight-bearing exercises between 0° and 60° are recommended to minimize complaints of patellofemoral symptoms. These exercises include for example wall slides, partial squats with symmetric weight distribution on both legs, weight-bearing terminal knee extension (with therapeutic tubing or other form of external resistance), and low-resistance, limited-arc leg press with a functional progression to step-up activities. Progressing from double-leg to single-leg extension activities aids in avoiding compensation using the nonsurgical extremity. After 3 to 4 months, the ROM for CKC exercises may be progressed to 75° to 90° of knee flexion. At this point during the rehabilitation program, CKC exercises may include double-leg and single-leg squats and leg press, lunges, and higher-level step-up/step-down exercises. As part of the strengthening progression, the eccentric component of exercises should be emphasized. Eccentric exercises have been found to be effective in increasing muscle strength and functional performance after ACL reconstruction.[22,23]

Activities and exercises emphasizing hip and lumbopelvic stabilization are also suggested. The role of appropriate hip abductor and external rotator strength has been described in the literature.[24,25] Weakness of the hip abductors and external rotators has been found to be associated with valgus collapse of the knee and noncontact ACL injuries.[26–28] Exercises including side-lying hip abduction and extension, lateral side support, resisted hip rotation, and lateral and diagonal walking against elastic bands for resistance are used to strengthen the hip abductors and external rotators. Weakness of the core trunk stabilizers has also been found to contribute to the risk of ACL injury. Therefore, rehabilitation after ACL reconstruction should include exercises that include activities that focus on transverse abdominus contraction, pelvic tilts, bridging, lateral side support, and activities that use the multifidus muscle group and paraspinal musculature. An advancement of these exercises with more functional approach is recommended.

Early in the strengthening and neuromuscular control stage, patients may begin to perform low-impact aerobic exercise. Appropriate activities include exercise on a stepper, pedaling a stationary bicycle ergometer, walking on an elliptical machine or treadmill, and aquatic jogging or swimming. As endurance activities are progressed, the patient should be monitored for the presence of swelling, pain, or other signs of inflammation.

As part of the functional progression, balance and perturbation activities should also be included. Two of the main impairments that patients may experience after ACL injury are lack of muscle strength and neuromuscular control of the lower extremity.[29] Evidence has shown that patients with ACL injury may develop an adaptive motor pattern and coping mechanism that cause biomechanical alterations, which increase dynamic stability and improve function of the knee.[30,31] Therefore, emphasis is placed on developing compensatory lower extremity muscle activity patterns that promote functional stability.

Perturbation training techniques have been found to be effective in enhancing neuromuscular control in patients undergoing nonoperative treatment after ACL injury.[32] We believe that perturbation training techniques are also beneficial after ACL reconstruction. Such techniques include the use of a roller board and tilt board, with application of controlled perturbation forces, which are progressed to random perturbations over time (**Fig. 1**). These techniques can also be modified so that patients can experience the perturbations during performance of activity-related tasks, which may enhance carry-over of learned protective responses to functional performance situations. Several studies have shown that hamstring reaction time and functional ability were improved after training with these techniques.[33,34] Reflex activity of the hamstring muscles after a direct stress placed on the ACL has been found to be a critical factor for dynamic knee stabilization.[35]

Balance training progression guidelines have been described in the literature.[36–38] Initially, tasks should be introduced in a predictable fashion on a stable surface. Over time, balance activities should be progressed to more complex tasks, with minimal cues. Increased task complexity can be achieved by changing surface variability through the use of foam surfaces or a tilt board. Positional cues can be given

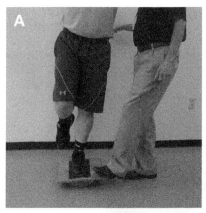
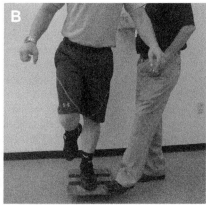
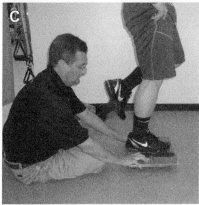

Fig. 1. Tilt board (*A* and *B*) and roller board (*C*) perturbations. Patient stands with operated leg over the tilt board or roller board. The therapist applies controlled perturbation forces that are progressed to random perturbations over time.

less often, and additional activities such as throwing and catching objects ensure an increase in task difficulty. Appropriate strength, ROM, and stability during basic perturbation and balance activities help ensure an adequate foundation on which more advanced functional activities can be built.

At the end of the strengthening and neuromuscular control stage, any residual strength and flexibility deficits that remain should be resolved. Progression with running may be initiated at this point, provided the patient meets specific strength requirements to advance with specific functional activities. Quadriceps strength should be assessed quantitatively. This assessment may include isometric testing with a hand-held dynamometer or isokinetic dynamometer, isokinetic testing, or a single-repetition maximum quadriceps strength test. Minimum quadriceps strength index values of 70% to 75% for running, 80% for submaximal agility training, and 85% for sport-specific skill training are recommended. In addition, to begin a jogging program, the patient should have full, pain-free ROM with no pain or swelling or evidence of patellofemoral symptoms and should be able to walk briskly for 15 minutes without gait deviations or symptoms.

When the patient meets these criteria, they can begin a jogging program. We recommend starting to run at a slow pace on a treadmill or over ground for 5 to 10 minutes every other day. The running program is gradually increased and progressed by 10% to 15% per week if the patient does not develop pain, swelling, or gait asymmetries. During this time, the patient can also be progressed to low-level submaximal (less than 50% effort) agility drills, including side-to-side shuffling, forward and backward running, and jumping and landing on both limbs simultaneously from distances less than 50% of the individual's height. These activities can be progressed to carioca drills and cone drills, which involve changing directions at various angles. Once proficiency of jogging and submaximal agility drills is shown, the patient should be evaluated to determine if they are a candidate for progressing toward a return to full activity and sport.

After successful completion of these activities, the individual should have no difficulty with daily activities. All strength and flexibility exercises should be tolerated without evidence of joint pain or inflammation. The patient should be able to jog 3.2 km (2 miles) (if possible previous to injury) and tolerate submaximal multidirectional functional activities (see **Table 2**).

RETURN TO ACTIVITY AND SPORTS STAGE

The final stage of rehabilitation after ACL reconstruction is the stage of returning to full activity and sports participation. The time to return to full activity and sport is variable and depends on several factors. Some of these factors are graft type, graft healing and maturation, the concomitant surgical procedures, individual patient tolerance for the activities, surgeon preferences, and the physical demands of the sport. The primary goals during this final stage (see **Table 1**) are to complete the entire functional rehabilitation spectrum and make a full return to the patient's previous level of daily, occupational, and athletic activity, and sports participation. During this stage of rehabilitation, emphasis is placed on a gradual increase in function that culminates in return to sport. Strengthening exercises through the full ROM and activities to enhance neuromuscular control are also continued to ensure full recovery and maintenance of strength and dynamic stability. Once the patient has achieved a quadriceps index of 85% or greater and has satisfied all the previous criteria (appropriate ROM, strength, proprioception, and endurance) for functional progression, they can begin full-effort sprinting, cutting, and plyometric activities. These activities may then be integrated into a sport-specific training program.

Plyometric activities should be prescribed in a manner that allows the patient to improve power and performance in relation to their sport and ensure an appropriate level of safety. Initially, activities focusing on landing and the appropriate attenuation of force through the lower extremity should be used. Such activities include double-leg jumping, single-leg jumping, and stepping off plyometric drill boxes. Activities can be made more challenging by changing height and distance of jump, time of drills, direction, and combining multiple tasks.

Once the patient is able to tolerate full-effort sprinting, cutting, pivoting, jumping, and hopping drills, return to sport can be considered (see **Table 2**). A functional brace may be considered for those individuals returning to strenuous sports. The use of a functional brace has been found to be beneficial in decreasing the risk of subsequent knee injury compared with not using them for patients with high-demand sports after ACL reconstruction.[39] However, the use of functional bracing after ACL reconstruction is still a source of debate. During this time, the patient can also be progressed to more specific sport-related exercises. Initially, training should begin with unopposed components of the individual's athletic activity. As the patient becomes proficient and can perform these tasks safely, speed and complexity should be increased. Opposition from other players should be introduced as tolerated. To return to full participation in sports, the patient should be progressed from partial return to practice to full return to practice, followed by return to competition.

SUMMARY

Rehabilitation after ACL reconstruction is one of the main factors that contributes to safe and full return of the individual to functional activities and sports participation after ACL injury. An appropriate rehabilitation program should reflect the advancement and changes in the surgical procedures of ACL reconstruction. There is no consensus in the literature regarding the optimal rehabilitation program and time to return to sports after ACL reconstruction. However, established rehabilitation guidelines for graft protection and functional progression should be followed.

REFERENCES

1. Van Eck CF, Lesniak BP, Schreiber VM, et al. Anatomic single-and double-bundle anterior cruciate ligament reconstruction flowchart. Arthroscopy 2010;26:258–68.
2. Kato Y, Ingham SJ, Kramer S, et al. Effect of tunnel position for anatomic single-bundle ACL reconstruction on knee biomechanics in a porcine model. Knee Surg Sports Traumatol Arthrosc 2010;18:2–10.
3. Paulos L, Noyes FR, Grood ES, et al. Knee rehabilitation after anterior cruciate ligament reconstruction and repair. Am J Sports Med 1981;9:140–9.
4. Steadman JR. Rehabilitation of acute injuries of the anterior cruciate ligament. Clin Orthop 1983;172:129–32.
5. Sheloborne KD, Nitz P. Accelerated rehabilitation after anterior cruciate ligament reconstruction. Am J Sports Med 1990;18:292–9.
6. Beynnon BD, Uh BS, Johnson RJ, et al. Rehabilitation after anterior ligament reconstruction: a prospective, randomized, double-blind comparison of programs administered over two different time intervals. Am J Sports Med 2005;33:347–59.
7. Wright RW, Preston E, Fleming BC, et al. A systematic review of anterior cruciate ligament reconstruction rehabilitation: part II: open versus closed kinetic chain exercises, neuromuscular electrical stimulation, accelerated rehabilitation, and miscellaneous topics. J Knee Surg 2008;21(3):225–34.
8. Raynor MC, Pietrobon R, Guller U, et al. Cryotherapy after ACL reconstruction: a meta-analysis. J Knee Surg 2005;18(2):123–9.
9. Starke C, Kopf S, Petersen W, et al. Meniscal repair. Arthroscopy 2009;25: 1033–44.
10. Wright RW, Preston E, Fleming BC, et al. A systematic review of anterior cruciate ligament reconstruction rehabilitation: part I: continuous passive motion, early weight bearing, postoperative bracing, and home-based rehabilitation. J Knee Surg 2008;21:217–24.
11. Smith T, Davies L. The efficacy of continuous passive motion after anterior cruciate ligament reconstruction: a systematic review. Phys Ther Sport 2007;8: 141–52.
12. Fitzgerald GK, Piva SR, Irrgang JJ. A modified neuromuscular electrical stimulation protocol for quadriceps strength training following anterior cruciate ligament reconstruction. J Orthop Sports Phys Ther 2003;33:492–501.
13. Snyder-Mackler L, Delitto A, Bailey SL, et al. Strength of the quadriceps femoris muscle and functional recovery after reconstruction of the anterior cruciate ligament. A prospective, randomized clinical trial of electrical stimulation. J Bone Joint Surg Am 1995;77:1166–73.

14. Kim KM, Croy T, Hertel J, et al. Effects of neuromuscular electrical stimulation after anterior cruciate ligament reconstruction on quadriceps strength, function, and patient-oriented outcomes: a systematic review. J Orthop Sports Phys Ther 2010;40:383–91.

15. Beynnon BD, Johnson RJ, Fleming BC, et al. The measurement of elongation of anterior cruciate ligament grafts in vivo. J Bone Joint Surg Am 1994;76A:511–9.

16. Perry MC, Morrissey MC, King JB, et al. Effects of closed versus open kinetic chain knee extensor resistance training on knee laxity and leg function in patients during the 8- to 14-week post-operative period after anterior cruciate ligament reconstruction. Knee Surg Sports Traumatol Arthrosc 2005;13(5):357–69.

17. Trees AH, Howe TE, Dixon J, et al. Exercise for treating isolated anterior cruciate ligament injuries in adults. Cochrane Database Syst Rev 2005;(4):CD005316.

18. Beynnon BD, Johnson RJ, Fleming BC, et al. The strain behavior of the anterior cruciate ligament during squatting and active flexion-extension. A comparison of an open and a closed kinetic chain exercise. Am J Sports Med 1997;25:823–9.

19. Fitzgerald GK. Open versus closed kinetic chain exercises: issues in rehabilitation after anterior cruciate ligament. Phys Ther 1997;77(12):1747.

20. Mikkelsen C, Werner S, Eriksson E. Closed kinetic chain alone compared to combined open and closed kinetic chain exercises for quadriceps strengthening after anterior cruciate ligament reconstruction with respect to return to sports: a prospective matched follow-up study. Knee Surg Sports Traumatol Arthrosc 2000;8:337–42.

21. Glass R, Waddell J, Hoogenboom B. The effects of open versus closed kinetic chain exercises on patients with ACL deficient or reconstructed knees: a systematic review. North Am J Sports Phys Ther 2010;5(2):74–84.

22. Gerber JP, Marcus RL, Dibble LE, et al. Effects of early progressive eccentric exercise on muscle size and function after anterior cruciate ligament reconstruction: a 1-year follow-up study of a randomized clinical trial. Phys Ther 2009;89:51–9.

23. Gerber JP, Marcus RL, Dibble LE, et al. Safety, feasibility, and efficacy of negative work exercise via eccentric muscle activity following anterior cruciate ligament reconstruction. J Orthop Sports Phys Ther 2007;37:10–8.

24. Hewett TE, Myer GD, Ford KR. Reducing knee and anterior cruciate ligament injuries among female athletes: a systematic review of neuromuscular training interventions. J Knee Surg 2005;18(1):82–8.

25. Leetun DT, Ireland ML, Willson JD, et al. Core stability measures as risk factors for lower extremity injury in athletes. Med Sci Sports Exerc 2004;36(6):926–34.

26. Powers CM. The influence of abnormal hip mechanics on knee injury: a biomechanical perspective. J Orthop Sports Phys Ther 2010;40:42–51.

27. Hewett TE, Ford KR, Myer GD. Anterior cruciate ligament injuries in female athletes: part 2, a meta-analysis of neuromuscular interventions aimed at injury prevention. Am J Sports Med 2006;34:490–8.

28. Hewett TE, Myer GD, Ford KR, et al. Biomechanical measures of neuromuscular control and valgus loading of the knee predict anterior cruciate ligament injury risk in female athletes: a prospective study. Am J Sports Med 2005;33:492–501.

29. Risberg MA, Lewek M, Snyder-Mackler L. A systematic review of evidence for anterior cruciate ligament rehabilitation: how much and what type? Phys Ther Sport 2004;5:125–45.

30. Riemann BL, Lephart SM. The sensorimotor system, part II: the role of proprioception in motor control and functional joint stability. J Athl Train 2002;37(1):80–4.

31. Tibone JE, Antich TJ. Electromyographic analysis of the anterior cruciate ligament-deficient knee. Clin Orthop Relat Res 1993;288:35–9.
32. Fitzgerald GK, Axe MJ, Snyder-Mackler L. The efficacy of perturbation training in nonoperative anterior cruciate ligament rehabilitation programs for physically active individuals. Phys Ther 2000;80(2):128–40.
33. Ihara H, Nakayama A. Dynamic joint control training for knee ligament injuries. Am J Sports Med 1986;14(4):309–15.
34. Beard DJ, Kyberd PJ, Fergusson CM, et al. Proprioception after rupture of the anterior cruciate ligament. An objective indication of the need for surgery? J Bone Joint Surg Br 1993;75(2):311–5.
35. Solomonow M, Baratta R, Zhou BH, et al. The synergistic action of the anterior cruciate ligament and thigh muscles in maintaining joint stability. Am J Sports Med 1987;15:207–13.
36. Irrgang JJ, Whitney S, Cox ED. Balance and proprioceptive training for rehabilitation of the lower extremity. J Sport Rehabil 1994;3:68–83.
37. Olsen OE, Mykleburst L, Holme I, et al. Exercises to prevent lower limb injuries in youth sports: cluster randomized controlled trial. BMJ 2005;330(7489):449.
38. Lephart SM, Pinicivero DM, Giraldo JL, et al. The role of proprioception in the management and rehabilitation of athletic injuries. Am J Sports Med 1997; 25(1):130–7.
39. Sterett WI, Briggs KK, Farley T, et al. Effect of functional bracing on knee injury in skiers with anterior cruciate ligament reconstruction: a prospective cohort study. Am J Sports Med 2006;34(10):1581–5.

Failure of Anterior Cruciate Ligament Reconstruction

Timothy S. Whitehead, FRACS[a,b,c,]*

KEYWORDS

- Anterior cruciate ligament • Graft failure • Loss of motion
- Extensor mechanism dysfunction • Osteoarthritis • Infection
- Anatomic ACL reconstruction • Extensor mechanism dysfunction

KEY POINTS

- Failure after anterior cruciate ligament (ACL) reconstruction is a potentially devastating event that affects a predominantly young and active population.
- This review article provides a comprehensive analysis of the potential causes of failure, including graft failure, loss of motion, extensor mechanism dysfunction, osteoarthritis, and infection.
- The etiology of graft failure is discussed in detail with a particular emphasis on failure after anatomic ACL reconstruction.

Injuries to the Anterior Cruciate Ligament (ACL) are becoming more frequent. Correspondingly there has been an increase in the number of ACL reconstructions performed, with more than 150,000 procedures documented annually in the United States.[1] This increase in primary ACL reconstructions almost certainly will lead to an increase in the number of revision procedures. A successful outcome after revision ACL reconstruction depends on many factors, including a comprehensive knowledge of the etiology of failure.

There is no universally accepted definition of failure after ACL reconstruction. In most cases, however, the cause of failure may be grouped into one or a combination of the following:

1. Graft failure
   a. Pathologic laxity
   b. Clinical instability
   c. Nonfunctional or detrimental graft
2. Loss of motion

---

[a] OrthoSport Victoria, Epworth Richmond, Level 5, 89 Bridge Road, Richmond, VIC 3121, Australia;
[b] Musculoskeletal Research Centre, Faculty of Health Sciences, LaTrobe University, Bundoora VIC 3086, Australia; [c] Austin Health, Orthopaedic Department, 145 Studley Road, Heidelberg, VIC, 3084, Australia
* OrthoSport Victoria, Epworth Richmond, Level 5, 89 Bridge Road, Richmond, VIC 3121, Australia.
E-mail address: tswhitehead@osv.com.au

Clin Sports Med 32 (2013) 177–204
http://dx.doi.org/10.1016/j.csm.2012.08.015
0278-5919/13/$ – see front matter © 2013 Elsevier Inc. All rights reserved.

    a. Arthrofibrosis

    b. Poor preoperative range of motion

    c. Prolonged postoperative immobilization

    d. Nonanatomic graft placement

    e. Excessive graft tension

    f. Intercondylar notch scar formation/cyclops lesion

    g. Complex regional pain syndrome

3. Extensor mechanism dysfunction

    a. Quadriceps muscle inhibition/weakness

    b. Loss of patellar mobility

    c. Patella fracture (post–bone-tendon-bone [BTB] harvest)

4. Osteoarthritis

    a. Influence of initial injury

    b. Postmeniscectomy

    c. Chondral lesions

    d. Loss of motion—in particular terminal extension

    e. Intrinsic factors—cartilage breakdown products, inflammatory mediators

5. Infection

The University of Pittsburgh has created a classification system that combines objective and subjective factors to further elucidate the reason for failure.[2] Although multifactorial and subject to significant overlap, recurrent instability can further be categorized into early (<6 months from surgery) or late (>6 months from surgery) failure. Early failures are usually secondary to poor operative technique, failure of graft incorporation, premature return to high-demand activities, or aggressive rehabilitation. Late failures may also be due to poor operative technique or graft malposition as well as repeat trauma to the graft; associated pathology, such as malalignment or collateral ligament injury; and generalized factors, such as ligamentous laxity. Incomplete biologic incorporation may also contribute to late failures.

GRAFT FAILURE

The true incidence of graft failure is unknown at present. Although graft failure is often defined as a combination of pathologic laxity and clinical instability due to graft rupture or elongation, it is well documented that objective laxity or graft rupture on MRI scan does not always correlate to subjective symptoms of instability.[3] Also the degree of laxity that defines graft failure is not universally accepted, with some studies allowing 3 mm of anterior translation (side-to-side difference using an instrumented laxity device)[4–7] whereas others accept 5 mm.[8–11] In addition, many studies only record failures as those requiring a revision procedure, not including those patients who decline further surgery or have no instability symptoms. Failure rate analysis should include all graft failures from the study institutions that occur during the defined study period, including those reviewed before subsequent graft failure; that were not reviewed because of graft failure; or that were not included because of a failure to satisfy study inclusion criteria.

Although failure rates as high as 24% have been reported,[12] most studies have reported graft failure rates in the range of 0.7% to 14%.[5,13–22] Several recent systematic reviews by Spindler and colleagues,[23] Lewis and colleagues,[24] and Wright and colleagues,[25] have reported failure rates of 3.6%, 4%, and 5.8%, respectively.

There has been a recent focus on anatomic ACL reconstruction, which has been defined as the "functional restoration of the ACL to its native dimensions, collagen orientation and insertion sites," independent of whether a single-bundle or double-bundle technique is used.[26] Several studies have demonstrated that anatomic procedures better control laxity and knee kinematics.[27-30] Most studies, however, comparing single-bundle and double-bundle techniques have not demonstrated a difference in failure rates.[31-37] Perhaps surprisingly, the failure rate after anatomic ACL reconstruction has not been shown significantly lower than the failure rate of nonanatomic procedures. A recent study by van Eck and colleagues[38] reported a failure rate for the double-bundle technique of 13%, which is at the upper border of failure rates published in the literature. The same study reported an anatomic single-bundle failure rate of 11%, although a possible confounding variable was the use of allograft material. A similar failure rate (12.3%) after double-bundle reconstructions using autograft hamstrings has been reported in a separate study.[39] Potential reasons for these findings are discussed later; however, this area requires additional research.

The pattern of ACL graft rupture is different for double-bundle and single-bundle techniques. In a recent study by van Eck and colleagues[40] that examined the pattern of rupture for double-bundle grafts, the anteromedial (AM) bundle was ruptured in all cases. The most common patterns were either midsubstance rupture of both AM and posterolateral (PL) bundles or midsubstance AM bundle rupture with elongation of the PL bundle. The same investigators in a separate study examined the pattern of rupture after single-bundle reconstruction and demonstrated the most common pattern in 58% of cases was graft elongation.[41] Both differ from the rupture pattern of the native ACL, which tends to demonstrate a proximal AM bundle rupture in combination with a proximal or midsubstance PL bundle injury.[42] These studies also showed, however, that with increasing time from surgery to reinjury, the pattern of graft rupture became more proximal or similar to the native ACL rupture pattern.[40,41] This is suggestive that the observed injury pattern may closely correlate with the degree of graft healing and ligamentization, which may be enhanced with time.

It is also possible for a graft to be intact but nonfunctional or detrimental to the function of the knee. Nonfunctional intact grafts may allow excessive laxity, particularly in the case of a poorly positioned vertical graft that is able to control anterior translation but not tibiofemoral rotation. Graft malposition may also lead to restriction of knee motion, especially terminal extension, which has been associated with increased rates of long-term osteoarthritis.[43]

Although multifactorial, the following factors are important to consider when investigating the cause of graft failure (**Fig. 1**):

1. Patient factors
2. Surgical technique
3. Graft incorporation/biologic factors
4. Rehabilitation
5. Trauma

Patient Factors

Certain factors inherent to patients, such as age, gender, activity profile, and generalized ligamentous laxity, have been associated with increased failure rates after ACL reconstruction.[12,44-51] Other factors involving the initial mechanism of injury[47] and preoperative condition of the knee have also been investigated.[52,53]

Age at the time of failure

Several investigators have observed higher graft failure rates in younger patients. Barrett and colleagues,[45] in a study that evaluated both autograft and allograft reconstructions, reported a failure rate of 16.5% in patients under 25 years of age compared with 8.3% in those over 25. Shelbourne and colleagues[54] reported similar results after

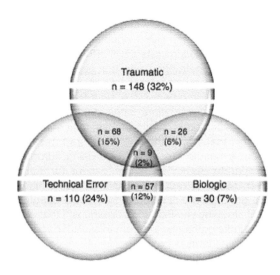

In addition, "other" = 12 (3%)

Fig. 1. Mode of failure (MARS Group 2010)[69].

BTB autograft reconstructions. Although the reasons are unclear, it is possible that return to a higher level of activity in the younger age group may be partly responsible. Hewett and Myer[55] have postulated a theory proposing a mismatch between neuromuscular adaptation and skeletal growth, which may contribute to ACL injury. These factors when present may persist post–ACL reconstruction in this younger population.

Gender
Although it has been well established that women are 2 to 8 times more likely to suffer an ACL injury than men,[56–58] a similar gender difference has not been clearly demonstrated for ACL graft ruptures. In a study performed by Noojin and colleagues,[46] women had a clinical failure rate of 23% compared with 4% in men after ACL reconstruction using hamstring tendons. The investigators did not control, however, for confounding variables, such as meniscal or chondral pathology, and included as failures those with a grade 1+ pivot shift (pivot glide). When only patients with at least a grade 2 pivot shift were analyzed, the failure rate in women was reduced to 10%. This compared favorably with the results reported by Salmon and colleagues,[48] which excluded those with significant meniscal and chondral pathology and demonstrated no gender difference in graft failure rates (10% in women and 11% in men), a finding supported by several other published studies.[54,59,60]

Activity profile
Return to a high activity level after ACL reconstruction has been established as an independent risk factor for ACL graft failure. Borchers and colleagues[44] demonstrated a higher failure rate with an odds ratio of 5.53 for those patients who returned to a high activity level. In a study by Salmon and colleagues,[47] return to competitive sidestepping, pivoting, or jumping sports was associated with an increased risk of ACL injury.

Generalized ligamentous laxity
Generalized joint laxity and specific knee hyperlaxity have been positively correlated with noncontact ACL injuries.[50,61–63] It has been hypothesized that excessive knee joint laxity after ACL reconstruction may lead to an increased risk of ACL failure in

these patients. Although the exact mechanism is unknown, it has been postulated that hyperlax connective tissues (secondary restraints) and excessive knee hyperextension with secondary graft impingement may contribute to graft failure.

Other factors

Meniscal injury and subsequent meniscectomy at the time of initial ACL surgery have been associated with increased postoperative laxity and, in a cadaveric study, increased in situ graft forces.[53,64] Theoretically, this should lead to increased graft failure rates, although this has not been documented in the literature. A contact mechanism of injury at the time of the original ACL disruption was found a risk factor for graft failure in a study of BTB and hamstring autograft ACL reconstructions.[47] Finally, higher body weight was associated with graft failure in a prospective analysis of failure rate after anatomic ACL reconstruction using allograft.[38]

Surgical Technique

Several studies have identified errors in surgical technique as the most common cause of graft failure, with between 50% and 88% of failures believed secondary to technical issues.[9,65–68] A recent study, however, from the Multicenter ACL Revision Study (MARS) Group attributed only 24% cases of graft failure requiring revision to technical error alone[69] (see **Fig. 1**).This difference may be attributed to a recently acquired increase in awareness of ACL anatomy and tunnel position, because all patients were enrolled in the MARS study after 2006. This may have reduced the impact of tunnel malposition as a cause of graft failure (see **Fig. 1**).

In the overall analysis of surgical technique as a possible cause of graft failure, the following factors are considered important:

1. Tunnel malposition
2. Graft impingement
3. Improper graft tensioning
4. Inadequate graft fixation
5. Graft material/quality
6. Failure to address concomitant factors

Tunnel malposition

Nonanatomic graft placement may lead to excessive length changes of the graft as the knee moves throughout a range of motion.[68,70] This in turn may produce secondary graft elongation or rupture, with likely resultant pathologic laxity and instability. If plastic deformation, however, of the graft does not occur, a nonanatomic graft may result in loss of knee motion or excessive compressive forces through articular cartilage and menisci.[43,71]

Most errors in tunnel position occur on the femoral side. A recent study reported femoral tunnel malposition in 80% of cases where surgical error was believed the primary cause of failure.[69] Because the femoral insertion of the ACL is closer to the axis of rotation of the knee, small changes in the femoral ACL attachment may have a significant effect on knee biomechanics. The most common surgical error is an excessively anterior or central tunnel position. An anterior femoral tunnel causes excessive graft tension with increasing knee flexion resulting in loss of flexion, stress at the graft fixation site or eventual plastic deformation of the graft, and pathologic laxity. A central femoral tunnel positioned along the intercondylar roof produces a vertical graft that may be able to control anterior tibial translation but not tibiofemoral rotation. This vertical graft position is also prone to graft impingement against the anterior aspect of the intercondylar notch, which may lead to loss of terminal extension and eventual attritional graft failure (**Fig. 2**).[72,73]

Despite less commonly recognized as a cause of failure, accurate placement of the tibial tunnel is critical. A recent study from the MARS Group reported tibial tunnel malposition in 37% of cases where surgical error was believed the primary cause of failure leading to a revision procedure.[69] An excessively anterior or lateral placement may lead to notch or lateral condyle impingement as the knee approaches terminal extension.[74] To avoid impingement, many investigators previously advocated a posterior tibial tunnel position.[72,74,75] This has been shown to cause excessive graft strain in extension as well as posterior cruciate ligament impingement with increasing degrees of flexion, particularly when coupled with a central femoral tunnel position.[71] A loss of flexion or progressive graft elongation and failure may result. Although graft obliquity in the sagittal plane largely depends largely on femoral tunnel position, it also depends on the position of the tibial tunnel. A recent study by Bedi and colleagues[76] demonstrated that a posterior tibial tunnel produced a vertical graft angle despite being coupled with an anatomic femoral tunnel, which led to an inability to adequately control anterior tibial translation and knee rotation.

Double-bundle procedures are technically demanding and subject to an increased risk of tunnel malposition, because 3 or 4 tunnels are created instead of 2. Although the AM and PL bundles of the ACL function synergistically throughout a range of motion to control anterior tibial translation and tibiofemoral rotation, under loaded conditions both bundles are stretched at low flexion angles.[77–79] A recent study by Zantop and colleagues[70] demonstrated that a nonanatomic femoral PL graft position resulted in rotatory instability. Several studies have reported increasing in situ forces in the PL bundle or graft as the knee moves from 30° to full extension (**Fig. 3**A).[80–82] Therefore, even small errors of femoral or tibial graft placement may lead to PL bundle overload and failure. Commonly the tibial AM bundle is positioned to avoid anterior impingement, which may influence the creation of a malpositioned posterior tibial PL bundle, which reflects the need to allow an adequate bone bridge. This posterior

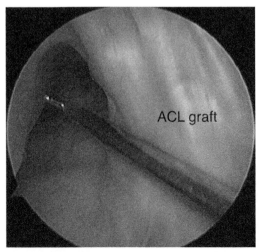

Fig. 2. Arthroscopic view (right knee) from the anterolateral portal demonstrating a nonanatomic vertical ACL graft (labeled) caused by an anterior and central femoral tunnel position. Metal probe is identifying the anatomic femoral tunnel position.

tibial PL tunnel may produce increased forces within the PL bundle as the knee moves into extension but also hyperflexion, as the length of the PL bundle increases with high degrees of flexion.[83] Zantop and colleagues[79] demonstrated that PL bundle failure may lead to excessive anterior tibial translation and increased strain on the remaining AM bundle, with overall graft failure a possible outcome (see **Fig. 3B**).

Graft impingement

ACL grafts may impinge against either soft tissue or bone. The most common soft tissue impingement occurs when a vertically orientated graft with a posteriorly positioned tibial tunnel impinges against the posterior cruciate ligament (described previously). An ACL graft may also impinge against the anterior aspect of the intercondylar

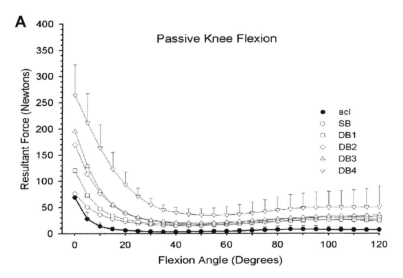

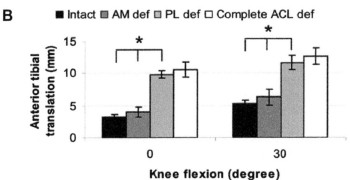

Fig. 3. (*A*) Mean curves of resultant force versus knee flexion angle for passive knee flexion with no applied tibial force. The mean curves are shown for intact knees and after single-bundle (SB) and double-bundle (DB) reconstructions. The mean forces with all DB reconstructions were significantly different ($P<.05$) from native ACL forces at all flexion angles. There was a sharp increase in forces from 30° to 0°. (*B*) Anterior tibial translation in response to a combined rotatory load of 10 Nm valgus and 4 Nm internal tibial torque. The increase in anterior tibial translation after transection of the PL bundle was statistically significantly higher when compared with the AM-deficient and intact knee. In the ACL reconstructed knee, this may lead to sequential AM bundle failure and graft rupture.

notch or the medial aspect of the lateral femoral condyle, particularly as the knee approaches terminal extension. This impingement may lead to focal areas of graft necrosis, inadequate biologic incorporation, and subsequent attritional graft failure.[74,84]

Most current graft materials have a greater cross-sectional area in their midsection than the original ACL. The native ACL is narrowest in this region, with insertion site areas more than 3.5 times greater than the middle section of the ligament.[85–87] This confers a long hourglass configuration to the native ACL, which allows physiologic impingement to occur where the ACL fibers course distally around the anterior aspect of the intercondylar notch. Current graft materials, however, are uniform in shape and often cylindrical. Therefore, impingement may occur when these grafts are positioned too close to the perimeter of the anatomic insertion sites.[88] An excessively large tibial tunnel positioned within the anterior aspect of the AM insertion site is the most commonly reported error, which may lead to pathologic graft impingement against the anterior aspect of the intercondylar notch.[76] Recent studies have also highlighted the important role of an anatomic femoral tunnel position in preventing graft impingement. This anatomic position produces a more oblique graft orientation in both coronal and sagittal planes, which in turn may reduce the risk and magnitude of graft impingement.[89]

Improper graft tensioning
The optimal amount of tension that should be applied to an ACL graft has not been identified. It depends on several factors, including the type and size of graft material used, graft placement, type of graft fixation, and the degree of knee flexion at the time of graft tensioning.[90–92] The aim of graft tensioning should be to eliminate pathologic laxity without increasing joint contact pressures or producing excessive in situ graft forces, while allowing adequate biologic incorporation of the graft. Yoshiya and colleagues[93] in a canine model, reported that highly tensioned patellar tendon grafts demonstrated areas of focal myxoid degeneration with loss of the normal parallel collagen fiber architecture. These grafts also showed areas of poor vascularity.

Other investigators have demonstrated that overtensioning may be associated with overconstraint of the joint, subsequent loss of joint motion, and increased joint contact pressures.[94,95] The ideal amount of tension required for a single-bundle graft has not been established, although the degree of tension may be graft type and size dependent.[96] Values ranging from 20 N to 80 N have been recommended in published literature.[91,97] The most appropriate angle of knee flexion for graft tensioning has also not been established; however, most studies recommend somewhere between 0° and 30°.[98] In situ ACL and graft forces, however, particularly within the PL fibers, increase significantly as the knee moves from 30° to terminal extension. More anatomically positioned single-bundle grafts may, therefore, be subjected to excessive graft force if tensioned at 30°, which has led several investigators to recommend tensioning in extension.[26,98]

The most appropriate graft tensioning technique for double-bundle procedures is controversial. Each technique should recognize and respect the individual tension pattern of the AM and PL bundle as the knee moves through a range of motion. In a recent literature review, van Eck and colleagues[99] reported that most investigators (57%) implemented a different tension pattern for the AM and PL graft with the AM bundle tensioned between 30° and 90° and the PL bundle between 0° and 30° flexion. When both bundles were tensioned at the same angle of flexion (27%), the angle ranged from 15° to 60°. A recent cadaveric study by Vercillo and colleagues[100] examined various outcomes after the tensioning of the AM and PL bundles at different knee flexion angles. The safest combination was a fixation protocol with the AM bundle tensioned at 45° and the PL bundle at 15°. This combination provided excellent restoration of knee kinematics with graft in situ forces approximating the intact knee. A comprehensive surgical technique article by Karlsson and colleagues[98] recommended a similar tensioning technique with the AM bundle tensioned at 45° and the PL bundle in full extension.

Inadequate graft fixation

The fixation should be strong enough to allow immediate weight bearing and range of motion as well as participation in an appropriate rehabilitation program. Bone-to-bone healing is usually complete by 8 weeks and tendon-to-bone healing should be completed by 8 to 12 weeks.[101] Failure to achieve this may lead to pathologic laxity and graft failure. Available fixation devices can be divided into extracortical, crosspin, or intratunnel (interference screw) fixation.[102,103]

Tibial fixation has long been considered more problematic than femoral fixation partly due to the bone quality of the tibial metaphysis but also the effect of parallel forces acting along the ACL graft and tibial tunnel.[104,105] The aim of tibial fixation should be to avoid early graft creep and slippage, and several factors, including length of screw, type of screw composition and design, concentric or eccentric screw placement, tunnel dilation, additional extracortical fixation, and graft preparation (whip stitch) have been investigated.[103,106,107] Pinczewski and colleagues[108] reported that female patients after hamstring reconstruction secured on the tibial side with an interference screw demonstrated greater anterior tibial translation than male subjects. This difference was eliminated with the addition of an extracortical staple, suggesting perhaps a gender differences in bone density and, therefore, fixation strength.[109]

Lehmann and colleagues[110] investigated the impact of the width of the femoral bridge between tunnels had on the structural properties of the graft-tunnel complex after double-bundle reconstruction in cadaveric knees. A cortical bridge of 1 mm between the tunnels produced inferior structural properties compared with a 2-mm or 3-mm bridge. When performing a double-bundle reconstruction, consideration needs to be given to the size of the femoral insertion area, which must be large enough to accommodate both tunnels with at least a 2-mm cortical bridge to reduce the risk of early graft failure.

Graft material/quality

The use of allograft tissue to perform an ACL reconstruction has increased over the past decade. Although satisfactory outcomes have been reported, concerns exist regarding disease transmission, slower biologic incorporation, incomplete ligamentization, and possible immunogenicity.[111–114] Several studies have reported high failure rates after allograft reconstructions when performed in young (<25 years) active patients and in those making an early often unsanctioned return to sport.[38,45] The allograft source and graft preparation method may be important, with irradiated grafts demonstrating a higher early failure rate (33%) than nonirradiated grafts (2.4%).[115] Recent systematic reviews by Carey and colleagues[114] and Foster and colleagues,[116] however, comparing outcomes after allograft and autograft reconstructions reported no significant differences in failure rates.

Most outcome studies investigating various autografts have failed to demonstrate a difference in graft failure rates. A systematic literature review by Spindler and colleagues[23] showed no difference in failure rates between BTB and hamstring grafts and concluded that autograft type may not be the primary determinant for successful ACL reconstruction. This finding was supported by Magnussen and colleagues,[117] who conducted a systematic review of studies with a minimum 5 years' follow-up. They reported no difference in failure rates between those graft choices. A level 1 systematic review by Reinhardt and colleagues,[118] however, which applied strict inclusion criteria and classified graft failure as those having undergone a revision procedure or with a documented positive pivot shift, reported a higher failure rate (15.8%) in the hamstring group compared with BTB reconstructions (7.2%).

Most hamstring double-bundle techniques recommend using the gracilis tendon to reconstruct the PL bundle.[33,34,119] The size of this tendon is reported in the literature as between 5 mm and 7 mm in diameter. Most graft sizing sets, however, have a minimum diameter of 5 mm, which may introduce a degree of measurement error. The doubled gracilis tendon often slides easily through the 5-mm sizing cylinder; therefore, unless the gracilis tendon is tripled, it may often be less than 5 mm in diameter. This combination of inadequate tissue and increased in situ forces in the PL bundle may lead to increased PL bundle rupture rates. In support, Kondo and Yasuka,[120] in a second-look arthroscopy study of double-bundle reconstructions where gracilis was used to create the PL bundle, graded the PL bundle as of intermediate or poor quality in 24% cases.

Failure to address concomitant factors

Failure to recognize and correct concomitant factors before ACL reconstruction may lead to increased tensile forces placed through the ACL graft, which may result in graft failure. Gersoff and colleagues[121] reported unrecognized PL laxity in 10% to 15% cases of chronic ACL deficiency. Graft failure secondary to untreated ligamentous laxity was reported in 15% revision cases by Getelman and colleagues[122] whereas in a recent study by the MARS Group at least 7% of technical errors were attributed to failure to treat malalignment or ligamentous laxity.[69] The following factors have been recognized as important secondary stabilizers:

- Lateral collateral ligament or PL corner instability
- Medial collateral ligament (MCL) injury, posteromedial structures
- Coronal malalignment, most commonly varus malalignment
- Increased tibial slope
- Posteromedial meniscal injury

LaPrade and colleagues,[123] in a controlled cadaveric biomechanical study, demonstrated that ACL graft forces are increased with sequential sectioning of the PL structures. In a study performed by Zantop and colleagues,[124] both single-bundle and double-bundle reconstructions were unable to restore normal knee kinematics in the presence of an absent lateral collateral ligament. Careful assessment of the PL structures should be part of a routine knee examination after ACL injury. In the presence of significant laxity the PL structures should be repaired and reconstructed if necessary. An assessment of coronal plane alignment is also critical. If varus malalignment and PL laxity are present in combination, particularly in the presence of a varus thrust, consideration should be given to performing a high tibial osteotomy to correct the varus deformity.[125]

The management of significant MCL injuries in the presence of an acute ACL disruption is controversial. Many MCL injuries heal sufficiently with appropriate nonoperative management. If persistent medial laxity is observed, however, it may be necessary to repair or reconstruct the medial structures, including the deep and superficial layers of the MCL, posterior oblique ligament, and potentially the posterior horn of the medial meniscus if avulsed.[126,127] Anatomic repair and early postoperative range of motion are necessary to reduce the incidence of postoperative stiffness.

Various investigators have demonstrated that varus malalignment, particularly in the presence of a clinically detectable varus thrust, may result in excessive forces in the ACL graft.[125,128,129] Careful clinical and radiologic assessment is required to make this diagnosis. If present, consideration should be given to performing a high tibial osteotomy, to unload the medial compartment, either in combination with the ACL reconstruction or as a staged procedure.

Giffin and colleagues[130] examined the effect of increasing tibial slope on knee kinematics and in situ ACL forces. They reported that small increases in tibial slope had little effect on anteroposterior translations or ACL forces. The tibial resting position, however, was shifted anteriorly with increasing tibial slope and was accentuated with the application of axial load. It was suggested that decreasing the tibial slope may be protective in an ACL-deficient knee.

The role of the medial meniscus as an important secondary restraint to anterior tibial translation has been well documented.[53] The status of the medial meniscus at the time of ACL reconstruction and the resultant risk of developing osteoarthritis has been previously reported.[131] It seems reasonable to preserve meniscal tissue when possible, by performing meniscal repair if indicated or a partial meniscectomy when repair is not possible. The role of meniscal allograft transplantation in the presence of ACL reconstruction is controversial, although it may have a role in restoring the important brake stop mechanism that is deficient in cases where a total or subtotal meniscectomy has been performed.[126]

Graft Incorporation/Biologic Factors

Successful ACL reconstruction ultimately depends on complete biologic incorporation of the graft material. In humans, biologic incorporation can only be assessed with MRI scans or biopsies that do not affect the integrity of the ACL graft.[132–135] It is difficult, therefore, to measure biologic failure, which makes it hard to define and often a diagnosis of exclusion. It is considered when other measurable causes of failure, such as poor surgical technique, aggressive rehabilitation, and trauma, have been excluded. The true incidence of biologic failure is difficult to ascertain but as tunnel positions become more anatomic, failure of biologic incorporation may be recognized more frequently. In support of this theory, a recent study by the MARS Group recognized biologic failure in combination with technical error and trauma in 20% cases and as the primary mode of failure in 7%.[69]

Several studies have investigated the process and stages of graft incorporation commonly referred to as ligamentization[84,136,137]:

1. Graft necrosis
2. Revascularization
3. Cellular repopulation and proliferation
4. Collagen remodeling and maturation

Graft necrosis
All grafts undergo a process of avascular necrosis, particularly in the central portion, during the first 3 to 4 weeks after implantation. This process produces several cytokines that initiate and guide various biologic processes, including revascularization and cell migration and proliferation.

Revascularization
The process of revascularization is critical to successful graft incorporation, because viable cells are introduced that release various growth factors responsible for collagen

and matrix production. Revascularization begins at 3 weeks and grafts are well perfused by 6 to 8 weeks.

Vascular supply to the graft originates from the infrapatellar fat pad distally and the posterior synovial tissues proximally. Care should be taken, therefore, during ACL reconstruction to avoid aggressive débridement of these structures. The following factors may lead to impairment of revascularization:

- Surgical factors, such as impingement and excessive graft tension, may cause focal graft necrosis and myxoid degeneration.
- Patient habits, such as smoking, or systemic disease, such as diabetes, may lead to vasoconstriction or small vessel vasculitis.
- Hypoxia during the process of avascular necrosis may, in theory, lead to a lack of stimulation of the revascularization process.

Graft choice may also be important. It has been established that allograft tissue compared with autograft tissue takes longer to revascularize and repopulate with viable cells and has been shown to remodel superficially with incomplete healing of the central area of the graft. This may partially explain the higher graft failure rates for allograft tissue demonstrated in several studies.[38,44,45]

Cellular repopulation and proliferation
Cellular repopulation with mesenchymal stem cells and fibroblasts is usually complete by 12 weeks. This process has been correlated with increased levels of growth factors, such as transforming growth factor β1, platelet-derived growth factor (PDGF)-AA, and PDGF-BB, deemed important for graft incorporation.

Collagen remodeling and maturation
Ligaments and tendons are fundamentally different with regard their structure and mechanical properties. Ligaments are predominantly composed of water (60%–80% net weight) and type 1 collagen (65%–80% dry weight) and are more cellular than tendons but have less overall collagen, whose fibrils are arranged with a different proportion of reducible intermolecular bonds.[84] With time, the grafted tendon undergoes a complex process of collagen production and remodeling known as ligamentization. Many factors may be detrimental to this process, including a lack of revascularization, inadequate release of growth factors, and insufficient mechanical forces.

It has been demonstrated that biologic graft incorporation is intimately linked to the biomechanical and biochemical environment of the knee. Nonanatomic graft placement produces nonparallel collagen fiber alignment within the graft, which may lead to collagen fragmentation and failure. Repeated microtrauma to the graft before complete graft maturation, which may result from an overly aggressive rehabilitation program, may lead to graft elongation or rupture.

It is currently not possible to accurately evaluate graft healing and maturation, although several promising studies using MRI as an evaluation tool have been published recently (**Fig. 4**).[133–135] Therefore, the time required to complete the ligamentization process is unknown. It is likely highly individualized but may take longer than 9 months, as reported in a study by van Eck and colleagues.[38] Other studies have reported that the pattern of ACL graft rupture becomes similar to the rupture pattern of the native ACL as the time from surgery increases.[40,41] This may indicate a time-dependent graft maturation process where ligament-like tissue with structural properties similar to the native ACL develops with time.

There has been a recent focus on investigating and developing methods to enhance biologic graft incorporation.[135,138] Several studies have demonstrated that ruptured

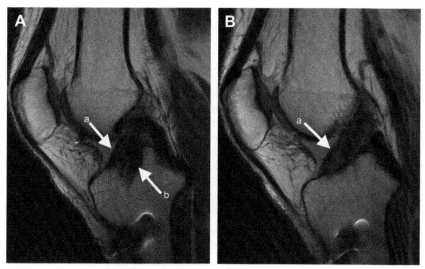

Fig. 4. (*A*) Sagittal MRI performed 8 months post–ACL reconstruction, demonstrating the remnant tibial stump of the native ACL positioned anterior to the hamstring ACL autograft. (*a arrow*) Remnant tibial stump of native ACL. (*b arrow*) Hamstring ACL autograft. (*B*) Sagittal MRI picture demonstrating incorporation of the remnant tibial stump with the ACL graft at 8 months post–ACL reconstruction (sequential MRI–same patient as depicted in **Fig. 4a**.

ACL tissue contains blood vessels and neural tissue.[139,140] Remnant preservation surgical techniques have been described and several investigators have demonstrated excellent early graft incorporation and restoration of proprioception (**Fig. 5**).[134,141] Biologic agents, such as fibrin clot and platelet-rich plasma, used to stimulate graft healing have also been investigated with promising early results.[135]

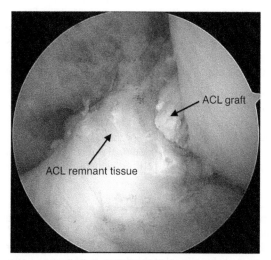

Fig. 5. An arthroscopic view (left knee) from the anterolateral portal demonstrating a surgical technique for ACL remnant preservation surgery. The hamstring autograft is almost completely covered by native ACL tissue.

Although further research is required, it is likely that greater attention to the biologic process may lead to a reduction in graft failure rates.

Rehabilitation

The aim of any rehabilitation program should be to facilitate a safe return to activities, including high-demand sport, by protecting a graft from early excessive loads and providing the neuromuscular support to prevent further injury secondary to trauma.[142] Studies have demonstrated graft strength and stiffness within the first year after surgery as only 30% to 50% of the original ACL.[143,144] In a study by van Eck and colleagues,[38] 50% graft failures occurred within 9 months of surgery and 22% between 9 and 12 months, leading the investigators to conclude that ACL grafts may require more than 9 months to fully heal.

Certain biomechanical and neuromuscular variables have been shown important in predicting second ACL injury after ACL reconstruction[145,146]:

- Increased net hip rotation moment impulse
- Abnormal frontal plane knee range of motion during landing
- Asymmetric sagittal plane knee moments at initial contact
- Abnormal postural stability

Rehabilitation programs should focus on recognizing and correcting these factors. Paterno and colleagues[146] recommended improving hip muscle strength (gluteus maximus strengthening) and plyometric training to improve frontal plane mechanics and gluteal muscle function and recruitment. Single-leg strengthening exercises to overcome asymmetry and routines to improve postural stability, such as double-leg and single-leg balance activities on stable and unstable surfaces, with and without perturbations, were also been recommended.

In a recent comprehensive systematic review of various rehabilitation programs, Wright and colleagues[147,148] made the following conclusions:

- Early weight bearing is beneficial and may reduce patellofemoral pain.
- Early motion is safe and may avoid late arthrofibrosis.
- Continuous passive motion offered no appreciable benefit.
- Supervised physical therapy is safe and beneficial for motivated patients.
- Closed chain exercises are recommended for the first 6 weeks after surgery.
- Postoperative bracing offers no significant advantage over no bracing.
- Accelerated rehabilitation programs are safe if conducted over 5 to 6 months.

Methods for noninvasive assessment of graft healing are required to guide postoperative rehabilitation. Currently, the intensity of rehabilitation programs and decisions regarding return to sport are based on parameters, such as time from surgery and various knee and lower limb strength and functional assessments. These assessments make the assumption that the graft has healed. The use of MRI to evaluate graft healing and maturation has been studied and is currently the focus of ongoing research.[134,135]

Trauma

Many studies have demonstrated that return to high-demand activities, including pivoting sports, increases the risk of reinjury to the ACL graft.[12,38,45,47] Traumatic failure of the graft is a well-recognized mode of failure.[149,150] In the absence of obvious technical error and a previously functional stable knee, the traumatic event is often considered the primary cause of failure. In a recent study, the MARS Group nominated trauma as the primary mode of failure in 32% cases, making it the most common individual cause.[69] That study allowed for multiple modes of failure to be documented and therefore a combination of causes was implicated in 35% cases.

FAILURE OF ANATOMIC ACL RECONSTRUCTION

There has been a recent focus on the anatomy of the ACL and a shift toward performing anatomic ACL reconstruction. Given that most available literature regarding modes of failure after ACL reconstruction predates this current paradigm shift, it is worth considering failure of anatomic ACL reconstructions separately.

In a recent study, van Eck and colleagues[38] reported failure rates of 13% and 11% for double-bundle and single-bundle anatomic reconstructions, respectively. Kato and colleagues[151] demonstrated that anatomically positioned grafts within the insertion sites of the ACL were subjected to high forces during knee motion. These forces were comparable to the native ACL and higher than those of nonanatomic grafts. Therefore, despite being able to better restore knee kinematics and function, anatomic grafts may be more prone to failure. This is particularly relevant for the PL bundle or single-bundle grafts positioned close to the PL insertion site.

In a recent study of 358 patients having undergone either an anatomic single-bundle or double-bundle procedure, the reported failure rates were 4.6% and 12.3%, respectively.[39] These failure rates were similar to those reported in the study by van Eck and colleagues. When considering the reasons for failure, the investigators identified the following factors as important, particularly when a the decision to perform a double-bundle or single-bundle reconstruction:

- Patient selection—insertion site size and anatomy, gender, skeletal maturity, activity profile, and pre-existing laxity
- Tunnel malposition
- Graft characteristics
- Biologic incorporation

The anatomy and dimensions of the insertion sites of the ACL are subject to extreme variability.[85,86] Failure to acknowledge and recognize this may lead to graft malposition and failure. Several investigators have recommended routine measurement of the insertion sites.[98] If the dimension of the insertion site is less than 14 mm, it may be more appropriate to perform a single-bundle procedure. A double-bundle procedure in this case may lead to crowding of the intercondylar notch, tunnel malposition, and possible graft impingement. Small errors in PL bundle position may have significant consequences, including PL bundle rupture and subsequent AM bundle failure (**Fig. 6**).[79,152]

Some investigators have used allograft tissue to increase the size of the implanted PL bundle when autologous hamstrings are small. There are still concerns, however, regarding allograft incorporation and possible increased failure rates. It may be more appropriate to perform a single-bundle reconstruction in this situation.

Biologic incorporation is critical to avoid graft failure but is difficult to measure (discussed previously). Preservation of the ACL remnants may be important. To visualize the footprint of the ACL during a double-bundle procedure, it has often been deemed necessary to débride much of the remnant ACL tissue, which may have a deleterious effect on graft healing.[39] Remnant preservation techniques have been described and if graft position is not compromised should be used.[153]

LOSS OF MOTION

Loss of motion after ACL reconstruction may involve either flexion or extension, although loss of extension is more problematic and functionally disabling.[154] It is

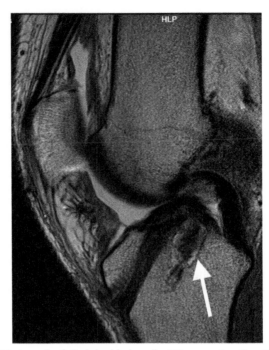

Fig. 6. Sagittal MRI view of a failed double-bundle ACL reconstruction. The tibial PL tunnel is too posterior (*arrow*) and may have been subjected to excessive in situ forces.

known that a loss of extension as small as 5° may impair athletic performance and significantly contribute to later osteoarthritis.[155] The exact incidence of motion loss is difficult to determine, although a range between 5.5% and 24% has been reported in the literature.[154,155] It is possible that with more anatomic procedures performed, the incidence of significant motion loss may decrease. Many possible causes of motion loss have been reported:

1. Postoperative swelling
2. Poor compliance with physical therapy
3. Immobilization
4. Concomitant ligament surgery
5. Surgical technique—impingement
6. Timing of surgery
7. Arthrofibrosis
8. Regional pain syndrome
9. Infection

Prevention is the best management of motion loss. The timing of surgery and status of the knee before surgery are critical. In many ways, the timing of surgery depends on the state of the knee and affected lower limb. Supervised physical therapy and a home exercise program are helpful in achieving the following prerequisites for surgery:

- Minimal swelling
- Full symmetric extension
- Flexion to at least 120°
- Functional quadriceps

Postoperative management is also important and should be aimed at regaining symmetric extension and quadriceps function immediately. Other factors shown to improve motion include cryotherapy for swelling reduction, patellar mobilization, and early weight bearing.[126]

Poor surgical technique may lead to motion loss. Tunnel placement is critical, because impingement or restricted motion secondary to nonanatomic graft position can occur. Patients with loss of extension need a thorough assessment of tunnel position. In some cases, after failure of more conservative measures, the graft may need to be débrided and a revision ACL reconstruction performed as a staged procedure after range of motion has been regained.[126]

Arthrofibrosis or capsulitis is defined as periarticular inflammation and swelling and results in adhesion and intra-articular scar tissue formation. Typically both flexion and extension are reduced and sequelae, such as quadriceps dysfunction, shortening of the patellar tendon, patella baja, and infrapatellar contracture syndrome, may result. In the early acute phase, the goal of treatment is to reduce the inflammation:

- Cryotherapy
- Anti-inflammatory medication
- Gentle stretching exercises
- Splinting to regain extension
- Avoidance of aggressive manipulation

Once the inflammatory phase settles, patients enter the fibrotic stage and arthroscopic débridement and lateral release may be considered. Arthrotomy with open releases and débridement may be necessary if infrapatellar contraction syndrome develops.[126]

EXTENSOR MECHANISM DYSFUNCTION

Multiple factors may contribute to extensor mechanism dysfunction after ACL reconstruction:

- Anterior knee pain
- Quadriceps muscle weakness and dysfunction
- Patellar tendonitis
- Graft harvest morbidity (patella fracture, tendonitis, patellar or quadriceps tendon rupture)
- Abnormal patellar tracking
- Patellar tendon contraction

Although the incidence of anterior knee pain has reduced due to improved surgical techniques and preoperative and postoperative rehabilitation, the reported incidence is between 3% and 47%.[126,156] Several factors may contribute to its onset, including preoperative anterior knee pain, patellofemoral joint chondral damage, flexion deformity, quadriceps weakness, ACL graft source, postoperative immobilization, graft impingement, and aggressive open chain exercises.[126] There is considerable overlap in the etiology of extensor mechanism dysfunction and loss of motion.

Correct surgical technique and attention to postoperative rehabilitation protocols may reduce the incidence of extensor mechanism dysfunction. Noyes and colleagues[157] recommended avoiding the use of patellar tendon grafts in patients with a narrow patellar tendon, severe patellofemoral osteoarthritis, patellofemoral malalignment, or a history of previous patellar tendon graft harvest from the same knee. Careful harvest of the patellar tendon and bone blocks is critical and care should be taken to avoid an excessively tight closure of the patellar tendon, so as to reduce the risk of patellar tendon contracture. Perhaps the most important factor is adherence to a postoperative rehabilitation program that encourages immediate symmetric extension, quadriceps control, and early weight bearing and avoids early open chain exercises.

OSTEOARTHRITIS

The reported incidence of osteoarthritis after ACL reconstruction is disturbingly high, with rates as high as 51% to 78% reported in the literature.[158,159] Unfortunately, a similar incidence has been observed in ACL-deficient patients managed nonoperatively.[160] The role of the menisci as important secondary stabilizers has been well established; however, many other factors may be important, including[161,162]

- Chondral and subchondral damage at the time of injury—70%–80% patients have bone bruises on MRI after initial injury[163,164]
- Surgical technique—graft type and orientation; incidence of osteoarthritis has been reported higher with the use of patellar tendon grafts[159]
- Lower limb alignment
- Postoperative strength and neuromuscular control
- Postoperative range of motion—in particular, extension
- Intrinsic tendency toward inflammatory response and articular cartilage breakdown

INFECTION

Septic arthritis after ACL reconstruction is uncommon, with a reported incidence between 0.3% and 1.7%, although most studies have documented rates less than 1%.[69,165] Risk factors include previous surgery to the same knee and concomitant surgery. Although there is concern regarding risk of disease transmission after allograft use, a recent literature review demonstrated no difference in infection rates for allograft or autograft ACL reconstructions.[166]

The ACL graft can be salvaged in most cases of septic arthritis but depends on an early diagnosis and aggressive management. Mouzopoulos and colleagues[165] recommended the following principles of management:

- Baseline white blood cell count, C-reactive protein, and erythrocyte sedimentation rate
- Collection of knee fluid for microscopy and culture
- Immediate arthroscopic lavage and débridement
- Repeat arthroscopy if septic presentation persists
- Intravenous antibiotics for 6 to 8 weeks—altered if necessary once organism identified
- Oral antibiotics for a further 2 to 4 weeks

The ACL graft may need to be removed if the graft is considered nonfunctional or lax or is covered in tenacious purulent material that necessitates extensive graft débridement or if there has been a significant delay in diagnosis or failure to respond to the graft retention protocol. Possible complications include loss of motion, cartilage degeneration, osteomyelitis, graft failure, and inferior outcome scoresl.[167]

SUMMARY

The true failure rate after ACL reconstruction is unknown and likely under-reported. Many possible factors may contribute to an unsatisfactory outcome after ACL reconstruction, including graft failure, motion loss, extensor mechanism dysfunction, osteoarthritis, and infection.

Graft failure may result in laxity and clinical instability. Several causes of graft failure have been reported, including various patient factors, surgical technique issues, trauma, aggressive rehabilitation, and failure of biologic incorporation. The absolute contribution of each of these factors is often difficult to quantify and in many cases they may act in combination.

Modes of failure after anatomic ACL reconstruction are increasingly recognized although more research is required. The role of biologic incorporation seems important, particularly in the setting of anatomically positioned grafts that may be subjected to greater in situ forces than nonanatomic grafts. A gradually progressive, targeted rehabilitation program and careful return to sport are also critical. Finally, an individual approach to anatomic ACL reconstruction, which involves recognizing each person's individual anatomy and includes modification of the surgical procedure accordingly, may lead to a reduction in failure rates.

REFERENCES

1. Busam ML, Fulkerson JP, Gaskill TR, et al. Technical aspects of anterior cruciate ligament reconstruction for the general orthopaedic surgeon. Instr Course Lect 2011;60:485–97.
2. Harner CD, Giffin JR, Dunteman RC, et al. Evaluation and treatment of recurrent instability after anterior cruciate ligament reconstruction. Instr Course Lect 2001; 50:463–74.
3. Kocher MS, Tucker R, Briggs KK. Relationship between subjective and objective assessment of outcomes after anterior cruciate ligament reconstruction. J Knee Surg 2005;18(1):73–81.
4. Anderson AF, Snyder RB, Lipscomb AB Jr. Anterior cruciate ligament reconstruction. A prospective randomized study of three surgical methods. Am J Sports Med 2001;29(3):272–9.
5. Beynnon BD, Johnson RJ, Fleming BC, et al. Anterior cruciate ligament replacement: comparison of bone-patellar tendon-bone grafts with two-strand hamstring grafts. A prospective, randomized study. J Bone Joint Surg Am 2002;84(9): 1503–13.
6. Brandsson S, Faxen E, Eriksson BI, et al. Reconstruction of the anterior cruciate ligament: comparison of outside-in and all-inside techniques. Br J Sports Med 1999;33(1):42–5.
7. Weiler A, Schmeling A, Stohr I, et al. Primary versus single-stage revision anterior cruciate ligament reconstruction using autologous hamstring tendon grafts: a prospective matched-group analysis. Am J Sports Med 2007;35(10):1643–52.
8. Noyes FR, Barber-Westin SD. Revision anterior cruciate surgery with use of bone-patellar tendon-bone autogenous grafts. J Bone Joint Surg Am 2001; 83(8):1131–43.
9. Diamantopoulos AP, Lorbach O, Paessler HH. Anterior cruciate ligament revision reconstruction: results in 107 patients. Am J Sports Med 2008;36(5):851–60.
10. Ahn JH, Lee YS, Ha HC. Comparison of revision surgery with primary anterior cruciate ligament reconstruction and outcome of revision surgery between different graft materials. Am J Sports Med 2008;36(10):1889–95.
11. Ferretti A, Conteduca F, Monaco E, et al. Revision anterior cruciate ligament reconstruction with doubled semitendinosus and gracilis tendons and lateral extra-articular reconstruction. J Bone Joint Surg Am 2006;88(11):2373–9.

12. Barrett GR, Luber K, Replogle WH, et al. Allograft anterior cruciate ligament reconstruction in the young, active patient: tegner activity level and failure rate. Arthroscopy 2010;26(12):1593–601.

13. Zaffagnini S, Marcacci M, Lo Presti M, et al. Prospective and randomized evaluation of ACL reconstruction with three techniques: a clinical and radiographic evaluation at 5 years follow-up. Knee Surg Sports Traumatol Arthrosc 2006;14(11):1060–9.

14. Fu FH, Shen W, Starman JS, et al. Primary anatomic double-bundle anterior cruciate ligament reconstruction: a preliminary 2-year prospective study. Am J Sports Med 2008;36(7):1263–74.

15. Colombet P, Robinson J, Jambou S, et al. Two-bundle, four-tunnel anterior cruciate ligament reconstruction. Knee Surg Sports Traumatol Arthrosc 2006; 14(7):629–36.

16. Mascarenhas R, Tranovich M, Karpie JC, et al. Patellar tendon anterior cruciate ligament reconstruction in the high-demand patient: evaluation of autograft versus allograft reconstruction. Arthroscopy 2010;26(Suppl 9):S58–66.

17. Wagner M, Kaab MJ, Schallock J, et al. Hamstring tendon versus patellar tendon anterior cruciate ligament reconstruction using biodegradable interference fit fixation: a prospective matched-group analysis. Am J Sports Med 2005;33(9):1327–36.

18. Aune AK, Holm I, Risberg MA, et al. Four-strand hamstring tendon autograft compared with patellar tendon-bone autograft for anterior cruciate ligament reconstruction. A randomized study with two-year follow-up. Am J Sports Med 2001;29(6):722–8.

19. Zaffagnini S, Bruni D, Marcheggiani Muccioli GM, et al. Single-bundle patellar tendon versus non-anatomical double-bundle hamstrings ACL reconstruction: a prospective randomized study at 8-year minimum follow-up. Knee Surg Sports Traumatol Arthrosc 2011;19(3):390–7.

20. Siebold R, Webster KE, Feller JA, et al. Anterior cruciate ligament reconstruction in females: a comparison of hamstring tendon and patellar tendon autografts. Knee Surg Sports Traumatol Arthrosc 2006;14(11):1070–6.

21. Isberg J, Faxen E, Brandsson S, et al. Early active extension after anterior cruciate ligament reconstruction does not result in increased laxity of the knee. Knee Surg Sports Traumatol Arthrosc 2006;14(11):1108–15.

22. Poehling GG, Curl WW, Lee CA, et al. Analysis of outcomes of anterior cruciate ligament repair with 5-year follow-up: allograft versus autograft. Arthroscopy 2005;21(7):774–85.

23. Spindler KP, Kuhn JE, Freedman KB, et al. Anterior cruciate ligament reconstruction autograft choice: bone-tendon-bone versus hamstring: does it really matter? A systematic review. Am J Sports Med 2004;32(8):1986–95.

24. Lewis PB, Parameswaran AD, Rue JP, et al. Systematic review of single-bundle anterior cruciate ligament reconstruction outcomes: a baseline assessment for consideration of double-bundle techniques. Am J Sports Med 2008;36(10): 2028–36.

25. Wright RW, Magnussen RA, Dunn WR, et al. Ipsilateral graft and contralateral ACL rupture at five years or more following ACL reconstruction: a systematic review. J Bone Joint Surg Am 2011;93(12):1159–65.

26. van Eck C, Working Z, Fu F. Current concepts in anatomic single- and double-bundle anterior cruciate ligament reconstruction. Phys Sportsmed 2011;39(2):140–8.

27. Tashman S, Collon D, Anderson K, et al. Abnormal rotational knee motion during running after anterior cruciate ligament reconstruction. Am J Sports Med 2004; 32(4):975–83.

28. Yamamoto Y, Hsu WH, Woo SL, et al. Knee stability and graft function after anterior cruciate ligament reconstruction: a comparison of a lateral and an anatomical femoral tunnel placement. Am J Sports Med 2004;32(8):1825–32.

29. Yagi M, Wong EK, Kanamori A, et al. Biomechanical analysis of an anatomic anterior cruciate ligament reconstruction. Am J Sports Med 2002;30(5): 660–6.

30. Woo SL, Kanamori A, Zeminski J, et al. The effectiveness of reconstruction of the anterior cruciate ligament with hamstrings and patellar tendon. A cadaveric study comparing anterior tibial and rotational loads. J Bone Joint Surg Am 2002;84(6):907–14.

31. Aglietti P, Giron F, Cuomo P, et al. Single-and double-incision double-bundle ACL reconstruction. Clin Orthop Relat Res 2007;454:108–13.

32. Jarvela T, Moisala AS, Sihvonen R, et al. Double-bundle anterior cruciate ligament reconstruction using hamstring autografts and bioabsorbable interference screw fixation: prospective, randomized, clinical study with 2-year results. Am J Sports Med 2008;36(2):290–7.

33. Jarvela T. Double-bundle versus single-bundle anterior cruciate ligament reconstruction: a prospective, randomize clinical study. Knee Surg Sports Traumatol Arthrosc 2007;15(5):500–7.

34. Siebold R, Dehler C, Ellert T. Prospective randomized comparison of double-bundle versus single-bundle anterior cruciate ligament reconstruction. Arthroscopy 2008;24(2):137–45.

35. Muneta T, Koga H, Mochizuki T, et al. A prospective randomized study of 4-strand semitendinosus tendon anterior cruciate ligament reconstruction comparing single-bundle and double-bundle techniques. Arthroscopy 2007; 23(6):618–28.

36. Kondo E, Yasuda K, Azuma H, et al. Prospective clinical comparisons of anatomic double-bundle versus single-bundle anterior cruciate ligament reconstruction procedures in 328 consecutive patients. Am J Sports Med 2008;36(9): 1675–87.

37. Streich NA, Friedrich K, Gotterbarm T, et al. Reconstruction of the ACL with a semitendinosus tendon graft: a prospective randomized single blinded comparison of double-bundle versus single-bundle technique in male athletes. Knee Surg Sports Traumatol Arthrosc 2008;16(3):232–8.

38. van Eck CF, Schkrohowsky JG, Working ZM, et al. Prospective analysis of failure rate and predictors of failure after anatomic anterior cruciate ligament reconstruction with allograft. Am J Sports Med 2012;40(4):800–7.

39. Whitehead TS. Albert Trillat young investigator award, ISAKOS 2011. Double versus single bundle ACL reconstruction - Does it really matter? ISAKOS 2011. Rio De Janeiro; 2011.

40. van Eck CF, Kropf EJ, Romanowski JR, et al. ACL graft re-rupture after double-bundle reconstruction: factors that influence the intra-articular pattern of injury. Knee Surg Sports Traumatol Arthrosc 2011;19(3):340–6.

41. van Eck CF, Kropf EJ, Romanowski JR, et al. Factors that influence the intra-articular rupture pattern of the ACL graft following single-bundle reconstruction. Knee Surg Sports Traumatol Arthrosc 2011;19(8):1243–8.

42. Zantop T, Brucker PU, Vidal A, et al. Intraarticular rupture pattern of the ACL. Clin Orthop Relat Res 2007;454:48–53.

43. Shelbourne KD, Urch SE, Gray T, et al. Loss of normal knee motion after anterior cruciate ligament reconstruction is associated with radiographic arthritic changes after surgery. Am J Sports Med 2012;40(1):108–13.

44. Borchers JR, Pedroza A, Kaeding C. Activity level and graft type as risk factors for anterior cruciate ligament graft failure: a case-control study. Am J Sports Med 2009;37(12):2362–7.

45. Barrett AM, Craft JA, Replogle WH, et al. Anterior cruciate ligament graft failure: a comparison of graft type based on age and tegner activity level. Am J Sports Med 2011;39(10):2194–8.

46. Noojin FK, Barrett GR, Hartzog CW, et al. Clinical comparison of intraarticular anterior cruciate ligament reconstruction using autogenous semitendinosus and gracilis tendons in men versus women. Am J Sports Med 2000;28(6):783–9.

47. Salmon L, Russell V, Musgrove T, et al. Incidence and risk factors for graft rupture and contralateral rupture after anterior cruciate ligament reconstruction. Arthroscopy 2005;21(8):948–57.

48. Salmon LJ, Refshauge KM, Russell VJ, et al. Gender differences in outcome after anterior cruciate ligament reconstruction with hamstring tendon autograft. Am J Sports Med 2006;34(4):621–9.

49. Kim SJ, Kumar P, Kim SH. Anterior cruciate ligament reconstruction in patients with generalized joint laxity. Clin Orthop Surg 2010;2(3):130–9.

50. Kim SJ, Kim TE, Lee DH, et al. Anterior cruciate ligament reconstruction in patients who have excessive joint laxity. J Bone Joint Surg Am 2008;90(4):735–41.

51. Kim SJ, Moon HK, Kim SG, et al. Does severity or specific joint laxity influence clinical outcomes of anterior cruciate ligament reconstruction? Clin Orthop Relat Res 2010;468(4):1136–41.

52. Shelbourne KD, Gray T. Results of anterior cruciate ligament reconstruction based on meniscus and articular cartilage status at the time of surgery. Five- to fifteen-year evaluations. Am J Sports Med 2000;28(4):446–52.

53. Papageorgiou CD, Gil JE, Kanamori A, et al. The biomechanical interdependence between the anterior cruciate ligament replacement graft and the medial meniscus. Am J Sports Med 2001;29(2):226–31.

54. Shelbourne KD, Gray T, Haro M. Incidence of subsequent injury to either knee within 5 years after anterior cruciate ligament reconstruction with patellar tendon autograft. Am J Sports Med 2009;37(2):246–51.

55. Hewett TE, Myer GD. The mechanistic connection between the trunk, hip, knee, and anterior cruciate ligament injury. Exerc Sport Sci Rev 2011;39(4):161–6.

56. Arendt E, Dick R. Knee injury patterns among men and women in collegiate basketball and soccer. NCAA data and review of literature. Am J Sports Med 1995;23(6):694–701.

57. Anderson AF, Dome DC, Gautam S, et al. Correlation of anthropometric measurements, strength, anterior cruciate ligament size, and intercondylar notch characteristics to sex differences in anterior cruciate ligament tear rates. Am J Sports Med 2001;29(1):58–66.

58. Gwinn DE, Wilckens JH, McDevitt ER, et al. The relative incidence of anterior cruciate ligament injury in men and women at the United States Naval Academy. Am J Sports Med 2000;28(1):98–102.

59. Barber-Westin SD, Noyes FR, Andrews M. A rigorous comparison between the sexes of results and complications after anterior cruciate ligament reconstruction. Am J Sports Med 1997;25(4):514–26.

60. Ferrari JD, Bach BR Jr, Bush-Joseph CA, et al. Anterior cruciate ligament reconstruction in men and women: an outcome analysis comparing gender. Arthroscopy 2001;17(6):588–96.

61. Kim SJ, Chang JH, Kim TW, et al. Anterior cruciate ligament reconstruction with use of a single or double-bundle technique in patients with generalized ligamentous laxity. J Bone Joint Surg Am 2009;91(2):257–62.
62. Myer GD, Ford KR, Paterno MV, et al. The effects of generalized joint laxity on risk of anterior cruciate ligament injury in young female athletes. Am J Sports Med 2008;36(6):1073–80.
63. Ramesh R, Von Arx O, Azzopardi T, et al. The risk of anterior cruciate ligament rupture with generalised joint laxity. J Bone Joint Surg Br 2005;87(6):800–3.
64. Shelbourne KD, Carr DR. Meniscal repair compared with meniscectomy for bucket-handle medial meniscal tears in anterior cruciate ligament-reconstructed knees. Am J Sports Med 2003;31(5):718–23.
65. Carson EW, Anisko EM, Restrepo C, et al. Revision anterior cruciate ligament reconstruction: etiology of failures and clinical results. J Knee Surg 2004; 17(3):127–32.
66. Johnson DL, Swenson TM, Irrgang JJ, et al. Revision anterior cruciate ligament surgery: experience from Pittsburgh. Clin Orthop Relat Res 1996;(325):100–9.
67. Denti M, Lo Vetere D, Bait C, et al. Revision anterior cruciate ligament reconstruction: causes of failure, surgical technique, and clinical results. Am J Sports Med 2008;36(10):1896–902.
68. Marchant BG, Noyes FR, Barber-Westin SD, et al. Prevalence of nonanatomical graft placement in a series of failed anterior cruciate ligament reconstructions. Am J Sports Med 2010;38(10):1987–96.
69. Wright RW, Huston LJ, Spindler KP, et al. Descriptive epidemiology of the multi-center ACL revision study (MARS) cohort. Am J Sports Med 2010;38(10): 1979–86.
70. Zantop T, Diermann N, Schumacher T, et al. Anatomical and nonanatomical double-bundle anterior cruciate ligament reconstruction: importance of femoral tunnel location on knee kinematics. Am J Sports Med 2008;36(4):678–85.
71. Howell SM, Gittins ME, Gottlieb JE, et al. The relationship between the angle of the tibial tunnel in the coronal plane and loss of flexion and anterior laxity after anterior cruciate ligament reconstruction. Am J Sports Med 2001;29(5):567–74.
72. Howell SM, Clark JA. Tibial tunnel placement in anterior cruciate ligament reconstructions and graft impingement. Clin Orthop Relat Res 1992;(283):187–95.
73. Howell SM, Taylor MA. Failure of reconstruction of the anterior cruciate ligament due to impingement by the intercondylar roof. J Bone Joint Surg Am 1993;75(7): 1044–55.
74. Muneta T, Yamamoto H, Ishibashi T, et al. The effects of tibial tunnel placement and roofplasty on reconstructed anterior cruciate ligament knees. Arthroscopy 1995;11(1):57–62.
75. Howell SM, Barad SJ. Knee extension and its relationship to the slope of the intercondylar roof. Implications for positioning the tibial tunnel in anterior cruciate ligament reconstructions. Am J Sports Med 1995;23(3):288–94.
76. Bedi A, Maak T, Musahl V, et al. Effect of tibial tunnel position on stability of the knee after anterior cruciate ligament reconstruction: is the tibial tunnel position most important? Am J Sports Med 2011;39(2):366–73.
77. Kurosawa H, Yamakoshi K, Yasuda K, et al. Simultaneous measurement of changes in length of the cruciate ligaments during knee motion. Clin Orthop Relat Res 1991;(265):233–40.
78. Chhabra A, Starman JS, Ferretti M, et al. Anatomic, radiographic, biomechanical, and kinematic evaluation of the anterior cruciate ligament and its two functional bundles. J Bone Joint Surg Am 2006;88(Suppl 4):2–10.

79. Zantop T, Herbort M, Raschke MJ, et al. The role of the anteromedial and posterolateral bundles of the anterior cruciate ligament in anterior tibial translation and internal rotation. Am J Sports Med 2007;35(2):223–7.

80. Markolf KL, Park S, Jackson SR, et al. Contributions of the posterolateral bundle of the anterior cruciate ligament to anterior-posterior knee laxity and ligament forces. Arthroscopy 2008;24(7):805–9.

81. Markolf KL, Park S, Jackson SR, et al. Anterior-posterior and rotatory stability of single and double-bundle anterior cruciate ligament reconstructions. J Bone Joint Surg Am 2009;91(1):107–18.

82. Seon JK, Gadikota HR, Wu JL, et al. Comparison of single- and double-bundle anterior cruciate ligament reconstructions in restoration of knee kinematics and anterior cruciate ligament forces. Am J Sports Med 2010;38(7):1359–67.

83. Yoo YS, Jeong WS, Shetty NS, et al. Changes in ACL length at different knee flexion angles: an in vivo biomechanical study. Knee Surg Sports Traumatol Arthrosc 2010;18(3):292–7.

84. Menetrey J, Duthon VB, Laumonier T, et al. "Biological failure" of the anterior cruciate ligament graft. Knee Surg Sports Traumatol Arthrosc 2008;16(3): 224–31.

85. Siebold R, Ellert T, Metz S, et al. Femoral insertions of the anteromedial and posterolateral bundles of the anterior cruciate ligament: morphometry and arthroscopic orientation models for double-bundle bone tunnel placement– a cadaver study. Arthroscopy 2008;24(5):585–92.

86. Siebold R, Ellert T, Metz S, et al. Tibial insertions of the anteromedial and posterolateral bundles of the anterior cruciate ligament: morphometry, arthroscopic landmarks, and orientation model for bone tunnel placement. Arthroscopy 2008;24(2):154–61.

87. Odensten M, Gillquist J. Functional anatomy of the anterior cruciate ligament and a rationale for reconstruction. J Bone Joint Surg Am 1985; 67(2):257–62.

88. Yasuda K, van Eck CF, Hoshino Y, et al. Anatomic single- and double-bundle anterior cruciate ligament reconstruction, part 1: basic science. Am J Sports Med 2011;39(8):1789–99.

89. Maak TG, Bedi A, Raphael BS, et al. Effect of femoral socket position on graft impingement after anterior cruciate ligament reconstruction. Am J Sports Med 2011;39(5):1018–23.

90. Andersen HN, Amis AA. Review on tension in the natural and reconstructed anterior cruciate ligament. Knee Surg Sports Traumatol Arthrosc 1994;2(4): 192–202.

91. Amis AA, Jakob RP. Anterior cruciate ligament graft positioning, tensioning and twisting. Knee Surg Sports Traumatol Arthrosc 1998;6(Suppl 1):S2–12.

92. Mae T, Shino K, Nakata K, et al. Optimization of graft fixation at the time of anterior cruciate ligament reconstruction. Part I: effect of initial tension. Am J Sports Med 2008;36(6):1087–93.

93. Yoshiya S, Andrish JT, Manley MT, et al. Graft tension in anterior cruciate ligament reconstruction. An in vivo study in dogs. Am J Sports Med 1987;15(5): 464–70.

94. Melby A 3rd, Noble JS, Askew MJ, et al. The effects of graft tensioning on the laxity and kinematics of the anterior cruciate ligament reconstructed knee. Arthroscopy 1991;7(3):257–66.

95. Nabors ED, Richmond JC, Vannah WM, et al. Anterior cruciate ligament graft tensioning in full extension. Am J Sports Med 1995;23(4):488–92.

96. Jaureguito JW, Paulos LE. Why grafts fail. Clin Orthop Relat Res 1996;(325): 25–41.
97. Yasuda K, Tsujino J, Tanabe Y, et al. Effects of initial graft tension on clinical outcome after anterior cruciate ligament reconstruction. Autogenous doubled hamstring tendons connected in series with polyester tapes. Am J Sports Med 1997;25(1):99–106.
98. Karlsson J, Irrgang JJ, van Eck CF, et al. Anatomic single- and double-bundle anterior cruciate ligament reconstruction, part 2: clinical application of surgical technique. Am J Sports Med 2011;39(9):2016–26.
99. van Eck CF, Schreiber VM, Mejia HA, et al. "Anatomic" anterior cruciate ligament reconstruction: a systematic review of surgical techniques and reporting of surgical data. Arthroscopy 2010;26(Suppl 9):S2–12.
100. Vercillo F, Woo SL, Noorani SY, et al. Determination of a safe range of knee flexion angles for fixation of the grafts in double-bundle anterior cruciate ligament reconstruction: a human cadaveric study. Am J Sports Med 2007;35(9): 1513–20.
101. Rodeo SA, Kawamura S, Kim HJ, et al. Tendon healing in a bone tunnel differs at the tunnel entrance versus the tunnel exit: an effect of graft-tunnel motion? Am J Sports Med 2006;34(11):1790–800.
102. Kousa P, Jarvinen TL, Vihavainen M, et al. The fixation strength of six hamstring tendon graft fixation devices in anterior cruciate ligament reconstruction. Part I: femoral site. Am J Sports Med 2003;31(2):174–81.
103. Kousa P, Jarvinen TL, Vihavainen M, et al. The fixation strength of six hamstring tendon graft fixation devices in anterior cruciate ligament reconstruction. Part II: tibial site. Am J Sports Med 2003;31(2):182–8.
104. Brand J Jr, Weiler A, Caborn DN, et al. Graft fixation in cruciate ligament reconstruction. Am J Sports Med 2000;28(5):761–74.
105. Brand JC Jr, Pienkowski D, Steenlage E, et al. Interference screw fixation strength of a quadrupled hamstring tendon graft is directly related to bone mineral density and insertion torque. Am J Sports Med 2000;28(5):705–10.
106. Selby JB, Johnson DL, Hester P, et al. Effect of screw length on bioabsorbable interference screw fixation in a tibial bone tunnel. Am J Sports Med 2001;29(5): 614–9.
107. Nurmi JT, Kannus P, Sievanen H, et al. Interference screw fixation of soft tissue grafts in anterior cruciate ligament reconstruction: part 1: effect of tunnel compaction by serial dilators versus extraction drilling on the initial fixation strength. Am J Sports Med 2004;32(2):411–7.
108. Pinczewski LA, Deehan DJ, Salmon LJ, et al. A five-year comparison of patellar tendon versus four-strand hamstring tendon autograft for arthroscopic reconstruction of the anterior cruciate ligament. Am J Sports Med 2002;30(4):523–36.
109. Hill PF, Russell VJ, Salmon LJ, et al. The influence of supplementary tibial fixation on laxity measurements after anterior cruciate ligament reconstruction with hamstring tendons in female patients. Am J Sports Med 2005;33(1):94–101.
110. Lehmann AK, Osada N, Zantop T, et al. Femoral bridge stability in double-bundle ACL reconstruction: impact of bridge width and different fixation techniques on the structural properties of the graft/femur complex. Arch Orthop Trauma Surg 2009;129(8):1127–32.
111. Barber FA. Should allografts be used for routine anterior cruciate ligament reconstructions? Arthroscopy 2003;19(4):421.
112. Jackson DW, Corsetti J, Simon TM. Biologic incorporation of allograft anterior cruciate ligament replacements. Clin Orthop Relat Res 1996;(324):126–33.

113. Jackson DW, Grood ES, Goldstein JD, et al. A comparison of patellar tendon autograft and allograft used for anterior cruciate ligament reconstruction in the goat model. Am J Sports Med 1993;21(2):176–85.
114. Carey JL, Dunn WR, Dahm DL, et al. A systematic review of anterior cruciate ligament reconstruction with autograft compared with allograft. J Bone Joint Surg Am 2009;91(9):2242–50.
115. Rappe M, Horodyski M, Meister K, et al. Nonirradiated versus irradiated Achilles allograft: in vivo failure comparison. Am J Sports Med 2007;35(10):1653–8.
116. Foster TE, Wolfe BL, Ryan S, et al. Does the graft source really matter in the outcome of patients undergoing anterior cruciate ligament reconstruction? An evaluation of autograft versus allograft reconstruction results: a systematic review. Am J Sports Med 2010;38(1):189–99.
117. Magnussen RA, Carey JL, Spindler KP. Does autograft choice determine intermediate-term outcome of ACL reconstruction? Knee Surg Sports Traumatol Arthrosc 2011;19(3):462–72.
118. Reinhardt KR, Hetsroni I, Marx RG. Graft selection for anterior cruciate ligament reconstruction: a level I systematic review comparing failure rates and functional outcomes. Orthop Clin North Am 2010;41(2):249–62.
119. Aglietti P, Giron F, Losco M, et al. Comparison between single-and double-bundle anterior cruciate ligament reconstruction: a prospective, randomized, single-blinded clinical trial. Am J Sports Med 2010;38(1):25–34.
120. Kondo E, Yasuda K. Second-look arthroscopic evaluations of anatomic double-bundle anterior cruciate ligament reconstruction: relation with postoperative knee stability. Arthroscopy 2007;23(11):1198–209.
121. Gersoff WK, Clancy WG Jr. Diagnosis of acute and chronic anterior cruciate ligament tears. Clin Sports Med 1988;7(4):727–38.
122. Getelman MH, Friedman MJ. Revision anterior cruciate ligament reconstruction surgery. J Am Acad Orthop Surg 1999;7(3):189–98.
123. LaPrade RF, Resig S, Wentorf F, et al. The effects of grade III posterolateral knee complex injuries on anterior cruciate ligament graft force. A biomechanical analysis. Am J Sports Med 1999;27(4):469–75.
124. Zantop T, Schumacher T, Schanz S, et al. Double-bundle reconstruction cannot restore intact knee kinematics in the ACL/LCL-deficient knee. Arch Orthop Trauma Surg 2010;130(8):1019–26.
125. Noyes FR, Barber SD, Simon R. High tibial osteotomy and ligament reconstruction in varus angulated, anterior cruciate ligament-deficient knees. A two- to seven-year follow-up study. Am J Sports Med 1993;21(1):2–12.
126. Brown CH Jr, Carson EW. Revision anterior cruciate ligament surgery. Clin Sports Med 1999;18(1):109–71.
127. Allen CR, Giffin JR, Harner CD. Revision anterior cruciate ligament reconstruction. Orthop Clin North Am 2003;34(1):79–98.
128. Noyes FR, Schipplein OD, Andriacchi TP, et al. The anterior cruciate ligament-deficient knee with varus alignment. An analysis of gait adaptations and dynamic joint loadings. Am J Sports Med 1992;20(6):707–16.
129. Noyes FR, Barber-Westin SD, Hewett TE. High tibial osteotomy and ligament reconstruction for varus angulated anterior cruciate ligament-deficient knees. Am J Sports Med 2000;28(3):282–96.
130. Giffin JR, Vogrin TM, Zantop T, et al. Effects of increasing tibial slope on the biomechanics of the knee. Am J Sports Med 2004;32(2):376–82.
131. Gillquist J, Messner K. Anterior cruciate ligament reconstruction and the long-term incidence of gonarthrosis. Sports Med 1999;27(3):143–56.

132. Alm A, Gillquist J, Stromberg B. The medial third of the patellar ligament in reconstruction of the anterior cruciate ligament. A clinical and histologic study by means of arthroscopy or arthrotomy. Acta Chir Scand Suppl 1974;445: 5–14.

133. Muramatsu K, Hachiya Y, Izawa H. Serial evaluation of human anterior cruciate ligament grafts by contrast-enhanced magnetic resonance imaging: comparison of allografts and autografts. Arthroscopy 2008;24(9):1038–44.

134. Gohil S, Annear PO, Breidahl W. Anterior cruciate ligament reconstruction using autologous double hamstrings: a comparison of standard versus minimal debridement techniques using MRI to assess revascularisation. A randomised prospective study with a one-year follow-up. J Bone Joint Surg Br 2007;89(9): 1165–71.

135. Radice F, Yanez R, Gutierrez V, et al. Comparison of magnetic resonance imaging findings in anterior cruciate ligament grafts with and without autologous platelet-derived growth factors. Arthroscopy 2010;26(1):50–7.

136. Slauterbeck JR, Hickox JR, Beynnon B, et al. Anterior cruciate ligament biology and its relationship to injury forces. Orthop Clin North Am 2006;37(4):585–91.

137. Deehan DJ, Cawston TE. The biology of integration of the anterior cruciate ligament. J Bone Joint Surg Br 2005;87(7):889–95.

138. Weiler A, Forster C, Hunt P, et al. The influence of locally applied platelet-derived growth factor-BB on free tendon graft remodeling after anterior cruciate ligament reconstruction. Am J Sports Med 2004;32(4):881–91.

139. Arnoczky SP, Tarvin GB, Marshall JL. Anterior cruciate ligament replacement using patellar tendon. An evaluation of graft revascularization in the dog. J Bone Joint Surg Am 1982;64(2):217–24.

140. Murray MM, Martin SD, Martin TL, et al. Histological changes in the human anterior cruciate ligament after rupture. J Bone Joint Surg Am 2000;82(10):1387–97.

141. Locherbach C, Zayni R, Chambat P, et al. Biologically enhanced ACL reconstruction. Orthop Traumatol Surg Res 2010;96(7):810–5.

142. Barber-Westin SD, Noyes FR. Objective criteria for return to athletics after anterior cruciate ligament reconstruction and subsequent reinjury rates: a systematic review. Phys Sportsmed 2011;39(3):100–10.

143. Clancy WG Jr, Narechania RG, Rosenberg TD, et al. Anterior and posterior cruciate ligament reconstruction in rhesus monkeys. J Bone Joint Surg Am 1981;63(8):1270–84.

144. Drez DJ Jr, DeLee J, Holden JP, et al. Anterior cruciate ligament reconstruction using bone-patellar tendon-bone allografts. A biological and biomechanical evaluation in goats. Am J Sports Med 1991;19(3):256–63.

145. Myer GD, Ford KR, Hewett TE. New method to identify athletes at high risk of ACL injury using clinic-based measurements and freeware computer analysis. Br J Sports Med 2011;45(4):238–44.

146. Paterno MV, Schmitt LC, Ford KR, et al. Biomechanical measures during landing and postural stability predict second anterior cruciate ligament injury after anterior cruciate ligament reconstruction and return to sport. Am J Sports Med 2010; 38(10):1968–78.

147. Wright RW, Preston E, Fleming BC, et al. A systematic review of anterior cruciate ligament reconstruction rehabilitation: part II: open versus closed kinetic chain exercises, neuromuscular electrical stimulation, accelerated rehabilitation, and miscellaneous topics. J Knee Surg 2008;21(3):225–34.

148. Wright RW, Preston E, Fleming BC, et al. A systematic review of anterior cruciate ligament reconstruction rehabilitation: part I: continuous passive motion, early

weight bearing, postoperative bracing, and home-based rehabilitation. J Knee Surg 2008;21(3):217–24.

149. Kamath GV, Redfern JC, Greis PE, et al. Revision anterior cruciate ligament reconstruction. Am J Sports Med 2011;39(1):199–217.

150. George MS, Dunn WR, Spindler KP. Current concepts review: revision anterior cruciate ligament reconstruction. Am J Sports Med 2006;34(12):2026–37.

151. Kato Y, Ingham SJ, Kramer S, et al. Effect of tunnel position for anatomic single-bundle ACL reconstruction on knee biomechanics in a porcine model. Knee Surg Sports Traumatol Arthrosc 2010;18(1):2–10.

152. Markolf KL, Jackson SR, McAllister DR. Single- versus double-bundle posterior cruciate ligament reconstruction: effects of femoral tunnel separation. Am J Sports Med 2010;38(6):1141–6.

153. Ahn JH, Lee YS, Ha HC. Anterior cruciate ligament reconstruction with preservation of remnant bundle using hamstring autograft: technical note. Arch Orthop Trauma Surg 2009;129(8):1011–5.

154. Irrgang JJ, Harner CD. Loss of motion following knee ligament reconstruction. Sports Med 1995;19(2):150–9.

155. Shelbourne KD. Range of motion loss will cause osteoarthritis. Arthroscopy 2011;27(4):451–2.

156. Aglietti P, Buzzi R, D'Andria S, et al. Patellofemoral problems after intraarticular anterior cruciate ligament reconstruction. Clin Orthop Relat Res 1993;(288):195–204.

157. Noyes FR, Barber SD, Mangine RE. Bone-patellar ligament-bone and fascia lata allografts for reconstruction of the anterior cruciate ligament. J Bone Joint Surg Am 1990;72(8):1125–36.

158. Lohmander LS, Ostenberg A, Englund M, et al. High prevalence of knee osteoarthritis, pain, and functional limitations in female soccer players twelve years after anterior cruciate ligament injury. Arthritis Rheum 2004;50(10):3145–52.

159. Hui C, Salmon LJ, Kok A, et al. Fifteen-year outcome of endoscopic anterior cruciate ligament reconstruction with patellar tendon autograft for "isolated" anterior cruciate ligament tear. Am J Sports Med 2011;39(1):89–98.

160. von Porat A, Roos EM, Roos H. High prevalence of osteoarthritis 14 years after an anterior cruciate ligament tear in male soccer players: a study of radiographic and patient relevant outcomes. Ann Rheum Dis 2004;63(3):269–73.

161. Louboutin H, Debarge R, Richou J, et al. Osteoarthritis in patients with anterior cruciate ligament rupture: a review of risk factors. Knee 2009;16(4):239–44.

162. Li RT, Lorenz S, Xu Y, et al. Predictors of radiographic knee osteoarthritis after anterior cruciate ligament reconstruction. Am J Sports Med 2011;39(12):2595–603.

163. Fowler PJ. Bone injuries associated with anterior cruciate ligament disruption. Arthroscopy 1994;10(4):453–60.

164. Bui KL, Ilaslan H, Parker RD, et al. Knee dislocations: a magnetic resonance imaging study correlated with clinical and operative findings. Skeletal Radiol 2008;37(7):653–61.

165. Mouzopoulos G, Fotopoulos VC, Tzurbakis M. Septic knee arthritis following ACL reconstruction: a systematic review. Knee Surg Sports Traumatol Arthrosc 2009;17(9):1033–42.

166. Greenberg DD, Robertson M, Vallurupalli S, et al. Allograft compared with autograft infection rates in primary anterior cruciate ligament reconstruction. J Bone Joint Surg Am 2010;92(14):2402–8.

167. McAllister DR, Parker RD, Cooper AE, et al. Outcomes of postoperative septic arthritis after anterior cruciate ligament reconstruction. Am J Sports Med 1999;27(5):562–70.

Index

Note: Page numbers of article titles are in **boldface** type.

A

Clin Sports Med 32 (2013) 205–210
http://dx.doi.org/10.1016/S0278-5919(12)00093-2
0278-5919/13/$ – see front matter © 2013 Elsevier Inc. All rights reserved.

sportsmed.theclinics.com

Moving?

Make sure your subscription moves with you!

To notify us of your new address, find your **Clinics Account Number** (located on your mailing label above your name), and contact customer service at:

Email: journalscustomerservice-usa@elsevier.com

800-654-2452 (subscribers in the U.S. & Canada)
314-447-8871 (subscribers outside of the U.S. & Canada)

Fax number: 314-447-8029

Elsevier Health Sciences Division
Subscription Customer Service
3251 Riverport Lane
Maryland Heights, MO 63043

*To ensure uninterrupted delivery of your subscription, please notify us at least 4 weeks in advance of move.

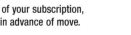

Printed and bound by CPI Group (UK) Ltd, Croydon, CR0 4YY

03/10/2024

01040441-0003